Herbal-Drug Interactions and Adverse Effects

NOTICE

Herbal-Drug Interactions and Adverse Effects

An Evidence-based
Quick Reference Guide

RICHARD B. PHILP, DVM, PhD
*Emeritus Professor and former Chair
Department of Pharmacology and Toxicology
Adjunct Professor
Department of Physiology and Pharmacology
Faculty of Medicine and Dentistry
The University of Western Ontario
London, Ontario, Canada*

PROPERTY OF
CLACKAMAS COMMUNITY COLLEGE
LIBRARY
WITHDRAWN

McGRAW-HILL
Medical Publishing Division

New York Chicago San Francisco Lisbon London Madrid Mexico City
Milan New Delhi San Juan Seoul Singapore Sydney Toronto

Herbal–Drug Interactions and Adverse Effects:
An Evidence-based Quick Reference Guide

Copyright © 2004 by The McGraw-Hill Companies, Inc. All rights reserved.
Printed in the United States of America. Except as permitted under the United
States Copyright Act of 1976, no part of this publication may be reproduced
or distributed in any form or by any means, or stored in a data base or
retrieval system, without the prior written permission of the publisher.

1 2 3 4 5 6 7 8 9 0   DOC/DOC   0 9 8 7 6 5 4 3

ISBN 0-07-142153-X

This book was set in Minion by Joanne Morbit of McGraw-Hill
Professional's Hightstown, NJ composition unit.
The editor was Andrea Seils.
The production supervisor was Phil Galea.
The index was prepared by Benjamin Tedoff.
RR Donnelley was printer and binder.

This book is printed on acid-free paper.

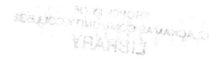

Cataloging-in-Publication data is on file for this title at the Library of
Congress.

To the docs who kept my motor running so I could do this,
to my family for their support,
and especially to my wife, Joan, for putting up with me meanwhile,
and keeping me sane in the process.

Contents

Preface

Public interest in alternative remedies, especially herbal ones that can be obtained without a visit to a physician or a prescription, continues to rise. This rise will be accompanied by an increased incidence of herb-related adverse reactions. There is a need for the medical profession to be increasingly vigilant for this and for possible untoward consequences resulting from herb-drug interactions.

There are many good texts on the market that deal with herbal remedies, but they tend to be therapeutic guides, educational texts, or extensive reference works. I felt there was a need for a quick reference text that would allow physicians and other health professionals to rapidly access essential information regarding a particular herb or nutriceutical.

I hope that this text will help to fill that need.

Richard B. Philp

Section 1

Overview and General Principles

Conventions and Special Tables

Plants have always provided an important source of medicines. These generally were used first in aboriginal or folk medicine and later adopted by conventional western medicine as their efficacy was confirmed. Thus, the muscle relaxant d-tubocurine came from the poisonous plant *Strychnos toxifera* and related species, used by Amazon natives to tip their arrows and darts. Related species of *Strychnos* in the eastern hemisphere are rich in strychnine-like alkaloids. Quinine, the antimalarial and antipyretic drug, comes from the bark of the cinchona tree. This bark was brought to Europe from South America by the Jesuits and became known as Jesuit bark. The story of William Withering's report, in 1885, of the use of foxglove to treat heart ailments and edema is well known. He had observed its use by English folk herbalists for "dropsy." Digoxin, one active principal of *Digitalis purpurea* and *D. lanata,* is still used. Many plants are rich in cardiac glycosides, including oleander, star-of-Bethlehem, and lily-of-the-valley. Colchicine (from the autumn crocus, *Colchicum autumnale),* used for acute gouty arthritis, was known as a poison to the ancient Greeks and is purported to have been introduced into the United States by Ben Franklin, himself a sufferer from gout. The list is a long one: Atropine from deadly nightshade (*Atropa belladonna*), also found in Jimson weed (*Datura stramonium*); scopolamine from henbane (*Hyoscyamus niger*); the salicylates from willow bark (various species of *Salix*); morphine from the opium poppy (*Papaver somniferum*); the antihypertensive reserpine from *Rauwolfia serpentina.* Most antibiotics were first isolated from saprophytic soil bacteria, members of the plant kingdom. For further information on the history of these botanical agents see reference 1.

The evolution from folk remedy to pharmaceutical agent generally followed a predictable path once science and medicine began to merge. Early on it became evident that standardization of dosage was dependent on standardization of the preparation. Because the active ingredient was generally not known, standardization of the process of preparation or extraction of the plant source, and of the horticultural practices, served as a substitute. Where possible, bioassays were used to assess potency. With the emergence of more sophisticated knowledge of chemistry and pharmacology, the final step was the extraction and identification of the active agent(s) and possibly even of its (their) synthesis. It was now possible to assess potency on the basis of chemical purity and to adjust dosage accordingly. Some biological agents are, of course, still administered by international units, with potency determined by bioassay.

The 16th-century Swiss physician Paracelsus is remembered for his statement that only the dose separates a poison from a remedy. This was possibly the first formal recognition of the fact that all medicines have a therapeutic range and a toxic range. These ranges may vary with the species, the individual, and the route of administration (portal of entry, in toxicological terms).

The realization that medications may have serious side effects was brought home forcefully by the thalidomide tragedy of the 1960s. This experience resulted in extensive modification of the legal requirements for safety testing by the pharmaceutical industry before a drug could be introduced onto the market. Developed countries now require animal and cell testing for mutagenicity and carcinogenicity as well as organ system toxicity before human testing can begin. If a substance passes these tests, an application is made for investigational new drug (IND) status. If this status is received, there are then three phases of human testing. Phase I involves the administration of the drug to healthy volunteers or a small number of patients and the accumulation of data regarding the pharmacokinetics of absorption, metabolism, distribution, and excretion. It is designed primarily to gather information about appropriate dosages as well as to identify any side effects that might arise. Phase II is a randomized, controlled, double-blind study of a relatively small number of patients looking for evidence of therapeutic efficacy as well as accumulating knowledge of side effects. If the results to date justify it, a new drug application (NDA) is sought and a multi-center, randomized, controlled, double-blind study (phase III) is conducted on a large number of patients. The final stage, phase IV, is a post-marketing, open-label study using family practitioners and clinics to accumulate further data on efficacy and side effects. It has been estimated that to develop a chemical from initial synthesis or identification to final approval requires $50 to $80 million and about 10 years.

Doubtless there are many herbal agents that possess significant pharmacological properties. Indeed, a plethora of active agents often is present in a single herb. This raises the possibility that synergism could occur if two such agents have similar actions, possibly by different mechanisms. It also means that antagonism could result if two or more agents have opposing effects. This possibility emphasizes the necessity of conducting controlled, clinical trials as is done for prescription pharmaceuticals, and laboratory research to identify, and possibly purify, the active principles. In short, the principle of evidence-based medicine must prevail.

Herbal preparations may take many forms. Drying is always the first stage in preparation, because fresh herbs are not readily available. The dried plant, leaves, or root may be used as teas and infusions (steeped in hot water), extracts and decoctions (soaked in alcohol, vinegar), or powdered in capsules. Freeze-dried preparations have appeared more recently.

One might wonder why so many substances that are biologically active for mammals should have evolved in plants. There is no doubt that many of these serve as chemical defenses against predators. If the substances render the plant bitter, as do the alkaloids, foragers will learn to avoid the plant. If they are toxic to herbivores, natural selection will eliminate those individuals with a taste for the plants. A mammal that becomes stupefied by a psychoactive agent in a plant will become easy prey for carnivores. Natural selection may thus wean out herbivores with a predilection for that plant. Bacteria and fungi have been conducting chemical warfare for eons. Mycotoxins are a source of increasing concern for human health. The ergot fungus *Claviceps purpurea* is a source of many pharmacological agents that taught us much about the sympathetic nervous system. It should thus come as no surprise that most, if not all, botanicals possess pharmacologically active agents in varying degrees.

The great 19th-century physician Sir William Osler once observed that "the desire to take medicine is perhaps the greatest feature which distinguishes man from animals."[2] The progress of pharmacology in the 20th century created the misconception that there is a pill for every ill, while at the same time faith in science was undermined by disasters such as the thalidomide tragedy. The cult of youth promoted the desire for an elixir of youth, and a mistaken belief emerged that all that is natural is superior to all that is synthetic. The age of the herbal remedy had arrived in the west. Many commercial herb suppliers list in excess of 800 preparations in their website catalogs. It would be impossible to deal with all of them here. An effort has been made to concentrate on those in common use or those that have significant toxicity.

The problems associated with the use of herbal remedies are the same ones that beset botanical source medicines in the early days. The concentration of the active ingredient may vary widely from one preparation to the next. More than one active ingredient, with quite different pharmacological profiles, may be present. In some cases there may be no active ingredient at all. Perhaps most important of all, the evidence for efficacy of a particular product may be scanty and wholly anecdotal. A new term, *evidence-based medicine,* has entered the lexicon of medical science. This term recognizes that before any therapeutic measure is embraced by the medical profession, there must be convincing evidence that it works in a significant number of cases. This kind of evidence is largely lacking for most herbal remedies. Indeed, some proponents of alternative remedies claim that they are not amenable to the customary test procedures applied to standard pharmacological agents because their effectiveness is based on the natural mixture of several ingredients that must all be present in the correct proportions. Because not all of the natural ingredients, or their correct proportions, are known, laboratory tests and clinical trials would be meaningless, according to these individuals. The specious nature of this argument should be apparent from the historical evolution of botanical source medicines discussed earlier. A truism that seems to have escaped the attention of the public at large is that, if an herbal remedy actually possesses the therapeutic benefits claimed for it, it is in fact, a drug, with everything that implies.

Governments are beginning to come to grips with the question of herbal and other alternative remedies. In May of 2000, Health Canada created the Office of Natural Health Products with an Expert Advisory Committee. In the words of the Minister of Health, "Our goal is to give Canadians the ability to choose natural health products with confidence, knowing they are safe, of high quality, and properly labeled." In the United States, the National Institutes of Health has an Office of Alternative Medicine. The Food and Drug Administration (FDA) has published a pamphlet, *An FDA Guide to Choosing Medical Treatments*, on the Internet at http://www.fda.gov/oashi/aids/fdaguide.html. In it, an alternative medicine is described as any medical practice that:

- Lacks sufficient documentation of its safety and effectiveness against specific diseases and conditions
- Is not generally taught in U.S. medical schools
- Is not generally reimbursable by health insurance providers

In both the United States and Canada, herbs are currently classified as dietary supplements; therefore, no claim can be made for therapeutic efficacy, and they are not subject to the regulations that apply to products for which such claims are made, whether prescription drugs or over-the-counter agents. Many government agencies, including the military, are publishing advisory pamphlets to guide their constituents in making informed choices about dietary supplements, including herbal remedies.

In the United States, the FDA defines a drug as "any substance or mixture of substances intended for the cure, mitigation, diagnosis or prevention of disease." Because the burden is on the manufacturer to provide proof of such claims, herbal remedies cannot generally qualify as drugs. In 1994, Congress sidestepped the issue by passing the Dietary Supplement and Health Act, which defined herbal remedies as "botanicals" rather than drugs and classified them as dietary supplements.[3]

The alternative medicine industry in the United States has been estimated to generate $3 billion annually in sales and to have a growth rate of about 20% per year.[4] Efforts to evaluate the safety of these agents are hampered by:

- The paucity of clinical trials
- The absence of definitive information regarding the pharmacology of the active principal
- The frequent presence of more than one active ingredient in one herb
- The practice of including several herbs in a single preparation
- Marked variations in the potency of various preparations

Efforts to evaluate safety are thus easy to criticize.

There are numerous ways in which pharmacologically active agents can interact, regardless of whether they are prescription medications, proprietary medicines or herbal preparations. Even nutrients can affect a therapeutic response in some cases. One agent may accelerate or retard the biotransformation of another by an effect on metabolizing enzymes. The effect on the response will depend on whether the second agent is activated (i.e., is a prodrug) or deactivated by the enzyme. One agent may impair the absorption of another from the gastrointestinal tract, or impair its renal excretion. Displacement from plasma protein binding sites may increase the availability of an agent to its active site. Active agents may compete for receptor sites, interfering with the pharmacological response. Agents with similar actions but by different mechanisms may be additive, whereas those with opposite actions by different mechanisms may be pharmacologically antagonistic. Given that most herbal remedies contain more than one pharmacologically active agent and that often little is known about their pharmacokinetics or interactions, it would seem best to err on the side of safety and avoid their use concomitantly with conventional drugs. It is important to remember that topical preparations, which are not usually considered to produce significant systemic effects, may do so when applied to skin that has lost epidermal integrity. If the affected area, such as an ulcer or burn, is large enough, absorption may result in systemic levels sufficient to produce interactions or adverse effects. Problems can arise when patients fail to inform their physicians about their use of herbal agents. As discussed in one editorial in the *Journal of the American Medical Association*,[5] the risks of embracing alternative medicine include unmonitored quality of care, lack of standardized quality of products, the possibility of adverse reactions, and lack of reliable proof of efficacy. In other words, much of alternative medicine is not evidence based.

According to one source, over 40% of Americans now use complementary and alternative medicine.[5] As of 1996, more than 5000 suspected herb-related adverse events were reported in the United States. From January 1993 to October 1998, 2621 adverse events and 101 deaths were associated with dietary supplements. In fairness, it must be noted that prescription medications are involved in far more deaths than herbal remedies and are involved in a significant percentage of in-hospital mortality. A recent report in the *New York Times* claimed that up to 10,000 deaths occurred annually in the United States because of prescription errors. One author estimated that 106,000 in-hospital deaths occurred annually in the United States as a result of appropriately prescribed prescription drugs.[6] A recent study indicates that the picture is no better for nonhospitalized patients. Over 30 patient-years of observation in a multispecialty group practice revealed 1523 adverse drug reactions of which 421 (27.6%) were deemed preventable. This rate was 50.1 events per 1000 person-years. Over half were attributed to prescribing errors.[7]

When one applies cost-benefit analysis to herbal remedies, however, they fare less well. For reasons noted earlier, the desired response is often lacking.[8] When properly controlled clinical trials are conducted, there is often little or no evidence of efficacy. Coon and Ernst[9] reviewed a number of controlled clinical trials of *Panax ginseng* and were not convinced that conclusive evidence was presented for clinical claims of benefit for vitality, immune function, cardiovascular disease, cancer, or cognitive, physical, and sexual performance. Conversely, some data have been interpreted as indicating benefit for other applications. See GINSENG.

Another problem that begs for legislative action is the occasional contamination of so-called herbal remedies with potentially toxic prescription drugs and even heavy metals.[8,10] This contamination has led to kidney damage and elevated blood levels of cadmium.[10] According to Mar and Bent,[11] the ten most commonly used herbs in the United States are echinacea, St.

John's wort, ginkgo biloba, garlic, saw palmetto, ginseng, Siberian ginseng, goldenseal, aloe, and valerian. The evidence for a beneficial effect was deemed absent or inconclusive for echinacea, ginseng, Siberian ginseng, goldenseal, aloe, and valerian, and modest for the others. When herbal use is viewed from the perspective of these problems, it seems the risks might well outweigh the benefits.

In a study of herbal use among patients presenting at an urban emergency department (Bellevue Hospital, New York), Hung and colleagues[12] found that the most frequently used herbs were goldenseal tea, garlic, and ginger. Women were almost twice as likely to have used herbs as men, and Asians users were at least twice as frequent as any other ethnic group.

Germany appears to be the only developed country to have established a comprehensive legislative body to deal with herbal remedies. The Federal Institute for Drugs and Medical Devices (formerly the German Federal Health Agency) has a special scientific body, Commission E, which evaluates data regarding the efficacy and safety of herbal remedies and publishes monographs on these judgments. Phytomedicines may be sold as either over-the-counter or prescription medications provided that there is proof of their safety and convincing evidence of efficacy.[13] No other developed country has such a comprehensive program.

Many factors can influence the response of an individual to a xenobiotic, whether its effect is beneficial or toxic. The expression of metabolizing enzymes often varies considerably from one individual to another. Hormonal influences may also affect this response. The degree and duration of the exposure may affect toxicity. The presence of other xenobiotics or even of nutrients may affect absorption from the gastrointestinal tract, binding to plasma proteins, metabolism (by inducing or inhibiting biotransforming enzymes), excretion, and so on. Pharmacological addition, potentiation, or antagonism can occur. Age is an important factor as all of the preceding factors can be quite different in the very young and the elderly as compared with young and middle-aged adults. Whether or not an individual is a smoker or a drinker can affect metabolizing liver enzymes and, hence, how xenobiotics are handled. Unidentified environmental factors, some likely related to nutrition, can affect an individual's health and possibly his or her susceptibility to environmental hazards. Prostate cancer is rare in Asian men but increases with time spent in North America.

It should be evident that herbal remedies will be with us for the foreseeable future, and the potential for adverse reactions and drug interactions will only increase. It would seem wise, therefore, to invoke the precautionary principal in dealing with herbal remedies, and there are some cautionary notes that can be applied generally.

1. Because it is rare to have any information on the effects of an herbal agent on the fetus, their use during pregnancy should be avoided.
2. Little is known about the transfer of active principles in mother's milk for most herbs, so their use in nursing mothers should be avoided.

3. In the absence of specific knowledge of an herb's interactions with prescription medications, concomitant use should be discouraged or monitored closely.

4. Except for agents with known estrogenic or androgenic properties, little is known about the effects of most herbs on fertility.

5. Oral anticoagulant therapy (OACT) has always been a concern regarding drug-drug interactions, and this is also true regarding herb-drug interactions. Heck and colleagues[14] identified more than 30 herbs that might interact with warfarin, based on laboratory studies and case reports. Concomitant use of most herbs with OACT should be avoided.

6. Generally, little is known about the effects of continued use over long periods of time. A periodic so-called herb holiday is probably a good idea, but how frequently this should occur, and how long it should be, are a matter of pure speculation given the lack of pharmacokinetic data in most cases.

7. There is some concern about the possibility that herbal medicines may create undue risk in the perioperative period. Withdrawal 7 to 10 days prior to surgery may be advisable for most herbs, but in some cases (e.g., valerian) a gradual reduction in dosage may be necessary.[8]

8. With respect to Chinese herbal medicines, there is a vast array of these, both as individual herbs and as mixtures. Some Chinese remedies have made their way into western herbalism; most have not. Only a few are covered in this text. An excellent text by Chan and Cheung[15] deals with 235 Chinese herbal medicines. Interactions with conventional drugs have been recorded for many, if not most of them.

9. Children are generally not good candidates for herbal therapy. They may have greater relative exposure, less well developed biotransforming enzymes, and a higher rate of cell division, making them more vulnerable to mutagenesis.

A few words about this text are in order. It is not intended to be a reference work for those contemplating the therapeutic use of herbs. Nor is it meant to provide a source of in-depth information for those seeking details concerning all aspects of a particular herb. Citations are not extensive, and reliance is placed on good review articles in reputable journals when such are available.

A new term has entered the lexicon of alternative medicine. A *nutriceutical* is a substance that is a normal dietary ingredient consumed in relatively pure form and in larger than normal quantities to achieve hoped-for prophylactic or therapeutic benefit. A number of such agents are included in this text. According to this definition, large doses of single vitamins would qualify as nutriceuticals. A discussion of vitamins is not included, however, as it is beyond the scope of this work and a voluminous literature is already available on this topic.

As the name implies, this text is intended to be a quick source of information for physicians and other health care professionals who wish to know something of the potential hazards associated with a particular herb or nutriceutical, especially as they relate to the concomitant use of conventional pharmaceuticals. It is my hope that it will fulfill this role to the reader's satisfaction.

■ REFERENCES

1. Hardman JG, Limbird L, Gilman AG, eds. *Goodman and Gilman's The Pharmacological Basis of Therapeutics.* 10th ed. New York, NY: McGraw-Hill; 2001.
2. Bartlett J. *Bartlett's Familiar Quotations.* 14th ed. Boston, Mass: Little, Brown; 1968:817.
3. Goldman P. Herbal medicines today and the roots of modern pharmacology. *Ann Intern Med* 2001;135:594.
4. Serrano E, Anderson J. Herbals for health? Colorado State University Cooperative Extension website. Available at: http://www.ext.colostate.edu/pubs/foodnut/09370.html.
5. Jonas WB. Alternative medicine—learning from the past, examining the present, advancing to the future. *JAMA* 1998;280:1616.
6. Lazzarou J, Pomeranz BH, Corey PN. Incidence of adverse drug reactions in hospitalized patients: A meta-analysis of prospective studies. *JAMA* 1998;279:1200.
7. Gurwitz JH, Field TS, Harrold, LR, et al. Incidence and preventability of adverse drug events among older patients in the ambulatory setting. *JAMA* 2003;289:1107.
8. Ang-Lee MK, Moss J, Yuan C-S. Herbal medicines and perioperative care. *JAMA* 2001;286:208.
9. Coon JT, Ernst E. Panax ginseng: A systematic review of adverse effects and drug interactions. *Drug Saf* 2002;25:323.
10. Philp RB. Toxicity of metals. In: Philp RB, ed. *Ecosystems and Human Health: Environmental Hazards and Toxicology.* Boca Raton, Fla: Lewis Publishers/CRC Press; 2001:161.
11. Mar C, Bent S. An evidence-based review of the 10 most commonly used herbs. *West J Med* 1999;171:168.
12. Hung OL, Shih RD, Chiang WD, Nelson LS, Hoffman RS, Goldfrank LR. Herbal preparation use amongst urban emergency department patients. *Acad Emerg Med* 1997;4:209.
13. Shulz V, Hansel R, Tyler VE. *Rational Phytotherapy: A Physician's Guide to Herbal Medicine.* New York, NY: Springer-Verlag; 1998:v.
14. Heck AM, Dewitt BA, Lukes AL. Potential interactions between alternative therapies and warfarin. *Am J Health Syst Pharm* 2000;57:1221.
15. Chan K, Cheung L. *Interactions Between Chinese Herbal Medicinal Products and Orthodox Drugs.* Amsterdam, Holland: Harwood Academic Publishers; 2000.

Section 2

Alphabetical Listing of Herb and Nutriceutical Monographs

ABSINTHE

See WORMWOOD.

ACONITE

■ SOURCE, DESCRIPTION, USES

The dried, powdered root of various *Aconitum* species is used in Chinese and Japanese herbal medicine, and formerly was used in European herbal medicine (until abandoned because of its toxicity), for analgesic and antirheumatic purposes, as a febrifuge, and for various neurological and other indications.[1,2] *A. napellus* is commonly used, but all species share the same toxic characteristics. The North American species is *A. uncinatum*, commonly called monkshood for the helmet-shaped purple flower[3] and also known as wolfsbane, friar's cap, and by other colloquialisms.[1] All are members of the Ranunculaceae (buttercup) family. Monkshood grows up to 1 m in height and has deeply indented leaves similar to those of a buttercup.

In Hong Kong the roots of *A. carmichaeli* (chuanwu) and *A. kusnezoffii* (caowu) are used for musculoskeletal, cardiovascular, and other disorders.[4]

■ PHARMACOLOGY

Aconitum root contains a number of alkaloid diterpenes, notably aconitine, mesaconitine, and hypaconitine, which are neurotoxins and cardiotoxins.[4,5] These have a variety of pharmacological properties that can be classified into three main groups. One group, with high toxicity, activates voltage-dependent sodium channels and inhibits noradrenaline uptake. The second group contains less toxic sodium channel blockers and possesses antinociceptive, antiarrhythmic, and antiepileptiform properties. The third group has markedly reduced toxicity, and lacks neuronal activity but has antiarrhythmic action.[1] These different properties are attributed to different binding characteristics at the alpha subunit of the sodium channel protein in neurons and myocardiocytes. Group 1 binds to the neurotoxin binding site 2.[1,6] One alkaloid, structurally similar to aconitine, is lappaconitine, an irreversible sodium channel blocker that binds to human heart hH1 sodium channels.[7] It, too, binds to the neurotoxin site 2, and it has antiepileptiform activity.

■ ADVERSE EFFECTS AND INTERACTIONS

There are numerous reports of aconite poisoning on record. Most of these come from Hong Kong, but they are also reported from Japan and western societies. Signs and symptoms include nausea, vomiting, diarrhea, numbness in the mouth and extremities, hypotension, ventricular tachyarrhythmias, and, in extreme cases, cardiac arrest and death.[4,5,8] In one fatal case (death occurred on day 6 after ingestion), most alkaloids were undetectable in blood taken 24 hours after ingestion but were readily detectable in urine.[8]

Although no drug interactions were detected in the literature, the potential for these would seem to be quite high, especially for cardiac and centrally acting drugs. Aconite is a botanical with high toxicity and should probably be avoided completely, especially because the incidence of toxic reactions is high even in societies where herbal therapists should be the most experienced and knowledgeable regarding the risks associated with its use. It may be that useful drugs will evolve from research into the actions of its various alkaloids, but this development is as yet in the future.

■ REFERENCES

1. Aconite. Available at: http://www.geocities.com/RainForest/Canopy/6901/herbs/aconite.html.

2. Ameri A. The effects of aconitum alkaloids on the central nervous system. *Prog Neurobiol* 1998;56:211.

3. Peterson RT, McKenny M. *Northeastern Wildflowers: Roger Tory Peterson Field Guides.* Norwalk, Conn: Easton Press; 1984:318.

4. Chan TY. Incidence of herb-induced aconitine poisoning in Hong Kong: Impact of publicity measures to promote awareness among the herbalists and the public. *Drug Saf* 2002:25:823.

5. Chan TY, Tomlinson B, Critchley JA. Aconitine poisoning following the ingestion of Chinese herbal medicines: A report of eight cases. *Aust N Z J Med* 1993;23:268.

6. Friese J, Gleitz J, Gutser UT, et al. Aconitum sp. alkaloids: The modulation of voltage-dependent Na^+ channels, toxicity and antinociceptive properties. *Eur J Pharmacol* 1997;337:165.

7. Wright SN. Irreversible block of human heart (hH1) sodium channels by the plant alkaloid lappaconitine. *Mol Pharmacol* 2002;59:193.

8. Yoshioka N, Gonmori K, Tagashira A, et al. A case of aconitine poisoning with analysis of aconitine alkaloids by GC/SIM. *Forensic Sci Int* 1996;81:117.

AGRIMONY

■ SOURCE, DESCRIPTION, USES

The herbaceous plant *Agrimonia eupatoria*, a member of the rose family Rosaceae, has small yellow flowers on a slender spike. One of several similar species that include *A. pilosa* and *A. procera*, it grows in woodlands and along fence rows throughout the northeastern United States and Canada as well as many parts of Europe. Because of the small hooked seed receptacles, it is also known as cockle burr and stickle wort or stick wort (various spellings for these). Other names include liverwort, church steeples, Hsian Ho Tsao, and Xian He Cao.[1] The herbal preparation includes the aerial parts of the plant with or without the flowers. These are dried, powdered, and taken as a tea, infusion, alcohol extract, tincture, or capsule.

This herb has been recommended for virtually every medical condition known to humankind. The list is exhaustive, according to lay sources, but attention seems to have been focused on the urogenital tract.[1,2]

■ PHARMACOLOGY

A number of compounds have been identified from the plant, including a new flavonol glycoside kaempferide (or kamferide) 3-rhamnoside, as well as kaempferide, kaempferol, kaempferol 3-rhamnoside, kaempferol 3-gluciside, and kaemperferol 3-rutoinoside.[3]

Recently, scientific interest has focused on the antidiabetic properties of the plant, stemming from its traditional use for this condition.[4] Using streptozotocin-induced diabetes in mice as a model, it was found that agrimony countered the weight loss, hyperphagia, polydipsia, and hyperglycemia associated with this condition.[4,5] A 1-mg/mL aqueous extract also stimulated glucose uptake and utilization in mouse abdominal muscle comparable to 0.1 µM of insulin.[4] It also stimulated insulin secretion from a pancreatic cell line.[4] Agrimony, along with numerous other herbal remedies, has been promoted for the treatment of perimenopausal urogenital atrophy, but there does not appear to be any convincing evidence in support of this claim.[6]

■ ADVERSE EFFECTS AND INTERACTIONS

One lay source[1] that does not provide references lists constipation, lactation, and pregnancy as contraindications to use of agrimony, as well as a number of incompatibilities with metals and proteins because of its high tannin content. A number of potential drug interactions also are listed, including antagonism of antihypertensive drugs, oral anticoagulants, and antidiabetic agents, and increased toxicity of diuretics and nonsteroidal anti-inflammatory drugs. The International Programme on Chemical Safety provides an extensive document on the toxicity of pyrrolizidine alkaloids (PAs).[7] *Eupatoriae* species are listed as potential sources of these substances. Evidence is cited that even a single exposure to PAs may progress "relentlessly" to advanced liver disease and cirrhosis. Synergism with aflatoxin also has been shown for PAs. Because of the long latency period of these substances and the reluctance of patients to provide a history of herbal use, underestimation of liver disease associated with use of herbs is a real possibility. PAs are eliminated within 24 *hours*; thus, laboratory tests may not be of much use. Although *Agrimonia eupatoria* is not specifically mentioned as a source of poisoning, the widespread distribution of PAs in flowering plants (perhaps in 3% of all these) and the paucity of reliable data on its toxicology suggest that extreme caution is indicated when agrimony use is suspected. Discouraging its use along with prescription medications, during pregnancy, in breast-feeding mothers, and in diabetic individuals is indicated. Long-term effects and effects on the reproductive process are unknown.

■ REFERENCES

1. Agrimony. NutritionFocus website. Available at: http://www.nutrition-focus.com.
2. Agrimony Available at: http://purplesage.org.uk/prfiles/agrimony.htm
3. Bilia AR, Palme E, Marsill A, et al. A flavonol glycoside from Agrimonia Eupatoria. *Phytochemistry-Oxford* 1993;32:1078.
4. Gray AM, Flatt PR. Actions of the traditional anti-diabetic plant, Agrimony eupatoria (agrimony): Effects on hyperglycemia, cellular glucose metabolism and insulin secretion. *Br J Nutr* 1998;80:109.
5. Swanston-Flatt SK, Day C, Bailey CJ, et al. Traditional plant treatments for diabetes. Studies in normal and streptozotocin diabetic mice. *Diabetologia* 1990;33:462.
6. Willhite LA, O'Connell MB. Urogenital atrophy: Prevention and treatment. *Pharmacotherapy* 2001;21:464.
7. Pyrrolizidine alkaloids. International Programme on Chemical Safety website. Available at: http://www.inchem.org/documents/ehc/ehc/ehc080.htm.

AKEE

■ SOURCE, DESCRIPTION, USES

The akee, or ackee, tree (*Blighia sapida*) was introduced in 1778 by Thomas Clarke to the island of Jamaica from West Africa, where it is known as ankye or ishin.[1] It has since spread throughout the West Indies and South America, where it has become plentiful. It was named after Captain William Bligh in the mistaken belief that he had introduced it, like the breadfruit, to Jamaica. For over a century it has been associated with a condition called the "vomiting sickness of Jamaica." Folklore and anecdotal reports attributed the condition to consuming unripe akee fruit. This fruit has been a cheap source of food for rural and economically depressed Africans and Jamaicans. In 1976, Tanaka and colleagues described two fatal cases of this condition and elaborated the causative agents.[2] Akee has been used in folk medicine for the treatment of diabetes because of its hypoglycemic effect.[3]

■ PHARMACOLOGY

A water-soluble toxic principle, hypoglycin A, has been isolated from the unripe akee fruit, but it is not present in ripe fruit. In addition to inducing pronounced vomiting, hypoglycin A causes a marked hypoglycemia. Prior to the discovery of this fact, mortality often reached 80% in Africa and Jamaica.[1] The administration of intravenous glucose can prevent death if the hypoglycemia has not been too prolonged.[1]

The hypoglycemia appears to be the result of inhibition of gluconeogenesis by depletion of coenzyme A and carnitine, both of which are essential cofactors for the oxidation of long-chain fatty acids.[1,4] Hypoglycemia also has been induced in rats by hypoglycin A, and in both rats and humans, unusually high levels of metabolites have been isolated from the urine. These are eight and ten carbon dicarboxylic acids, including 2-ethylmalonic, 2-methylsuccinic, glutaric, and adipic acids.[2]

■ ADVERSE EFFECTS AND INTERACTIONS

Akee poisoning has not produced any documented drug interactions, probably because of the acute and severe nature of the toxicity. There is the theoretical possibility that milder intoxication could be exacerbated by the concomitant use of oral antidiabetic drugs or insulin. There does not seem to have been much interest in exploring the therapeutic usefulness of hypoglycin A, probably because of its toxicity.

Reports of serious and fatal intoxication continue to appear in the literature. Meda and colleagues[5] documented an extensive outbreak in the West African country of Burkina Faso. Seven fatalities occurred in preschool children aged 2 to 7 years. It was assumed that the children had picked up unripe fruit from the ground or picked it from low branches. By May 31, 1998, 29 cases had been identified since the beginning of the year. The seven fatal cases of encephalopathy involved hypotonia, convulsions, coma, hypoglycemia, and high urine levels of dicarboxylic acids. Fever developed in some cases. Other recent reports of poisonings have come from Haiti.[6] Typically in such cases, the local population was unaware of the toxic nature of unripe akee.

■ REFERENCES

1. Bressler R. The unripe akee—forbidden fruit. *N Engl J Med* 1976;295:500.
2. Tanaka K, Kean EA, Johnson B. Jamaican vomiting sickness: Biochemical investigation of two cases. *N Engl J Med* 1976;295:461.
3. Fisher CR, Veronneau JH. Herbal preparations: A primer for the aeromedical physician. *Aviat Space Environ Med* 2000;71:45.
4. Billington D, Osmundsen H, Sherratt HAS. The biochemical basis of Jamaican akee poisoning. *N Engl J Med* 1976;295:1482.
5. Meda HA, Diallo B, Buchet JP, et al. Epidemic of fatal encephalopathy in preschool children in Burkina Faso and consumption of unripe ackee (Blighia sapida) fruit. *Lancet* 1999;353:536.
6. Moya J. Ackee (Blighia sapida) poisoning in Northern Province, Haiti, 2001. *Epidemiol Bull* 2001;22:82.

ALFALFA

■ SOURCE, DESCRIPTION, USES

A cultivated forage plant (*Medicago sativa*), this low, clover-like plant often escapes to roadsides.

■ PHARMACOLOGY

See PHYTOESTROGENS AND PHYTOPROGESTINS.

ALOE VERA

■ SOURCES, DESCRIPTION, USES

The gel (mucilage) from the inner central zone of the leaves of *Aloe vulgari* and *A. barbadensis* has been used for generations as a topical treatment for wounds and burns and now appears as an ingredient in many skin creams and other cosmetics.[1] The plant, a native of Africa, is grown commercially in many locales, including the island of Aruba. Although contact allergic dermatitis is a theoretical possibility because of the presence of glycoprotein fractions,[2] this does not seem to be much of a problem.

PHARMACOLOGY

The healing properties of aloe vera may be a result of its ability, demonstrated experimentally, to facilitate dermal blood flow by inhibiting thromboxane synthase and the formation of the vasoconstrictor thromboxane A_2.[3] It also appears to facilitate the attachment of cultured human tumor and normal cells.[4] Gel polysaccharides may have an immunomodulatory effect.[2]

Aloe juice (latex) is a bitter, yellow liquid from pericyclic cells of the inner plant leaf,[1,5] possessing stimulant laxative properties. The purgative effect of aloe results from the presence of the anthraquinone glycoside 1,8-dihydroxyanthraquinone (danthron) and related compounds.[6] These are also present in other members of the Liliaceae, including senna, cascara, and rhubarb (family Polygonaceae). Bacteria in the colon remove the sugar from the anthraquinone glycoside to form anthrol, the active principal, which stimulates motility of the large bowel.

ADVERSE EFFECTS AND INTERACTIONS

Concern regarding the use of aloe vera relates to its internal use as a potent cathartic.[5] The use of danthron itself has been discontinued because of evidence that it can cause intestinal and hepatic tumors in laboratory animals.[6] This response has not been reported for botanical preparations; however, chronic use of aloe as a cathartic is not recommended. Similar to all strong cathartics, aloe may cause griping, colicky pain and excessive laxative effect.[6] Chronic use may lead to electrolyte imbalance, especially potassium depletion.[5] The active principal is secreted in mother's milk and may be in sufficient concentration to affect the nursing infant.[5] Clearly, this cathartic should not be given in conjunction with other laxatives. Potassium depletion may be exacerbated by thiazide diuretics, corticosteroids, or licorice root.[5] Potassium depletion may also potentiate the effects of cardiac glycosides and antiarrhythmics.[5,7] Aloe may cause pelvic engorgement and increase menstrual bleeding and the risk of spontaneous abortion. Aloe cathartic is contraindicated in pregnancy, nursing mothers, children younger than 12 years of age, and suspected intestinal obstruction. Large doses may produce nephritis. Emodin, one of the anthraquinones (1,6,8-trihydroxy-3-methylanthraquinone) found in this and related cathartic herbal preparations, has been shown to be mutagenic in the Ames *Salmonella*/mammalian microsomal assay. This effect was activation dependent and appeared to result from a stable, oxidized metabolite forming a physicochemical association with DNA.[8] This effect further supports the contraindication for use of aloe and related herbal preparations in pregnancy.

■ REFERENCES

1. Pribitkin E deA, Boger G. Herbal therapy: What every facial plastic surgeon must know. *Arch Facial Plast Surg* 2001;3:127.
2. Dweck RT. Aloe vera leaf gel: A review update. *J Ethnopharmacol* 1999;68:3.
3. Klein AD, Pennys NS. Aloe vera. *J Am Acad Dermatol* 1988;18:714.
4. Winters WD, Benavides R, Clouse WJ. Effect of aloe extracts on human normal and tumor cells in vitro. *Econ Botany* 1981;35:89.
5. Hadley SK, Petry JJ. Medicinal herbs: A primer for primary care. *Hosp Pract* 1999;34:105.
6. Brunton LL. Agents affecting gastrointestinal water flux and motility, digestants, and bile acids. In: Gilman AG, Rall TW, Nies AS, Taylor P, eds. *Goodman and Gilman's The Pharmacological Basis of Therapeutics.* 8th ed. New York, NY: Pergamon Press; 1990:921.
7. Herb/drug interactions. Space Coast Medical Associates website. Available at: http://spacecoastmedicalassociates.com/herbalsupplements/interactions.htm.
8. Bosch R, Freidrich U, Lutz WK, et al. Investigation on DNA binding in rat liver and in Salmonella and on mutagenicity in the Ames test by emodin, a natural anthraquinone. *Mutat Res* 1987;188:161.

AMMI

■ SOURCE, DESCRIPTION, USES

Ammi (*Ammi majus,* family Umbelliferae) is a native of the Nile valley and has been used in folk medicine in that region for centuries, principally for the treatment of vitiligo, or leukoderma (literally white skin), a condition in which there is depigmentation of patchy areas of the skin. Ammi is also called false Bishop's weed or false Queen Anne's lace. It should not to be confused with the North American version, also called wild carrot (*Daucus carota*),which is also a member of the family Umbelliferae. Ammi is still used today in Egyptian folk medicine for many purposes.[1,2]

■ PHARMACOLOGY

In the 1940s, Abdel Monem el Mofty, an Egyptian professor of dermatology, noted that the folk medicine practice of rubbing the juice of ammi on patches of vitiligo and having the individual lie in the sun resulted in repigmentation of the affected area. His observations resulted in the development of modern photochemotherapy, referred to as PUVA (psoralen-ultra-violet A). The process depends on the presence of psoralens, furocoumarins that sensitize the skin to the ultraviolet A (UVA) in sunlight or from an artificial source. El Mofty first crystallized 8-methoxypsoralen, or xanthotoxin, from ammi. It is still used as the psoralen in PUVA.[1]Psoralens are tricyclic compounds consisting of a furan ring linked to a coumarin. They are very hydrophobic compounds that, because of their planar structure, can intercalate with DNA bases. They have strong absorption bands in the 200 to 350 nm range, which is that of UVA. When thus excited, the molecule can bind covalently to DNA. The adducts so formed in melanocyte DNA promote increased mitosis, and melanocyte numbers can double or triple within a week.[1,3,4] PUVA is used to treat several skin conditions, including psoriasis.

■ ADVERSE EFFECTS AND INTERACTIONS

In common with other members of the Umbelliferae, ammi herb or plant can cause phytophotodermatitis. This is not a true allergic reaction, having no immunological component, and therefore it can affect anyone and is dose- and exposure-dependent.[1,5] Both the extent of UVA or sunlight exposure and the total psoralen load can affect the severity of the reaction. After a latent period of about 24 hours, unusual patterns of erythema, edema, and bullae appear. These manifestations generally are painful but not itchy and the reaction peaks in about 72 hours. Topical exposure can elicit a reaction within 15 minutes. Because ammi is used as an ornamental plant, contact exposure in gardeners is a possibility.

Although phytophotodermatitis is not a true allergic reaction, such reactions can occur with ammi as with other plants. In one report, a florist who developed immunoglobulin E–mediated rhinitis and contact dermatitis to ammi developed an 8-mm wheal when tested by skin prick using ammi (Bishop's weed) flowers.[6]

PUVA therapy has been associated with a significant increase in the incidence of squamous cell and basal cell carcinoma of the skin,[3,4] not surprising considering the DNA adduct-forming properties of psoralens. Hepatotoxicity also has been reported with PUVA, although infrequently.[4] The extent to which these adverse reactions represent risks following herbal use of ammi or accidental contact with psoralen-containing plants is presently unknown, but there is probably a similar exposure and dose relationship. Readers who wish to know more on this subject should refer to reference 1. See also Appendix XIII.

■ REFERENCES

1. Botanical dermatology: Phytophotodermatitis. Available at: http://www.telemedicine.org. Click on "electronic textbook," then on "phytophotodermatitis."

2. Singab ANB. Acetylated flavonol triglycosides from Ammi majus L. *Phytochemistry* 1998;7:2188.

3. Bethea D, Fullmer B, Syed S, et al. Psoralen photobiology and photochemotherapy: 50 years of science and medicine. *J Dermatol Sci* 1999;19:78.

4. Wyatt EL, Sutter SH, Drake LA. Dermatological pharmacology. In: Hardman JG, Limbird L, Gilman AG, eds. *Goodman and Gilman's The Pharmacological Basis of Therapeutics.* 10th ed. New York, NY: McGraw-Hill; 2001:1808.

5. Klaassen CD. Principles of toxicology and treatment of poisoning. In: Hardman JG, Limbird L, Gilman AG, eds. *Goodman and Gilman's The Pharmacological Basis of Therapeutics.* 10th ed. New York, NY: McGraw-Hill; 2001:67.

6. Kiistala R, Makinen-Kiljunen S. Occupational allergic rhinitis and contact urticaria caused by bishop's weed (Ammi majus). *Allergy* 1999;54:635.

ANGELICA (DAHURICA)

See BAI ZHI.

ANGELICA (SINENSIS)

See DONG QUAI.

ANISE

■ SOURCE, DESCRIPTION, USES

Anise is the essential oil of the ripe fruit (often called seeds) of *Pimpinella anisum* (family Umbelliferae or Apiaceae).[1] The plant is a native of southeastern Europe and Asia Minor and has been widely cultivated in England and throughout Europe.[2] Its use as a spice, flavoring agent, scent ingredient, and herbal medicine dates back centuries. It is used also in the preparation of liqueurs. Traditionally, anise was used as a carminative and expectorant. The seeds have even been smoked to obtain relief from cough.[2] In the past it was recommended for infant catarrh, a practice that has led to toxic reactions. See ANISE (STAR), immediately following.

Modern usage has changed little. Anise is still used as an expectorant for catarrhal diseases, four drops of anise oil, diluted, being the recommended dose.[1]

■ PHARMACOLOGY

The active principle of anise oil is anethole. It is obtained by freezing the oil, which causes anethole crystals to form.[1] Anethole is believed to stimulate ciliary activity in the bronchi. Anethole is rapidly absorbed from the gastrointestinal tract and rapidly eliminated in the urine and, to some extent, in the expired air. Some metabolites have been identified, such as 4-methoxyhippuric acid and 4-methoxybenzoic acid.[1] Anethole has been shown to possess anti-inflammatory and anticancer properties in laboratory rodents, possibly by blocking tumor necrosis factor–mediated responses.[3] A number of glycosides of 2-C-methyl-D-erythritol have also been identified in anise fruit[4] as have several sesquiterpenes.[5]

■ ADVERSE EFFECTS AND INTERACTIONS

The main concern regarding the use of anise and oil is allergic reactions, especially dermatitis.[1] Cross-reactivity has been demonstrated to coriander, fennel, and cumin (all Umbelliferae) and allergens include Bet v 1- and profilin-related ones and higher molecular weight allergens causing type I allergy.[6] Anethole also has been shown to be a constituent of fennel and camphor.[3] See also Appendix V.

Similar to other members of the Umbelliferae family, anise may contain psoralens and cause phytophotodermatitis, mostly on contact with the skin. This is a photochemical reaction and not a true antibody-based allergic reaction. For more details on phytophotodermatitis, see AMMI; see also Appendix XIII.

In rodent LD50 studies, cis-anethole has been shown to be 15 times more toxic than trans-anethole, and there are no restrictions limiting the amount of cis-anethole allowed in herbal preparations.[1]

Although animal studies have failed to demonstrate carcinogenicity for anise,[1] a more recent long-term study of rats and mice examined the carcinogenicity of methyleugenol, a constituent of anise oil and of many essential oils and foodstuffs.[7] Hepatic neoplasms occurred at all doses in rats and mice, and stomach and kidney tumors occurred in rats. All male rats receiving 150 or 300 mg/kg per day died before the study ended, and survival was decreased in female rats and mice. Although anise oil per se may not be a carcinogen, it could contribute to the total body exposure to methyleugenol if taken to excess.

In summary, anise oil seems to be a fairly innocuous herbal remedy for cough if not overdone and provided no allergic tendency is present. Its use in very young children is questionable. The situation with respect to star anise, however, is quite different (see next entry).

■ REFERENCES

1. Schulz V, Hansel R, Tyler VE. *Rational Phytotherapy: A Physician's Guide to Herbal Medicine.* New York, NY: Springer-Verlag; 1998:159.
2. Anise. In: Grieve M. *A Modern Herbal.* Botanical.com website. Available at: http://www.botanical.com/botanical/mgmh/a/anise040.html.
3. Chainy GB, Manna SK, Chaturvedi MM, Aggarwal BB. Anethole blocks both early and late cellular responses transduced by tumor necrosis factor: Effect on NF-kappaB, AP-1, JNK, MAPKK and apoptosis. *Oncogene* 2000;19:2943.
4. Kitajima J, Ishikawa T, Fujimatu E, Kondho K, Takayangi T. Glycosides of 2-C-methyl-D-erythritol from the fruits of anise, coriander and cumin. *Phytochemistry* 2003;62:115.
5. Burkhardt G, Reichling J, Martin R, Becker H. Terpene hydrocarbons in Pimpinella anisum L. *Pharm Weekbl Sci* 1986;8:190.
6. Jensen-Jarolim E, Gangleberger E, Leitner A, Radauer C, Scheiner O, Breiteneder H. Characterization of allergens in Apiaceae spices: Anise, fennel, coriander and cumin. *Clin Exp Allergy* 1997;27:1299.
7. Johnson JD, Ryan MJ, Toft JD II, et al. Two-year toxicity study of methyleugenol in F344/N rats and B6C3F mice. *J Agric Food Chem* 2000;48:3620.

ANISE (STAR)

■ SOURCE, DESCRIPTION, USES

The herbal form of star anise comes from the star-shaped fruit of a small tree native to the Far East (*Illicium verum*, family Magnoliaceae).[1] Traditionally, it has been used for colic and rheumatism and as a seasoning.[2] Currently, star anise oil is used in some parts of the world for digestive ailments and as a carminative, mild expectorant, and cough suppressant, as well as for diuresis.[2]

■ PHARMACOLOGY

Similar to anise, star anise contains anethole, which has been identified as benzene 1-methoxy-4-(1-propenyl).[2] Its useful properties are, therefore, similar to those of anise (see ANISE). Anethole also has been shown to possess antimicrobial activity against a variety of microorganisms.[2] The toxicity of star anise, however, is quite different from that of anise and potentially quite serious.

■ ADVERSE EFFECTS AND INTERACTIONS

In some parts of Spain (and probably elsewhere), the practice persists of giving infants infusions (teas) of star anise as a treatment for cholic. This has resulted in numerous cases of infants with acute neurological and gastrointestinal signs and symptoms.[3,4] In one study of 23 cases, the mean age was 39 days. Symptoms included irritability, abnormal movements, vomiting, and nystagmus.[4] Epileptiform seizures also have been reported.[3] In some cases contamination with *I. anisatum*, a related but more toxic species, was implicated. This also may have been the case in an outbreak of epileptic seizures in Holland. Sixty-three people reported symptoms of general malaise and vomiting 2 to 4 hours following consumption of an herbal tea. Sixteen developed generalized clonic-tonic seizures.[5] Contamination with *I. anisatum* was suspected but not proven. However, nuclear magnetic resonance analysis confirmed the presence of the neurotoxin anisatin, a noncompetitive γ-aminobutyric acid (GABA) antagonist that can cause hyperactivity.

Although *I. anisatum* may be more toxic than *I. verum*, neurotoxic sesquiterpenoids (veranisatins A, B, and C) have been isolated from the latter and have been shown to induce convulsions in mice.[6] The use of star anise oil in infants is contraindicated regardless of the source.

■ REFERENCES

1. Anise (star). In: Grieve M. *A Modern Herbal*. Available at: http://botanical.com/botanical/mgmh/a/anise041.html.
2. De M, De AK, Sen P, Banerjee AB. Antimicrobial properties of star anise (Illicium verum Hook f). *Phytother Res* 2002;16:93.
3. Gil Campos M, Perez Navero JL, Ibarra De la Rosa L. Convulsive status secondary to star anis poisoning in a neonate. *An Esp Pediatr* 2002;57:366.
4. Garzo Fernandez C, Gomez Pintado P, Barrasa Blanco A, Martinez Arrieta R, Ramirez Fernandez R, Ramon Rosa F. Cases of neurological symptoms associated with star anis consumption used as a carminative. *An Esp Pediatr* 2002;57:290.

5. Johanns ES, van der Kolk LE, van Gemert HM, Sijben AE, Peters PW, de Vries I. An epidemic of epileptic seizures after consumption of herbal tea [in Dutch]. *Ned Tijdschr Geneeskd* 2002;146:813, comment 808.

6. Nakamura T, Okuyama E, Yamakazi M. Neurotropic companents from star anise (Illicium verum Hook.fil). *Chem Parm Bull (Tokyo)* 1996;44:1908.

ARISTOLOCHIA

■ SOURCE, DESCRIPTION, USES

Members of the Aristolochiaceae family have a worldwide distribution, mostly tropical, but there are several species in North America and many have been used as herbal remedies. Various *Aristolochia* species have been used for centuries for arthritis, gout, rheumatism, festering wounds, and in obstetrics (hence the common name for the family, "birthwort"[1]). Another ancient use is for the treatment of snakebite; hence, the name of a common North American species, snakeroot (*A. serpentaria*).[1-4] Recent interest and concern regarding these herbs relates to their accidental incorporation into herbal slimming agents in Chinese herbal remedies.[5]

■ PHARMACOLOGY

There are probably several active ingredients in aristolochia, but it is generally conceded that most of its activity, and toxicity, is related to aristolochic acids I and II. These are mixtures of structurally related nitrophenanthrene carboxylic acids.[2] It appears that there is a biochemical basis for the use of *Aristolochia* species for treating snakebite. An aristolochic acid, 9-hydroxy-8-methoxy-6-nitrophenanthro(3,4-d)-1,3-dioxole-5-carboxylic acid, has been shown to interact with several components of snake venom and to inhibit one of these, phospholipase A_2 (PLA$_2$).[6] Mammalian PLA$_2$ mobilizes arachidonic acid from membrane lipids for the synthesis of leukotrienes and prostaglandins by lipoxygenases and cyclooxygenases.[7] These may be involved in inflammatory processes and even in carcinogenesis.[6] Hong and colleagues[8] examined a number of *Aristolochia* species used as Korean medicinal plants for ability to inhibit cyclooxygenase-2 (the inducible form) and inducible nitric oxide synthase and found that all exhibited some inhibitory activity and one, *A. debilis*, almost completely inhibited both enzymes. These results would suggest that some members of the Aristolochiaceae possess potential anti-inflammatory agents. Indeed, one group examining some Central American plants found that a chloroform extract of the leaves of *A. trilobata* was almost as potent as indomethacin as a topical anti-inflammatory agent in a mouse ear (croton oil) edema test.[9] This was one of several plants used in traditional medicine as poultices for topical inflammations and wounds.

■ ADVERSE EFFECTS AND INTERACTIONS

Several cases have been reported of end-stage renal failure and several of nephropathy associated with the use of Chinese herbal medicines for weight reduction. Unique histopathological changes in the kidneys (cortical interstitial fibrosis with relative preservation of the glomeruli) led to the coining of the term *Chinese herbal nephropathy*, or CHN, for this condition.[10] These accidental poisonings arose out of confusion over the Latin versus the Chinese names for some herbs. The herb intended for use in weight reduction was *Stephania tetranda*, the Chinese name for which is *fangchi* or *han-fangji*. Unfortunately *A. fangchi* was substituted in a number of preparations, and it is extremely toxic. Most western countries, including the United States, Canada, and Great Britain, have now banned the importation and sale of herbals containing *Aristolochia* plants or extracts. This herb also has been associated with urothelial carcinoma.[11] It is now apparent that both the fibrotic process in the kidneys and the carcinogenesis result from formation of DNA adducts by aristolochic acid.[2] Further confirmation that *A. fangchi* is the causative agent of CHN comes from a study of 44 cases of end-stage renal disease and 27 of chronic renal failure that determined a relationship between the cumulative dose of the herb and the progression rate to end-stage renal failure.[12]

There is obviously no place for this herb in any botanical pharmacy, but it is likely that it will continue to find its way into the homes of unsuspecting victims who purchase it over the Internet or from unscrupulous herbalists. Although no documented cases of drug interactions were found, the potential with any potent agent such as this is present.

■ REFERENCES

1. Peterson RT, McKenny M. *Northeastern Wildflowers: Roger Tory Peterson Field Guides*. Norwalk, Conn: Easton Press; 1984:xvii, 388.

2. M.Arlt V, Stiborova M, Schmeiser HH. Aristolochic acid as a probable human cancer hazard in herbal remedies: A review. *Mutagenesis* 2002;17:265.

3. Birthwort. In: Grieve M. *A Modern Herbal*. Botanical.com website. Available at: http://botanical.com/botanical/mgmh/b/birthw44.html.

4. Snakeroot. In: Grieve M. *A Modern Herbal*. Botanical.com website. Available at: http://www.botanical.com/botanical/mgmh/s/snaker56.html.

5. Ioset J-R, Raoelison GE, Hostettmann K. Detection of aristolochic acid in Chinese phytomedicines and dietary supplements used in slimming regimens. *Food Chem Toxicol* 2003;41:29.

6. Chandra V, Jayasankur J, Jasti J et al. Structural basis of phospholipase A2 inhibition by the plant alkaloid aristolochic acid from a 1.7 A° crystal structure. *Biochemistry* 2002;41:10914.

7. Morrow JD, Roberts LJ II. Lipid-derived autocoids: Eicosanoids and platelet-activating factor, In: Hardman JG, Limbird L, Gilman AG, eds. *Goodman and Gilman's The Pharmacological Basis of Therapeutics.* 10th ed. New York, NY: McGraw-Hill; 2001:669.

8. Hong CH, Hur SK, Oh OJ, Kim SS, Nam KA, Lee SK. Evaluation of natural products on inhibition of inducible cyclooxygenase (COX-2) and nitric oxide synthase (iNOS) in cultured mouse macrophage cells. *J Ethnopharmacol* 2002;83:153.

9. Sosa S, Balick MJ, Arvigo R, et al. Screening of the topical anti-inflammatory activity of some Central American plants. *J Ethnopharmacol* 2002;81:211.

10. Vanherweghem JL, Depierreux M, Tielemans C, et al. Rapidly progressive renal interstitial fibrosis in young women: Association with slimming regimen including Chinese herbs. *Lancet* 1993;341:387.

11. Nortier JL, Martinez MC, Schmeiser HH, et al. Urothelial carcinoma associated with the use of a Chinese herb (Aristolochia fangchi). *N Engl J Med* 2000;342:1686.

12 Martinez M-C, Nortier J, Vereerstaeten P, Vanherweghen JL. Progression rate of Chinese herb nephropathy: Impact of Aristolochia fangchi dose. *Nephrol Dial Transplant* 2002;17:408.

ARNICA

■ SOURCE, DESCRIPTION, USES

Arnica herb is prepared from the roots and aerial portions of a number of *Arnica* species. The European variety, *A. montana*, a tall plant bearing orange-yellow daisy-like flowers, is the principal source of the herb.[1] Other species that have been used include *A. chamissonis, A. fulgens, A. cordifolia,* and *A. sororia.*[2] Synonyms for arnica include mountain tobacco and leopard's bane.[1] Native North American species include *A. mollis* and *A. acaulis* (also called leopard's bane).[3] All are members of the daisy family (Compositae).[3] Traditional uses have included topical application for a variety of conditions such as sprains, bruises, wounds, and chilblains, and the herb also has been used internally to lower fever and as a stimulant and diuretic. Systemic toxicity was noted early on.[1] Arnica is used in a variety of homeopathic remedies, but the principal use is as a topical application for trauma-related conditions and for rheumatic conditions of the muscles and joints.[4] It is one of the topical herbs approved by the German Commission E.[4] Current approved use is for topical application, only.

PHARMACOLOGY

Arnica contains the sesquiterpene lactones helenalin, $11\alpha,13$-dihydrohelenalin, and chamissonolid, thought to be the active anti-inflammatory ingredients.[2] Experimental studies of these substances have shown activities (not all possessed by all of them) that include inhibition of the following: neutrophil migration and chemotaxis, prostaglandin synthase, and activation of the transcription factor NF-κB in T cells.[2,5] Inhibition of platelet aggregation also has been reported.[2] A study of arnica extract for antimicrobial properties found only slight activity.[6]

Well-controlled clinical studies have failed to yield convincing evidence for the efficacy of topical arnica. In a study of post–laser treatment bruises, no significant difference from controls was observed when arnica gel was compared with a vehicle gel.[2] Several studies have debunked the effectiveness of homeopathic arnica in several conditions, including muscle soreness in runners,[7] tissue trauma,[8] and postoperative hematomas.[9]

ADVERSE EFFECTS AND INTERACTIONS

Up to 20 different chemicals have been identified in arnica extracts, depending on the method of extraction, weather conditions, and growing locale.[10] Extracts generally were found to be nontoxic and nonirritant in animal tests, although mutagenesis was noted in the Ames test.[10] Conversely, ingestion of products containing A. montana has caused severe gastroenteritis, nervousness, tachycardia, muscle weakness, and even death.[10] Contact allergic dermatitis is widely recognized as a problem with arnica flowers, and cross-sensitivity with other members of the Compositae, such as marigolds, is common.[11,12] The allergenicity of this group seems to depend on their sesquiterpene lactone content.[13,14]

In view of the lack of proven efficacy and the potential for adverse reactions, the topical use of arnica is a questionable practice. Additional safety data are required,[10] and the plethora of active components, including coumarins,[10] creates a potential for drug interactions,[15] See also Appendices I and VIII.

■ REFERENCES

1. Arnica. In: Grieve M. *A Modern Herbal.* Botanical.com website. Available at: http://www.botanical.com/botanical/mgmh/a/arnic058.html.
2. Alonso D, Lazarus MC, Bauman L. Effects of topical arnica gel on post-laser treatment bruises. *Dermatol Surg* 2002;28:686.
3. Peterson RT, McKenny M. *Northeastern Wildflowers: Roger Tory Peterson Field Guides.* Norwalk, Conn: Easton Press; 1984:188.
4. Schulz V, Hansel R, Tyler VE. *Rational Phytotherapy: A Physician's Guide to Herbal Medicine.* New York, NY: Springer-Verlag; 1998:252.
5. Klaas CA, Wagner G, Laufer S, et al. Studies on the anti-inflammatory activity of phytopharmaceuticals prepared from arnica flowers. *Planta Med* 2002;68:385.
6. Koo H, Gomes BF, Rosalen PL, Ambrosano GM, Park YK, Cury JA. In vitro antimicrobial activity of propolis and Arnica montana against oral pathogens. *Arch Oral Biol* 2000;45:141.
7. Vickers AJ, Fisher P, Smith C, Wyllie SE, Rees R. Homeopathic arnica 30x is ineffective for muscle soreness after long distance running: A randomized, double-blind, placebo-controlled trial. *Clin J Pain* 1998;14:227.
8. Ernst E, Pittler MH. Efficacy of homeopathic arnica: A systematic review of placebo-controlled clinical trials. *Arch Surg* 1998;133:1187.
9. Ramelet AA, Buchheim G, Lorenz P, Imfeld M. Homeopathic arnica in postoperative hematomas: A double-blind study. *Dermatology* 2000;201:347.
10. Final report on the safety assessment of Arnica montana extract and Arnica montana. *Int J Toxicol* 2000;20(suppl 2):1.
11. Reider N, Komericki P, Hausen BM, Fritsch P, Aberer W. The seamy side of natural medicines: Contact sensitization to arnica (Arnica montana L.) and marigold Calendula officinalis L.). *Contact Dermatitis* 2001;45:269.
12. Paulson E, Andersen KE, Hausen BM. Sensitization and cross-reaction patterns in Danish Compositae-allergic patients. *Contact Dermatitis* 2001;45:197.
13. Spettoli E, Silvani S, Lucente P, Guerra L, Vincenzi C. Contact dermatitis caused by sesquiterpene lactones. *Am J Contact Dermat* 1998;9:49.
14. Kiken DA, Cohen DE. Contact dermatitis to botanical extracts. *Am J Contact Dermatol* 2002;13:148.
15. Heck AM, Dewitt BA, Lukes AA. Potential interactions between alternative therapies and warfarin. *Am J Health Syst Pharm* 2000;57:1221.

ASH BARK

■ SOURCE, DESCRIPTION, USES

The bark of ash species (*Fraxinus* spp) contains salicylates and has been used in the same way as willow bark. See WILLOW BARK for details; see also Appendix VIII.

AUTUMN CROCUS

See COLCHICUM.

AVENA SATIVA

■ SOURCE, DESCRIPTION, USES

Early interest in an alcoholic extract of oat straw, from the cereal grain oats (*Avena sativa*), stemmed from reports that it assisted smokers to break their addiction to nicotine.[1] More recently it has been touted as an alternative to sildenafil (Viagra) for erectile dysfunction in men.

■ PHARMACOLOGY

Connor and colleagues[1] conducted studies in experimental animals using a dried alcohol extract of oat straw redissolved in water and found that it antagonized the antinociceptive effects of morphine in mice and the pressor response to nicotine in anesthetized rats but did not affect the seizure threshold to nicotine. Subsequently, Schmidt and Geckeler,[2] in a double-blind study with the alcohol extract in smokers, found that both the extract and the placebo assisted 35% of smokers in quitting, more frequently in light smokers than in heavy ones. Thus, there does not appear to be any convincing evidence that this preparation is useful in this regard. No evidence for an aphrodisiac effect, nor for usefulness for erectile dysfunction, could be found. One website, which describes studies conducted at the Institute for Advanced Study of Human Sexuality, asserts that a double-blind study of green oats on sexual function purportedly found that sexual performance was improved in men, an effect ascribed to the release of testosterone from binding sites. A review of the Institute's website revealed that a dissertation, entitled "Aphrodisiacal Efficacy of Swissoats," was presented by W. R. Wiley in 1987; however, a search of the scientific literature failed to turn up any related publication.

■ ADVERSE EFFECTS AND INTERACTIONS

No evidence for these was found.

■ REFERENCES

1. Connor J, Connor T, Marshall PB, Reid A, Turnbull MJ. The pharmacology of Avena sativa. *J Pharm Pharmacol* 1975;27:92.
2. Schmidt K, Geckeler K. Pharmacotherapy with Avena sativa—a double blind study. *Int J Clin Pharmacol Biochem* 1976;14:214.

AVOCADO/SOYBEAN UNSAPONIFIABLES (ASU)

■ SOURCE, DESCRIPTION, USES

ASU is composed of the unsaponifiable fraction of one-third avocado oil and two-thirds soybean oil.[1] Experimental and clinical evidence suggests that it inhibits mediators of pain and inflammation and displays clinical efficacy in osteoarthritis.

■ PHARMACOLOGY

Studies with cultured chondrocytes indicate that ASU inhibits neutral metalloproteinases, proinflammatory cytokines such as interleukin (IL)-6 and IL-8, and inducible nitric oxide synthase and prostaglandin E_2. It also appears to stimulate matrix synthesis through stimulation of transforming growth factor-β_2 and plasminogen activator inhibitor 1.[2-4] Studies in rats have shown a cartilage-protecting effect that was better with the combination of avocado and soybean than with either alone.[5]

Several placebo-controlled, double-blind, clinical studies have been conducted with ASU with generally positive results.[6,7]. A Cochrane review found convincing evidence for efficacy of ASU in osteoarthritis with respect to functional index, pain, intake of nonsteroidal anti-inflammatory agents, and global evaluation.[8]

ADVERSE EFFECTS AND INTERACTIONS

No serious side effects were reported in any of the clinical trials. It appears that ASU constitutes a safe and effective alternative therapy for the treatment of mild to moderate osteoarthritis.

REFERENCES

1. Curatolo M, Bogduk N. Pharmacologic treatment of musculoskeletal disorders: Current perspectives and future prospects. *Clin J Pain* 2001;17:25.
2. Hauselmann HJ. Nutripharmaceuticals for osteoarthritis. *Best Pract Res Clin Rheum* 2001;15:595.
3. Kut-Lasserre C, Miller CC, Ejeil AL, et al. Effect of avocado and soybean unsaponifiables on gelatinase A (MMP-2) stromelysin 1 (MMP-3) and tissue inhibitors of matrix metalloproteinase (TIMP-1 and TIMP-2) secretion by human fibroblasts in culture. *J Periodontol* 2001;72:1685.
4. Henrotin YE, Labasse AH, Jaspar JM, et al. Effects of three avocado/soybean unsaponifiable mixtures on metalloproteinases, cytokinases and prostaglandin E2 production by human articular chondrocytes. *Clin Rheumatol* 1998;17:31.
5. Khayyal MT, el-Ghazaly MA. The possible "chondroprotective" effect of the unsaponifiable constituents of avocado and soya in vivo. *Drugs Exp Clin Res* 1998;24:41.
6. Maheu E, Mazieres B, Valat JP, et al. Symptomatic efficacy of avocado/soybean unsaponifiables in the treatment of osteoarthritis of the knee and hip: A prospective, randomized, double-blind, placebo-controlled, multicenter clinical trial with a six-month treatment period and a two-month followup demonstrating a persistent effect. *Arthritis Rheum* 1998;41:81.
7. Blotman F, Maheu E, Wulwik A, Caspard H, Lopez A. Efficacy and safety of avocado/soybean unsaponifiables in the treatment of symptomatic osteoarthritis of the knee and hip—a prospective, multicenter, three-month, randomized, double-blind, placebo-controlled trial. *Rev Rheum Engl Ed* 1997;64:825.
8. Little CV, Parsons T, Logan S. Herbal therapy for treating osteoarthritis (Cochrane Review). Available at: http://www.cochrane.org/cochrane/revabstr/ab002947.htm.

BAI ZHI

■ SOURCE, DESCRIPTION, USES

Bai zhi is the Chinese herbal name for *Angelica dahurica*. It is also referred to as Chinese angelica to distinguish it from *A. sinensis* (Dong quai). The dried root is used in a variety of Chinese and Japanese herbal remedies and is purported to be useful for many medical conditions, including acne and other skin eruptions; erythema; as a sedative, analgesic, and antipyretic; and to relieve headache and sinus congestion.[1,2] This perennial herb with pale green flowers is native to central Asia from Siberia to Japan and is widely cultivated in China.[1]

■ PHARMACOLOGY

Bai zhi is rich in coumarins and furocoumarins.[3,4] Over 20 of these have been isolated from the crude herb, including coumarin, scopoletin, psoralen, xanthotoxin, bergapten, and imperatorin.[3] A broad range of pharmacological properties has been demonstrated experimentally for these substances. One furocoumarin, phellopterin, has been shown to be a partial agonist for the benzodiazepine (GABA$_A$) receptor in rat brain slices.[3,5] Others have been shown to possess antibacterial and antifungal activity.[4] Still others (bergapten, oxypeucedanin hydrate, and byakangelicin) have been shown to prevent histamine release induced by compound 48/80 injected intraperitoneally into mice.[6] Angelica extract had antiatherogenic properties in a rat model by decreasing serum triglyceride levels[7] as well as protecting human umbilical vein endothelial cells from damage induced by oxidized low-density lipoproteins.[8]

■ ADVERSE EFFECTS AND INTERACTIONS

Coumarins and furocoumarins have been shown to inhibit many of the cytochrome P450 isozymes in animal studies. Rat studies showed inhibition by extract of *Angelica dahurica* of CYP2C, CYP3A, and CYP2D1, as well as potent inhibition of testosterone 2α- and 16α-hydroxylase.[9] The metabolism of tolbutamide, nifedipine, and burfuralol was inhibited as well. Byakangelicol has been shown to inhibit both the activity and the induction of cyclooxygenase-2 in human pulmonary epithelial cells.[10]

It should be evident that there is a significant potential for interactions with many pharmacological agents, both mechanistically and by alteration of their biotransformation. This herbal agent should be used very cautiously, if at all, in conjunction with prescription or over-the-counter medications.

Of particular concern are centrally acting agents such as the benzodiazepines and oral anticoagulants. See also Appendices I and VI.

■ REFERENCES

1. Available at: http://www.elixirfarm.com/images/Chinese/chinesea.htm.

2. KimuraY, Okuda H. Baba K. Histamine release effectors from Angelica dahurica var. dahurica root. *J Nat Prod* 1997;60:249.

3. Bergendorff O, Dekermendjian K, Nielsen M, et al. Furocoumarins with affinity to brain benzodiazepine receptors in vitro. *Phytochemistry* 1997;44:1121.

4. Kwon Y-S, Kobayashi A, Kajiyama S, Kawazu K, Kanzaki H, Kim CM. Antimicrobial constituents of Angelica dahurica roots. *Phytochemistry* 1997;44:887.

5. Dekermendjian K, Ai J, Nielsen M, Sterner O, Shan R, Witt MR. Characterisastion of the furanocoumarin phellopterin as a rat brain benzodiazepine receptor partial agonist in vitro. *Neurosci Lett* 1996;21:151.

6. Kimura Y, Okuda H, Baba K. Histamine-release effectors from Angelica dahurica var. dahurica root. *J Nat Prod* 1997;60:249.

7. Zhui Y, Jing-Ping OY, Yongming L, et al. Experimental study of the antiatherogenic effects of Chinese medicine angelica and its mechanisms. *Clin Hemorheol Microcirc* 2000;22:305.

8. Xiaohong Y, Jing-ping OY, Shuzheng T. Angelica protects the human vascular endothelial cell from the effects of oxidized low-density lipoprotein in vitro. *Clin Hemorheol Microcirc* 2000;22:317.

9. Ishihara K, Kushida H, Yuzurihara M, et al. Interaction of drugs and Chinese herbs: Pharmacokinetic changes of tolbutamide and diazepam caused by extract of Angelica dahurica. *J Pharm Pharmacol* 2000;52:1023.

10. Lin CH, Chang CW, Wang CC, Chang MS, Yang LL. Byakangelicol, isolated from Angelica dahurica, inhibits both the activity and induction of cyclooxygenase-2 in human pulmonary epithelial cells. *J Pharm Pharmacol* 2002;54:1271.

BALM

■ SOURCE, DESCRIPTION, USES

Balm (*Melissa officinalis*), also known as lemon balm, sweet balm, and bee balm, is a member of the mint (Labiatae) family. It is also classified as a member of the family Lamiaceae. It is a native of southern Europe favoring mountainous regions, but it has become common in parts of the eastern region of North America. The flowers are in loose, small bunches, white or yellowish, and the heart-shaped, toothed leaves emit a lemon scent when bruised and have a lemon taste.[1] The plant is very attractive to bees. Some other plants belonging to the mint family also are called bee balm.

Both the root and the aerial portion of the plant are used as an herb. Balm extract has been used traditionally as a diaphoretic, carminative, febrifuge for people with flu or colds, and as a sedative.[1] It also has been purported to enhance cognitive performance.

■ PHARMACOLOGY

Balm extract contains several flavonoids, the main one being luteolin 3'glucuronide.[2] An alcohol extract of the leaves has been shown to displace tritiated nicotine and scopolamine from nicotinic and muscarinic receptors in homogenized human brain tissue.[3]

In a double-blind, placebo-controlled trial of aromatherapy to manage agitation in severe dementia, oil of balm was compared with sunflower oil (placebo) for ability to exert a calming effect. Seventy-two patients were randomly assigned to the two treatment groups, and the oils were applied to the face and arms as a lotion twice daily. The Cohen-Mansfield Agitation Inventory (CMAI) and Dementia Care Mapping (a quality-of-life index) were used for assessment. After 4 weeks, 60% of the active treatment group versus 14% of the placebo group experienced a 30% reduction in the CMAI.[4] Quality-of-life scores also were significantly improved in the treatment group. In another double-blind, placebo-controlled, crossover study, 20 healthy young adults (15 females and 5 males) received various doses of *M. officinalis* extract or placebo at 7-day intervals, and cognitive performance was assessed by a standard method. Cognitive performance was improved as measured by the Accuracy of Attention factor, but memory performance was disrupted. Sedation also was significant, and self-assessed calmness was improved.[5] Binding to brain receptors also was studied; both nicotinic and muscarinic binding were demonstrated in homogenized human brain tissue, but the levels were much lower than reported by others.

A controlled study showed that a cream containing balm extract was beneficial in controlling the signs and symptoms of genital herpes in females and might also prolong the intervals between the acute attacks.[6]

■ ADVERSE EFFECTS AND INTERACTIONS

These small clinical studies did not report any adverse reactions associated with the use of balm extract. Given its central mechanism of action, there is a theoretical risk of interference with other centrally acting drugs, especially those involving acetylcholine receptors. Safety of systemic administration in children and pregnant women has not been established.

■ REFERENCES

1. Balm. In: Grieve M. *A Modern Herbal.* Botanical.com website. Available at: http://www.botanical.com/botanical/mgmh/b/balm—02.html
2. Heitz A, Carnat A, Fraisse D, Carnat AP, Lamaison JL. Luteolin 3' glucuronide, the major flavonoid from Melissa officinalis subsp. officinalis. *Fitoterapia* 2000;71:201.
3. Wake G, Court J, Pickering A, Lewis R, Wilkins R, Perry E. CNS acetylcholine receptor activity in European medicinal plants traditionally used to improve failing memory. *J Ethnopharmacol* 2000;69:105.
4. Ballard CG, O'Brien JT, Reichelt K, Perry EK. Aromatherapy as a safe and effective treatment for the management of agitation in severe dementia: The results of a double-blind, placebo-controlled trial with Melissa. *J Clin Psychiatry* 2002;63:553.
5. Kennedy DO, Scholey AB, Tildesley NT, Perry EK, Wesnes KA. Modulation of mood and cognitive performance following acute administration of Melissa officinalis (lemon balm). *Pharmacol Biochem Behav* 2002;72:953.
6. Koytchev R, Alken RG, Dundarov S. Balm mint extract (Lo-701) for topical treatment or recurring herpes labialis. *Phytomedicine* 1999;6:225.

BARBERRY

■ SOURCE, DESCRIPTION, USES

The common barberry (*Berberis vulgaris*) is a tall (to 3 m), bushy shrub with pale yellow flowers and red berries, native to most of Europe, North Africa, and temperate Asia.[1] It is a member of the Berberidaceae family, which includes, for technical reasons, such diverse species as may apple and blue cohosh.[2] Synonyms include berbery, pipperidge bush, and holy thorn.[1] Traditionally, it has been used as a tonic, purgative, carminative, and for jaundice. It also has been used as a lotion for skin conditions and orally as an antipyretic. Many other actions have been ascribed to members of this family.[3] Tinctures and extracts of bark and root bark are used. The fruit may be used in jams and jellies.

■ PHARMACOLOGY

The main active constituent of barberry appears to be an alkaloid called *berberine.* Animal studies have demonstrated a wide range of pharmacological activities for derivatives of various *Berberis* species. Although not all tests have been conducted in all species, evidence suggests that the pharmacological properties are generally shared, and the herbal preparations are collectively referred to as *barberry*. One source[3] reported that *B. oblongota* is used for lumbago in Uzbekistan, *B. vulgaris* for rheumatism and fever in Azerbaijan and Bulgaria, *B. lycium* for muscle and joint pain in Pakistan, and *B. asiatica* for fever and inflammation in Nepal. Studies in rats and mice demonstrated potent anti-inflammatory, analgesic, and antipyretic activity. Hot water, cold water, and ethanol extracts of *B. crataegina* root were prepared. All demonstrated anti-inflammatory and antipyretic activity, which varied depending on the model employed. The experimental evidence thus suggested a mechanism similar to that of nonsteroidal anti-inflammatory drugs (NSAIDs), possibly involving inhibition of prostaglandin synthesis.

Anti-inflammatory and immunomodulatory activity has been reported for bisbenzylisoquinolines from barberry,[3] and antihistaminic and anticholinergic activity in guinea pig ileum studies.[4]

Current medicinal use of berberine[5] is based on demonstrated activity as an antibacterial and antiparasitic agent. It has been used for bacterial diarrhea, intestinal parasites such as *Giardia* (where it has compared favorably with metronidazole), and for ocular trachoma. Antihypertensive activity also has been shown. Potential as an anticancer agent has been demonstrated experimentally.[5]

■ ADVERSE EFFECTS AND INTERACTIONS

Berberine (barberry) appears to be well tolerated at recommended doses. Excessive doses, however, have resulted in lethargy, nosebleeds, dyspnea, nephritis, gastrointestinal discomfort, hypotension, flu-like symptoms, and cardiac damage.[3,5] Berberine should be avoided in pregnancy as it may stimulate uterine contractions, and in neonates as it can displace bilirubin from albumin.[5] Little appears to be known about its effects on reproduction and development.

Although no drug interactions seem to have been reported, there is a strong possibility that barberry may interact with NSAIDs and should be used cautiously, if at all, in patients receiving antithrombotic or antirheumatic therapy. It should be noted that berberine is present in many botanicals, such as goldenseal and Oregon grape, so that there is a theoretical possibility that polyherbal remedies could lead to adverse reactions as a result of the high total content of berberine. See also Appendix VIII.

■ REFERENCES

1. Barberry, common. In: Grieve M. *A Modern Herbal*. Botanical.com website. Available at: http://botanical.com/botanical/mgmh/b/barcom12.html

2. Peterson RT, McKenny M. *Northeastern Wildflowers: Roger Tory Peterson Field Guides.* Norwalk, Conn: Easton Press; 1984:xix.
3. Yesilada E, Kupeli E. Berberis crataegina DC, root exhibits potent anti-inflammatory, analgesic and febrifuge effects in mice and rats. *J Ethnopharmacol* 2002;79:237.
4. Shamsa F, Ahmadiani A, Khosrokhavar R. Antihistaminic and anticholinergic activity of barberry fruit (Berberis vulgaris) in the guinea-pig ileum. *J Ethnopharmacol* 1999;64:161.
5. Berberine. *Altern Med Rev* 2000;5:175.

β-SITOSTEROL

■ SOURCE, DESCRIPTION, USES

β-Sitosterol is a phytosterol that is present in many botanicals. Most herbal preparations of it originate from African star grass tuber (*Hypoxis rooperi*) and species of pine (*Pinus*) and spruce (*Picea*).[1] It resembles cholesterol chemically and can interfere with the intestinal absorption of cholesterol.[2] It has been suggested that it might be useful in treating hypercholesterolemia.[2] β-Sitosterol (henceforth sitosterol) is extracted with organic solvents. β-Sitosterolin, a sitosterol glycoside, may also be an active principle.[2]

■ PHARMACOLOGY

The greatest interest in sitosterol centers on its potential for treating benign prostatic hyperplasia (BPH). Prostatic tissue binds sitosterol, which is claimed to inhibit both cyclooxygenase and lipoxygenase, and hence to have an anti-inflammatory effect.[1] It also has been shown to stimulate growth factor transforming growth factor-β,[1] which would have the effect of promoting apoptosis and potentially shrinking the prostate. The clinical significance of these theoretical mechanisms of action, however, has not been established.

There have been a number of double-blind, placebo-controlled, clinical trials that have been reviewed by several authors. A 1996 review noted that a β-D-glycoside of sitosterol failed to produce any clinically significant improvement after 6 months of treatment.[3] A German multicenter study of 200 patients used a preparation that was rich in sitosterol but that also had a number of other phytosterols present. Treatment continued for 6 months and follow-up for 18 months. The treated group showed significant improvement in both objective and subjective measures.[1,3] Another, more recent, study also used a preparation containing sitosterol and reported similar findings.[3] A Cochrane review of clinical data conducted in 2000 concluded that the nonglycosidic sitosterols improved urinary symptoms and flow measures in patients with BPH.[4] In a follow-up open-label study of one of these placebo-controlled, double-blind trials conducted that same year, patients with symptomatic BPH were treated for 6 months with sitosterol, followed for 18 months, and maintained beneficial effects during the observation period; 117 patients were eligible for the follow-up study.[5]

Another recent randomized, placebo-controlled study investigated an herbal mixture containing cernitin, saw palmetto, β-sitosterol, and vitamin E in 177 patients who took the mixture, or placebo, for 3 months. The treated group showed significant improvement in both objective and subjective measures.[6]

■ ADVERSE EFFECTS AND INTERACTIONS

None of the previously discussed clinical studies found any serious side effects to use of β-sitosterol. Withdrawals from the study did not appear to be related to treatment. Problems relating to clinical studies of sitosterol stem from their relatively short duration and from the lack of standardization of the preparations used. This effectively precludes meta-analysis. No information seems to be available regarding long-term effects or interactions with other medications. See also SAW PALMETTO.

■ REFERENCES

1. Dreikorn K. The role of phytotherapy in treating lower urinary tract symptoms and benign prostatic hyperplasia. *World J Urol* 2002;19:426.
2. Schulz V, Hansel R, Tyler VE. *Rational Phytotherapy: A Physician's Guide to Herbal Medicine.* New York, NY: Springer-Verlag; 1998:p 231.
3. Lowe FC, Ku JC. Phytotherapy in treatment of benign prostatic hyperplasia: A critical review. *Urology* 1996;48:12.
4. Wilt T, Ishani A, MacDonald R, Stark G, Mulrow C, Lau J. Beta-sitosterols for benign prostatic hyperplasia. *Cochrane Database Syst Rev* 2000;2:CD001043.
5. Berges RR, Kassen A, Senge T. Treatment of symptomatic benign prostatic hyperplasia with beta-sitosterol: An 18-month follow-up. *BJU* 2000;85:842.
6. Preuss HG, Marcusen C, Regan J, Klimberg IW, Welebir TA, Jones WA. Randomized trial of a combination of natural products (cernitin, saw palmetto, β-sitosterol, vitamin E) on symptoms of benign prostatic hyperplasia (BPH). *Internat Urol Nephrol* 2001;33:217.

BETEL NUT

■ SOURCE, DESCRIPTION, USES

Betel nut is from the fruit of the tropical palm tree *Areca catechu*. The dried, chopped nut is generally chewed wrapped in a leaf of the vine *Piper betle* (related to the pepper plant) mixed with lime obtained from seashells.[1] It has been estimated that up to 600 million people, or 10% of the world's population, chew betel for its euphoric effect. Its use is widespread in India, Taiwan, South Africa, and throughout Southeast Asia.[2] Strictly speaking, betel nut might be described more accurately as a recreational, psychoactive botanical rather than a true herbal remedy. It is often chewed along with tobacco.

■ PHARMACOLOGY

The main active principle of betel nut is the cholinergic agent arecoline. This tertiary amine alkaloid has both muscarinic and nicotinic agonist activity.[3] Arecoline can have effects on smooth muscle, the cardiovascular system, and the gastrointestinal tract in addition to its central effects. The betel leaf is purported to contain a volatile, phenolic oil with central nervous system–stimulating properties and an alkaloid with cocaine-like action.[4]

Pharmacological responses that have been observed in betel chewers include a sense of well-being, euphoria, heightened alertness, sweating, salivation, a hot sensation in the body, and increased capacity to work.[5] Many of these can be attributed to the cholinergic action of arecoline.[3] Betel chewing, however, can lead to habituation, addiction, and withdrawal symptoms.[5] In the presence of lime, arecoline and another alkaloid, guvacoline, are hydrolyzed to arecaidine and guvacine, which are inhibitors of γ-aminobutyric acid uptake. *P. betle* also has been shown to contain compounds that stimulate the release of catecholamines.[5] Betel chewing thus can have complex effects on both the central and peripheral nervous systems.

■ ADVERSE EFFECTS AND INTERACTIONS

One of the most dramatic and instantly observable side effects of betel chewing is the bright red staining of teeth, gums, and oral mucosa that it causes.[6] There are, however, considerably more serious risks associated with its use, most notably, carcinogenesis. Betel chewing has been identified as an independent risk factor for oral cancer.[7] The relative risk factor for oral squamous cell carcinoma associated with habitual use of betel chewing alone was estimated at 68.4 in the Taiwanese population.[7] When it is combined with tobacco the relative risk increases even more.[7] A study in northern India found that betel chewing was a significant risk factor for esophageal cancer, as well, and the risk was further increased if tobacco use was combined with betel chewing.[8] Other medical problems that occur more frequently in betel users include cardiovascular disease, diabetes mellitus, and asthma.[4,7] Betel chewing also is a major risk factor for oral submucous fibrosis, a precancerous condition that often precedes squamous cell carcinoma.[9] Betel nut has a high copper content, and high levels of copper have been detected in saliva and submucous tissues following 30 minutes of chewing. This is believed to be an initiating factor in the development of submucous fibrosis.[9] In one laboratory study, however, copper chelation failed to prevent unscheduled DNA synthesis induced by areca nut extract in cultured gingival keratinocytes, whereas vitamin C, glutathione, and N-acetyl-L-cysteine did so in a concentration-dependent fashion.[2]

Given the extensive effects of betel chewing on the central and peripheral nervous systems the potential for interactions with prescription and over-the-counter medications is very high. Deahl[1] reported two cases of an extrapyramidal syndrome involving rigidity, bradykinesia, jaw tremor, and akathisia. Both patients were Indian residents of Great Britain. One was receiving fluphenazine decanoate for schizophrenia and the other flupenthixol for schizoaffective disorder. Recent betel chewing was identified from the red dental staining. The extrapyramidal side effects gradually resolved when the betel chewing was discontinued.

Acute toxicity can occur as a result of betel chewing, although it is not common. Deng and colleagues[10] reviewed 17 cases from Taiwan. A wide range of signs and symptoms was observed, involving neurological, gastrointestinal, and cardiovascular manifestations. These included tachycardia, dyspnea, sweating, hypotension, vomiting, dizziness, colic, numbness, and coma. Although most patients recovered within 24 hours, one patient developed acute myocardial infarction with ventricular fibrillation and died despite resuscitative measures.

For cosmetic reasons alone, betel chewing is unlikely to gain much of a following in the general population in North America and other developed countries. It persists, however, in immigrant populations. Betel preparations are widely available on the Internet and may be brought in by family members from their homeland. The medical community will no doubt continue to see the consequences of this undesirable but culturally ingrained habit. It is obvious that the practice should be discouraged in pregnant women and younger adults, because the risk for the former is unknown but likely significant, and risk is known to increase with years of use. See also Appendix VII.

■ REFERENCES

1. Deahl M. betel nut-induced extrapyramidal syndrome: An unusual drug interaction. *Mov Disord* 1989;4:330.

2. Chang MC, Ho YS, Lee JJ, Kok SH, Hahn LJ, Jeng JH. Prevention of the arecanut extract-induced unscheduled DNA synthesis of gingival keratinocytes by vitamin V and thiol compounds. *Oral Oncol* 2002;38:258.

3. Brown JH, Taylor P. Muscarinic receptor agonists and antagonists. In: Hardman JG, Limbird L, Gilman AG, eds. *Goodman and Gilman's The Pharmacological Basis of Therapeutics*. 10th ed. New York, NY: McGraw-Hill; 2001:167.

4. Taylor RF, al-Jarad N, John LM, Conroy DM, Barnes NC. Betel-nut chewing and asthma. *Lancet* 1992;339:1134.

5. Chu NS. Effects of betel chewing on the central and autonomic nervous systems. *J Biomed Sci* 2001;8:229.

6. Yoganathan P. Betel chewing creeps into the New World. *N Z Dent J* 2002;98:40.

7. Warnakulasuriya S, Trivedy C, Peters TJ. Areca nut use: an independent risk factor for oral cancer. *BMJ* 2002;324:799.

8. Phukan RK, Ali MS, Chetia CK, Mahanta J. Betel nut and tobacco chewing: Potential risk factors of cancer of the oesophagus in Assam, India. *Brit J Cancer* 2001;85:661.

9. Celik N, Wei FC, Chang YM, Yang WG, Chen DJ, Tsai CY. Squamous cell carcinoma of the oral mucosa after release of submucous fibrosis and bilateral small radial forearm flap reconstruction. *Plast Reconstr Surg* 2002;110:34.

10. Deng JF, Ger J, Tsai WJ, Kao WF, Yang CC. Acute toxicities of betel nut: Rare but probably overlooked events. *J Toxicol Clin Toxicol* 2001;39:355.

BILBERRY

■ SOURCE, DESCRIPTION, USES

Bilberries are the dried fruit of *Vaccinium myrtillus*, also known as the European blueberry,[1] huckleberry, or whortleberry.[2] It is a member of the Ericaceae family and related to other *Vaccinium* species, including the cranberries. The shrub grows in mountains and forests of Europe and the northern United States.[2] It has been used traditionally for nonspecific diarrhea and inflammation of the oropharyngeal mucosa.[1] A number of other uses have been investigated recently with some promising results. Patients with retinitis pigmentosa and hemeralopia (inability to see well in bright light) showed a significant improvement in vision after being given bilberry extract.[2] Conversely, no improvement in night visual acuity could be demonstrated in healthy young men given bilberry extract.[3] Studies have shown clinical benefits in glaucoma, cataracts, and diabetic retinopathy, and bilberry has been proposed for a wide variety of other conditions, including dysmenorrhea, rheumatoid arthritis,[2] and chronic fatigue syndrome,[4] based on its pharmacological actions.

■ PHARMACOLOGY

Bilberry has been shown to contain a number of potential pharmacologically active compounds, including catechins, flavone glycosides, and anthocyanosides.[1,2] Attention has focused primarily on the anthocyanosides. Pharmacological actions that have been demonstrated include strong antioxidant properties, stabilization of collagen fibers and promotion of collagen biosynthesis, decreased capillary permeability and fragility, and inhibition of platelet function. Lowering of blood glucose also has been demonstrated, and the prevention of the release of proinflammatory compounds.[2]

■ ADVERSE EFFECTS AND INTERACTIONS

Only mild side effects, mostly gastrointestinal, have been reported. Based on the platelet-inhibiting properties of bilberry, there is a potential for an increased risk of bleeding or bruising if high doses are given to patients taking oral anticoagulants or platelet-inhibiting drugs.[2,5]

■ REFERENCES

1. Schulz V, Hansel R, Tyler VE. *Rational Phytotherapy: A Physician's Guide to Herbal Medicine.* New York, NY: Springer-Verlag; 1998:26, 193.
2. Vaccinium myrtillus (bilberry). *Altern Med Rev* 2001;6:500.
3. Muth ER, Laurent LM, Jasper P. The effect of bilberry nutritional supplementation on night visual acuity and contrast sensitivity. *Altern Med Rev* 2000;5:164.
4. Logan AC, Wong C. Chronic fatigue syndrome: Oxidative stress and dietary modifications. *Altern Med Rev* 2001;6:450.
5. Lambrecht JE, Hamilton W, Rabinovich A. A review of herb-drug interactions: Documented and theoretical. *US Pharmacist* 25:8. Available at: http://www.uspharmacist.com/NewLook/DisplayArticle.cfm?/item_num=566.

BIRCH (COMMON)

■ SOURCE, DESCRIPTION, USES

The bark of *Betula alba* (family Betulaceae), a European species of birch that has spread throughout northeastern North America, is used like that of its European relative. All species of birch contain salicylic acid–yielding alkaloids and are similar in usage to wintergreen oil.[1]

■ PHARMACOLOGY

See WILLOW BARK and WINTERGREEN OIL.

■ ADVERSE REACTIONS AND INTERACTIONS

The same concerns regarding interaction with oral anticoagulants pertain as with willow bark.[2] See also Appendices I and VIII.

■ REFERENCES

1. Birch, common. In: Grieve M. *A Modern Herbal.* Botanical.com website. Available at: http://www.botanical.com/botanical/mgmb/b/bircom43.html.
2. Pribitkin E deA, Boger B. Herbal therapy: What every facial plastic surgeon must know. *Arch Facial Plast Surg* 2001;3:127.

BITTER GOURD

See KARELA.

BITTERSWEET

■ SOURCE, DESCRIPTION, USES

Shoots and new twigs of *Solanum dulcamara* (wooded or woody nightshade) are extracted to yield bittersweet. Wooded nightshade is a member of the family Solanaceae, which includes deadly nightshade (*S. nigrum, Atropa belladonna*), tomato (*Lycopersicon esculentum*), and potato (*S. tuberosum*). Synonyms for bittersweet include dulcamara, felonwood, felonwort, scarlet berry, and violet bloom.[1] This slender vine with red berries and purple flowers grows widely throughout North America, favoring thickets and moist areas.[2] It also grows extensively in Europe. The name bittersweet comes from the fact that the root and stem, when chewed, taste bitter at first and then sweet.[1] Traditional uses, now largely abandoned, include as a restorative, for rheumatism, fever, and inflammation.[1]. Use now is largely restricted to topical application for skin conditions. It is one of several herbal preparations approved by the German Commission E for topical use, in this case for chronic eczema.[3]

■ PHARMACOLOGY

Several chemicals of plant origin have been shown to possess beneficial properties in treating skin conditions, including β-carotene, chrysarobin, anthralin, methoxalen, and salicylates.[3] In addition to whatever dermatologically beneficial substances are present, woody nightshade contains solanine, a glycoalkaloid related to atropine and scopolamine (from deadly nightshade). It differs pharmacologically, however, in possessing cholinesterase-inhibiting activity as well as positive inotropic activity.[4] It is structurally related to the cardiac glycosides. This may explain its positive inotropic activity.

■ ADVERSE EFFECTS AND INTERACTIONS

The topical use of bittersweet extract appears to be safe, at least when applied to intact skin. Transdermal absorption of belladonna alkaloids occurs, and skin patches of scopolamine have been used,[5] so the possibility of absorption from areas of damaged skin cannot be discounted. Poisoning with the berries, especially unripe ones, is fairly common in children,[4,6] and their toxicity has been confirmed experimentally in mice.[7]

New pharmacological and toxicological activities for bittersweet continue to emerge. Because various preparations of bittersweet have been used to treat inflammation, gout, and rheumatism in Swedish folk medicine, Tunon and colleagues[8] included bittersweet in a survey of the ability of botanicals to affect prostaglandin synthesis and exocytosis induced by platelet-activating factor (PAF). Although prostaglandin synthesis was inhibited by only 12%, PAF-induced exocytosis was completely blocked. In contrast, salix bark blocked both prostaglandin synthesis and exocytosis by over 85%. Keeler and colleagues[9] studied the toxicity of spirosolane-containing *Solanum* species using craniofacial deformities in newborn hamsters as the model. *S. dulcamara* contained appreciable amounts of an unknown spirosolane in addition to solasodine in the unhydrolyzed alkaloid fraction of the fruit. This fraction induced a 16.3% incidence of deformities ($p < .001$). Interestingly, potato sprouts (*S. tuberosum*) caused a 24% incidence of malformations at the same significance level. *Solanum* species have already yielded pharmacologically important agents (atropine, scopolamine) and may continue to do so.

■ REFERENCES

1. Nightshade, woody. In: Grieve M. *A Modern Herbal*. Botanical.com website. Available at: http://www.botanical.com/botanical/mgmh/n/nighwo06.html.
2. Peterson RT, McKenny M. *Northeastern Wildflowers: Roger Tory Peterson Field Guides*. Norwalk, Conn: Easton Press; 1984:324.
3. Schulz V, Hansel R, Tyler VE. *Rational Phytotherapy: A Physician's Guide to Herbal Medicine*. New York, NY: Springer-Verlag; 1998:251.
4. Ceha LJ, Presperin C, Young E, Allswede M, Erickson T. Anticholinergic toxicity from nightshade berry poisoning responsive to physostigmine. *J Emerg Med* 1997;15:65.
5. Brown JH, Taylor P. Muscarinic receptor agonists and antagonists. In: Hardman JG, Limbird L, Gilman AG, eds. *Goodman and Gilman's The Pharmacological Basis of Therapeutics*. 10th ed. New York, NY: McGraw-Hill; 2001:167.
6. Rubenfeld RS, Currie JN. Accidental mydriasis from blue nightshade "lipstick". *J Clin Neuroophthalmol* 1987;7:34.
7. Hornfeldt CS, Collins JE. Toxicity of nightshade berries (Solanum dulcamara) in mice. *J Toxicol Clin Toxicol* 1990;28:185.
8. Tunon H, Olavsdotter C, Bohlin L. Evaluation of anti-inflammatory activity of some Swedish medicinal plants. Inhibition or prostaglandin biosynthesis and PAF-induced exocytosis. *J Ethnopharmacol* 1995;48:61.
9. Keeler RF, Baker DC, Gaffield W. Spirosolane-containing Solanum species and induction of congenital craniofacial malformations. *Toxicon* 1990;28:873.

BLACK COHOSH

■ SOURCE, DESCRIPTION, USES

Black cohosh, from *Cimicifuga racemosa*, is also known as bugbane. It grows in wooded areas from Wisconsin and southern Ontario south to Georgia and Missouri. It is a member of the buttercup family.

■ PHARMACOLOGY

See PHYTOESTROGENS AND PHYTOPROGESTINS.

■ ADVERSE EFFECTS AND INTERACTIONS

There is one case report of a female who took black cohosh as a sole, herbal preparation for 1 week to relieve symptoms of menopause. She presented with clinical and laboratory evidence of acute hepatitis, subsequently developed fulminant hepatic failure, and required a liver transplant. No other potential cause of the liver failure could be demonstrated. There was no history of alcohol or drug abuse, and no prescription medications were involved. There was no family history of liver disease, and no hepatic or biliary tract disease was present. It was concluded that the black cohosh was the precipitating cause of the liver failure.[1] Tannin-containing herbs such as black cohosh may interfere with iron absorption.[2] This may not be a serious problem clinically but should be considered in anemic patients, and it is advisable to avoid taking iron and the herbal preparation together.

See PHYTOESTROGENS AND PHYTOPROGESTINS and Appendix IV.

■ REFERENCES

1. Whiting PW, Clouston A, Kerlin P. Black cohosh and other herbal remedies associated with acute hepatitis. *Med J Austral* 2002;177:440.
2. Miller LG. Herbal medicinals: Selected clinical considerations focusing on known or potential herb-drug interactions. *Arch Intern Med* 1998;158:2200.

BONESET

■ SOURCE, DESCRIPTION, USES

Boneset or thoroughwort (*Eupatorium perfoliatum*) is a perennial member of the Compositae or daisy family, which grows widely throughout the eastern half of North America. It is also known as feverwort. It is a tall (to 1 m) plant with opposing wrinkled, hairy leaves contiguous at the stem (hence perfoliate) and clusters of small, fuzzy white flowers at the top.[1] Boneset was used by North American natives as an herbal remedy for fever, aches, and pains. At one time it appeared in the U.S. Pharmacopoeia.[2] Traditional use included as a febrifuge, laxative, tonic, diaphoretic, and antirheumatic remedy.[2] Boneset is still used for colds and fevers. It is usually taken as a warm infusion of the leaves and flowers.

■ PHARMACOLOGY

Boneset contains several active principles, including flavonoids, sesquiterpene lactones, and polysaccharides with immunostimulant properties.[3] The precise constituents responsible for the herb's activity, however, have not been identified. An ethanol extract of boneset leaves has been shown to have weak antibacterial properties, about one order of magnitude less than that of penicillin G, against gram-positive but not gram-negative organisms.[3] Some clinical evidence for diaphoretic action has been obtained.[4] One German clinical trial compared boneset to acetylsalicylic acid in 53 randomly assigned patients with a common cold and found, on the basis of symptom checklists filled in by the patients, that there were no significant differences between the groups.[5] The authors interpreted this patient response as indicating that both treatments were equally effective.

■ ADVERSE EFFECTS AND INTERACTIONS

Neither contraindications nor drug interactions appear to have been reported. Nausea has been reported following ingestion.[3] Recent studies of the effects of an ethanol extract of leaves on several cultured mammalian cell lines found cytotoxicity equivalent in potency to that of chlorambucil.[3] Preliminary attempts to purify the responsible agent indicated that it is of medium polarity. The authors caution that care should be taken with this herbal remedy in view of its overt cytotoxicity.

As a member of the Compositae family, contact dermatitis and cross-reactivity with other Compositae are possible. See also Appendix IX.

■ REFERENCES

1. Peterson RT, McKenny M. *Northeastern Wildflowers: Roger Tory Peterson Field Guides*. Norwalk, Conn: Easton Press; 1984:46.
2. Boneset. In: Grieve M. *A Modern Herbal*. Botanical.com website. Available at: http://www.botanical.com/botanical/mgmh/b/bonese65.html.
3. Habtemariam S, Macpherson AM. Cytotoxicity and antibacterial activity of ethanol extract from leaves of an herbal drug, boneset (Eupatorium perfoliatum). *Phytother Res* 2000;14:575.
4. Fisher CR Jr, Veronneau SJ. Herbal preparations: A primer for the aeromedical physician. *Aviat Space Environ Med* 2000;71:45.
5. Gassinger CA, Wunstel G, Netter P. A controlled clinical trial for testing the efficacy of the homeopathic drug Eupatorium perfoliatum D2 in the treatment of the common cold. *Arznneimettelforschung* 1981;31:732.

BORAGE

■ SOURCE, DESCRIPTION, USES

Borage (*Borago officinalis*), also known as starflower, is a member of the Boraginaceae family and is related to forget-me-not.[1,2] It is naturalized throughout much of Europe and is a garden escapee in North America. It has star-shaped blue flowers much like forget-me-not, but the plant grows to 0.5 m in height and lower stems are covered with stiff hairs. It tends to grow on rough ground and in ditches. In addition to its use as a flavoring herb and in salads, the leaves and flowers of borage have been used traditionally as an infusion for fever and upper respiratory infections, as a diuretic, as a poultice for inflammation and swelling, as an expectorant, and for depression.[1,3] More recently borage oil has been taken, like evening primrose oil, as a source of gamolenic acid (γ-linolenic acid). γ–Linolenic acid, an omega-6 fatty acid, is a precursor for dihomo-γ-linolenic acid and arachidonic acid and, hence, for prostaglandin (PG) synthesis.[4,5] The multiplicity of actions of PGs forms the theoretical basis for using evening primrose oil in such conditions as cardiovascular disease because one PG, prostacyclin, inhibits platelet aggregation.[6]

■ PHARMACOLOGY

In one study in humans, borage oil was found to reduce cardiovascular reactivity associated with increased workload in the face of reduced systolic blood pressure and heart rate.[7] The mechanism of this effect is unclear. Borage seed oil may provide up to 3 g daily of gamolenic acid at recommended doses, which may, on theoretical grounds according to one German source, be useful in controlling arthritic pain.[8]

■ ADVERSE EFFECTS AND INTERACTIONS

Gamolenic acid appears to lower the seizure threshold; thus, borage may increase the dosage requirement for anticonvulsant drugs.[3] Borage also contains low concentrations of pyrrolizidine alkaloids that are known to be hepatotoxic; thus, this herb should not be used in conjunction with other hepatotoxic drugs or herbs.[3] Because of the effect of gamolenic acid on prostaglandin synthesis, there is a potential for interaction with oral anticoagulants[9] and platelet-inhibiting drugs. The use of borage in pregnant women is unwise.

A problem that may occur with any herbal preparation, but which in this case involves borage, is misidentification of a botanical. In one case from the German literature, a woman mistakenly picked leaves of purple foxglove (*Digitalis purpurea*), believing they were from borage plants. She

developed nausea, vomiting, diarrhea, palpitations, nystagmus, atrioven-
tricular block, and had blood digoxin and digitoxin levels of 3.93 and 133.5
ng/mL, respectively.[10]

■ REFERENCES

1. Borage. In: Grieve M. *A Modern Herbal*. Botanical.com website. Available   at: http://www.botanical.com/botanical/mgmh/b/borage66.html.
2. Peterson LA. *Edible Wild Plants: Roger Tory Peterson Field Guides*. Norwalk, Conn: Easton Press; 1985:xxv.
3. Miler LG. Herbal medicinals: Selected clinical considerations focusing on known or potential drug-herb interactions. *Arch Intern Med* 1998;158:2200.
4. Horrobin DF. Multiple sclerosis: The rational basis for treatment with colchicine and evening primrose oil. *Med Hypotheses* 1979;5:365.
5. Schulz V, Hansel R, Tyler VE. *Rational Phytotherapy: A Physician's Guide to Herbal Medicine*. New York, NY: Springer-Verlag; 1998:258.
6. Philp RB. *Methods of Testing Proposed Antithrombotic Drugs*. Boca Raton, Fla: CRC Press; 1981:44.
7. Mills DE. Dietary fatty acid supplementation alters stress reactivity and performance in man. *J Hum Hypertens* 1989;3:111.
8. Chrubasik S, Pollak S. Pain management with herbal antirheumatic drugs. *Wien Med Wochenscher* 2002;152:198.
9. Heck AM, Dewitt BA, Lukes AA. Potential interactions between alternative therapies and warfarin. *Am J Health Syst Pharm* 2000;57:1221.
10. Brustbauer R, Wenisch C. Bradycardiac atrial fibrillation after consuming herbal tea. *Dtsch Med Wochenschr* 1997;122:930.

BOSWELLIN

See SALAI GUGGAL.

BROMELAIN

■ SOURCE, DESCRIPTION, USES

Bromelain is a proteolytic enzyme obtained from the pineapple (*Ananas comosus*, family Bromeliaceae). Although the enzyme is present throughout the plant, the stem has the highest concentration and is used as the source. Indigenous people of Central and South America have used the pineapple as a medicinal plant for centuries.[1] Current interest centers on the use of bromelain as an anti-inflammatory agent.[2]

■ PHARMACOLOGY

Despite the fact that bromeain is a protein, there is evidence that some absorption from the gastrointestinal tract occurs, apparently via the lymphatic system.[1,2] Animal studies reported anti-inflammatory and antiedema activity in the rat paw edema model and prolongation of prothrombin time and bleeding time in rabbits and humans.[1] It has been proposed that bromelain favors the production of anti-inflammatory prostaglandin I_2 over proinflammatory prostaglandin E_2.[2] Bromelain also digests fibrin and inhibits the synthesis of bradykinin.[2] All of these activities would, in theory, contribute to an anti-inflammatory effect.

Numerous clinical studies of bromelain in various anti-inflammatory conditions have been performed. The German Commission E reviewed five of these suitable for statistical analysis in 1993; three studies had favorable results, and two, negative results.[1] The Commission concluded that efficacy had been established for "acute post operative and post traumatic swelling, especially of the nose and paranasal sinuses." It also recommended that treatment not exceed 10 days. Stone and colleagues[2] more recently reviewed existing clinical studies and found several flaws in them, including lack of objective measures to assess results, lack of proper controls, and inadequate statistical analysis. In their own study of delayed onset muscle soreness, they found that neither ibuprofen (400 mg three times daily) nor bromelain (300 mg three times daily) had any beneficial effects. Responses measured were elbow flexor pain, loss of range of motion, or loss of concentric peak torque as a result of an eccentric exercise regimen. In another study, 77 patients with mild, acute knee pain of less than 3 months' duration were randomly assigned to receive 200 or 400 mg of bromelain daily.[3] Using the WOMAC knee health index and the Psychological Wellbeing Index, the researchers found significant improvement after 1 month and concluded that the results justified a large-scale, double-blind, placebo-controlled clinical trial.

Another recent study[4] showed that bromelain alters adhesion surface proteins of leukocytes, thus affecting their migration and activation. This effect could play a role in reducing inflammation. If this property could also be demonstrated on cancer cells, bromelain could emerge as a useful adjunct to cancer therapy; however, this is pure speculation at present.

■ ADVERSE EFFECTS AND INTERACTIONS

Adverse effects are largely confined to the gastrointestinal tract, with dyspepsia and diarrhea reported. Allergic sensitivity to pineapple, and to bromelain, also occurs. Because of its anti-inflammatory activity and anti-coagulant action on prothrombin and fibrin, bromelain could potentiate oral anticoagulants and platelet-inhibiting drugs. See also Appendices I and VIII.

In summary it appears that bromelain may have potential as a useful treatment for inflammatory conditions, and experimental evidence supports this contention, but it is evident that better clinical trials are needed before definitive claims can be made regarding the anti-inflammatory efficacy of bromelain.

■ REFERENCES

1. Schulz V, Hansel R, Tyler VE. *Rational Phytotherapy: A Physician's Guide to Herbal Medicine*. New York, NY: Springer-Verlag; 1998:262.
2. Stone MB, Merrick MA, Ingersoll CD, Edwards JE. Preliminary comparison of bromelain and ibuprofen for delayed onset muscle soreness management. *Clin J Sport Med* 2002;12:373.
3. Walker AF, Bundy R, Hicks SM, Middleton RW. Bromelain reduces mild acute knee pain and improves well-being in a dose-dependent fashion in an open study of otherwise healthy adults. *Phytomedicine* 2002;9:681.
4. Hale LP, Greer PK, Sempowski GD. Bromelain treatment alters leukocyte expression of cell surface molecules involved in cellular adhesion and activation. *Clin Immunol* 2002;104:183.

BUCHU

■ SOURCE, DESCRIPTION, USES

Buchu (*Barosma betulina*, family Rutaceae) is a native of the Cape region of South Africa. It is a shrubby plant with pale green, leathery leaves with fine-toothed edges. It has white, five-petaled flowers and brown fruit.[1] Natives of the region have used the leaves for centuries as a treatment for a variety of bladder conditions, including stones and inflammation.[1] An essential oil is also now used as a diuretic; for stomachache, bladder and kidney infections, colds, rheumatic problems, cholera, and gout; and as a diaphoretic.[2,3]

■ PHARMACOLOGY

The plant contains volatile oil, mucilage, and diosphenol, to which antiseptic properties have been attributed. Other related species, also Rutaceae, are also called buchu and come from the same region. Two of these, *Agathosma betulina* and *A. crenulata,* were examined for pharmacological activity of their essential oils using the isolated guinea pig ileum.[3] At high concentrations they had initial spasmogenic activity followed by spasmolysis. This appeared to be a direct effect on smooth muscle. *A. betulina* displayed calcium channel blocking activity. Both species of *Agathosma* were also tested for antibacterial activity, but none was found. There appears to be little else known about the pharmacological activity of buchu. Chemical constituents that have been identified include menthone and isomenthone, diosphenol (to which diuretic action is attributed), limonine, pulegone (a known hepatotoxin), and isopulegone.[2]

■ ADVERSE EFFECTS AND INTERACTIONS

One reference[4] mentions the theoretical possibility that buchu might interact with other diuretics. There do not appear to be any reports of clinical trials. There is one reference to a dog that ate leaves of *A. crenulata,* a potent diuretic plant, and passed excessive amounts of clear urine.[2] In view of the lack of data, pregnant and lactating women should avoid buchu as should anyone with renal disease or infection. Long-term use should be avoided because of the presence of hepatotoxic components. See also Appendices III and XI.

■ REFERENCES

1. Buchu. In: Grieve M. *A Modern Herbal.* Botanical.com website. Available at: http://botanical.com/botanical/mgmh/b/buchu-78.html.
2. Simpson D. Buchu—South Africa's amazing herbal remedy. *Scott Med J* 1998;43:189.
3. Lis-Balchin M, Hart S, Simpson E. Buchu (Agathsoma betulina and A. crenulata, Rutaceae) essential oils: Their pharmacological action on guinea-pig ileum and antimicrobial activity on microorganisms. *J Pharm Pharmacol* 2001;53:579.
4. Fisher CR, Veronneau SJH. Herbal preparations: A primer for the aeromedical physician. *Aviat Space Environ Med* 2000;71:45.

CALENDULA (MARIGOLD)

■ SOURCE, DESCRIPTION, USES

Calendula officinalis, the common garden marigold, with pale green leaves and gold-orange flowers, has been used as an herbal remedy for centuries. The name *marigold* has been associated with the Virgin Mary and with the 17th-century English Queen Mary, but the name apparently derives from the Anglo-Saxon name for the marsh marigold *merso-meargealla*.[1] Originally associated with English herbal medicine, calendula has more recently made an appearance in European usage and is listed by the German Commission E.[2] Traditional uses include as a topical preparation for inflammation, bee stings, and so on; for sprains and bruises; as a diaphoretic; orally for inflammation of the oral and esophageal mucous membranes; and for chronic peptic ulcer.[1] Current practice still includes many of these applications. The marigold is a member of the large Asteraceae (Compositae) family, also known as the daisy family.[3] The flower heads are composed of clusters of many small flowers; hence, are composite. Calendula leaves and flowers have been used in infusions, tinctures, fluidextracts, oils, and ointments.[2]

■ PHARMACOLOGY

Many pharmacologically active principles have been identified in calendula, giving some credence to its multifunctional application in herbal medicine. The topical anti-inflammatory activity has been attributed to triterpenoid secondary metabolites, possibly through inhibition of inducible nitric oxide synthase.[4] Studies in rats and mice found that calendasaponins A, B, C, and D inhibited the increase in serum glucose following glucose loading of rats, and exhibited gastroprotective properties in indomethacin-challenged rats.[5]

The main flavonols in calendula are iorhamnetin, quercetin, and kaempferol. These have been shown to have antibacterial, anti-inflammatory, antiviral, antitumor, and antimutagenic activity.[6] Aqueous and aqueous-ethanol extracts of calendula flowers prevented the genotoxic effects of diethylnitrosamine in cultured rat liver cells, and the exposure required to induce mutagenic effects by the extracts alone was three orders of magnitude greater than the cytoprotective concentration.[6] An organic, but not an aqueous, extract demonstrated potent anti–human immunodeficiency virus (HIV)-1 replication in human Molt-4 lymphocytes.[7] A dose- and time-dependent reduction of reverse transcription activity was observed. A butanol extract has been shown to be noncytotoxic, to have antioxidant properties,[8] and to inhibit mitogen-induced lymphocyte proliferation.[9]

A recent, randomized, clinical trial was conducted in children aged 6 to 18 years with acute otitis media. Treatment was with eardrops consisting either of a topical anesthetic (ametocaine and phenazone in glycerin) or a mixture of herbal extracts (Otikon) containing *Allium sativum, Verbascum thapsus, Calendula flores,* and *Hypericum perforatum* in olive oil. Results indicated that the treatments were equally efficacious in relieving pain.[10] Antitumor activity also has been demonstrated in hepatoma cell lines.[11]

■ ADVERSE EFFECTS AND INTERACTIONS

Although some authors report that no adverse effects have occurred with calendula,[2] there are concerns, especially with respect to the occurrence of contact dermatitis. The large Compositae family, of which calendula is a member, is a common cause of plant-related contact dermatitis.[12] Other members include chamomile, arnica, echinacea, and many other plants used as herbal remedies (see Appendix IX). Sesquiterpene lactones seem to be the most important allergens, but others such as coumarins, may be involved.[12]

Calendula officinalis extract is reportedly used in over 200 cosmetic preparations. Additional data are required to evaluate such factors as ultraviolet absorption in the presence of these preparations, as well as data regarding dermal carcinogenicity and inhalation toxicity.[13] There is some evidence that skin testing with Compositae mix or sesquiterpene mix alone may not elicit a reaction in sensitized people, and inclusion of locally used species may be necessary.[14]

In summary, calendula (marigold) may be a useful agent for topical use in inflammatory conditions and may be of low toxicity. The frequency of contact dermatitis in members of the Compositae family, however, makes this a potential problem and the ubiquity of members of this species, including many garden ornamental flowers, raises the possibility of cross-sensitization. This herb may serve as a source of useful pharmacological agents pending further research.

■ REFERENCES

1. Marigold. In: Grieve M. *A Modern Herbal.* Botanical.com website. Available at: http://www.botanical.com/botanical/mgmh/m/marigo16.html
2. Schulz V, Hansel R, Tyler VE. *Rational Phytotherapy: A Physician's Guide to Herbal Medicine.* New York, NY: Springer-Verlag; 1998:259.
3. Peterson RT, McKenny M. *Northeastern Wildflowers: Roger Tory Peterson Field Guides.* Norwalk, Conn: Easton Press; 1984:xviii.
4. Dirsch VM, Kiemer AK, Wagner H, Vollmar AM. The triterpenoid quinonemethide pristimerin inhibits inducible nitric oxide synthase in murine macrophages. *Eur J Pharmacol* 1997;336:211.

5. Yoshikawa M, Murakami T, Kishi A, Kageura T, Matsuda H. Medicinal flowers III. Marigold (1): Hypoglycemic, gastric emptying inhibitory and gastroprotective principles and new oleanane-type triterpene oligoglycosides, calendasaponins A, B, C, and D, from Egyptian Calendula officinalis. *Chem Pharm Bull* 2001;49:863.

6. Perez-Carreon JI, Cruz-Jimenez G, Licea-Vega JA, Arce-Popoca E, Fattel Fazenda S, Villa-Trevino S. Genotoxic and anti-genotoxic properties of Calendula officinalis extracts in rat liver cell cultures treated with diethylnitrosamine. *Toxicol In Vitro* 2002;16:253.

7. Kalvatchev Z, Walder R, Garzaro D. Anti-HIV activity of extracts from Calendula officinalis flowers. *Biomed Pharmacother* 1997;51:176.

8. Cordova CA, Siqueira IR, Netto CA, et al. Protective properties of butanolic extract of the Calendula officinalis L. (marigold) against lipid peroxidation of rat liver microsomes and action as a free radical scavenger. *Redox Rep* 2002;7:95.

9. Amirghofran Z, Azadbakht M, Karimi M. Evaluation of the immunomodulatory effects of five herbal plants. *J Ethnopharmacol* 2000;72:167.

10. Sarrell EM, Mandelberg A, Cohen HA. Efficacy of naturopathic extracts in the management of ear pain associated with acute otitis media. *Arch Pediatr Adolesc Med* 2001;155:796.

11. Lin LT, Liu LT, Chiang LC, Lin CC. In vitro anti-hepatoma activity of fifteen natural medicines from Canada. *Phytother Res* 2002;16:440.

12. Paulsen E. Contact sensitization from Compositae-containing herbal remedies and cosmetics. *Contact Dermatitis* 2002;47:189.

13. Final report on the safety assessment of Calendula officinalis extract and Calendula officinalis. *Int J Toxicol* 2001;20(suppl 2):13.

14. Reider N, Komericki P, Hausen BM, Fritsch P, Aberer W. The seamy side of natural medicines: Contact sensitization to arnica (Arnica montana L.) and marigold (Calendula officinalis L.). *Contact Dermatitis* 2001;45:269.

CALAMUS

■ SOURCE, DESCRIPTION, USES

The herb calamus is prepared from the root of *Acorus calamus* (family Araceae), also known as sweetflag.[1] This semiaquatic plant has long, narrow leaves with parallel veins and a spiked head with tightly massed, tiny flowers.[1] It grows widely in northeastern North America and is also native to Europe and the Far East. In India, it is part of traditional Ayurvedic medicine for the treatment of epilepsy, hysteria, insomnia, neurosis,[2] and gastrointestinal disorders, especially diarrhea.[3]

■ PHARMACOLOGY

Aqueous and alcohol extracts of the root of calamus have been shown to possess pharmacological activity, including neuroprotective properties[2] and antidiarrheal action,[3] especially in the alcoholic (methanol) extract. Two active principles, alkylbenzenes, have been isolated from the essential oil, α-asarone and β-asarone. A transisomer of α-asarone, (E)-1,2,4-trimethoxy-5-(1-propenyl)benzene, has been shown to possess antilipidemic activiity.[4] It was isolated from a Mexican herb, *Guatteria gaumeri*.[4] The ethanolic extract also has been shown to inhibit growth in several human and mouse cell lines, to inhibit production of nitric oxide, interleukin-2, and tumor necrosis factor-α,[5] and to have immunosuppressive properties.

■ ADVERSE EFFECTS AND INTERACTIONS

The α- and β-asarones are hepatocarcinogenic in rodents, and are genotoxic in cultured rat hepatocytes by inducing unscheduled DNA synthesis, apparently through a cytochrome P450–dependent mechanism.[6] α-Asarone also has been shown to be toxic to mouse spermatozoa and to induce a dominant lethal mutation.[4]

No data were found relating to herb-drug interactions nor to effects on reproduction and growth. Given the demonstrated actions of calamus extract and the asarones, it would be unwise to mix this herb with prescription or over-the-counter drugs, especially centrally acting ones and antineoplastic agents. Its mutagenicity makes it a poor choice for use during pregnancy or for nursing mothers. See also Appendix II.

■ REFERENCES

1. Peterson RT, McKenny M. *Northeastern Wildflowers: Roger Tory Peterson Field Guides.* Norwalk, Conn: Easton Press; 1984:116.
2. Shukla PK, Khanna VK, Ali MM, Maurya RR, Handa SS, Srimal PC. Protective effect of Acorus calamus against acrylamide induced neurotoxicity. *Phytother Res* 2002;16:256.
3. Shoba FG, Thomas M. Study of antidiarrheal activity of four medicinal plants in castor-oil induced diarrhoea. *J Ethnopharmacol* 2001;76:73.
4. Chamorro G, Garduno L, Martinez E, Madrigal E, Tamariz J, Salazar M. Dominant lethality of α-asarone in male mice. *Toxicol Lett* 1998;99:71.
5. Mehrotra S, Mishra KP, Maurya R, et al. Anticellular and immunosuppressive properties of ethanolic extract of Acorus calamus rhizome. *Int Immunopharmacol* 2003;3:53.
6. Hasheminejad G, Caldwell J. Genotoxicity of the alkylbenzenes alpha- and beta-asarone, myristicin and elimicin in cultured rat hepatocytes. *Food Chem Toxicol* 1994;32:223.

CAPSAICIN

■ SOURCE, DESCRIPTION, USES

Derived from the pepper *Capsicum frutescens* (cayenne pepper), capsaicin is present in all *Capsicum* species (family Solanaceae) and is the ingredient that makes peppers hot. The capsaicin content varies greatly among peppers, being greatest in Thai, Jamaican, and chili peppers and lowest in bell peppers.[1] Cayenne has been used medicinally for centuries as a carminative orally and a rubefacient locally. It can produce a powerful local vasodilation without vesication.[2] Capsaicin is the active ingredient in pepper spray.

■ PHARMACOLOGY

Capsaicin enhances the release of substance P from neurons and prevents its reuptake. The resulting depletion of substance P from nerve endings in the skin desensitizes them from further pain stimuli. A commercial cream, Zostrix, has been approved for the relief of local pain of shingles (herpes zoster).[3]

■ ADVERSE EFFECTS AND INTERACTIONS

Individuals with peptic ulcer or reflux disease are obviously not good candidates for oral treatment with cayenne powder or herbal pills. Topical use has not been associated with untoward effects except local irritation. Application to open sores is ill advised. The greatest concern regarding cayenne/capsaicin relates to a significantly higher incidence of stomach and liver cancers in cultures that are noted for their spicy cooking.[4] There also has been experimental evidence of co-carcinogenicity in mice but, conversely, there is also experimental evidence of anticarcinogen activity by several mechanisms, such as prevention of apoptosis, prevention of DNA strand breaks, and other actions.[5] Capsaicin also has been shown to promote oxidative DNA damage in the presence of copper and the formation of hydroxyl radicals.[5] The question of capsaicin's carcinogenicity must remain open for now.

■ REFERENCES

1. Capsaicin. Available at: http://people.cornell.edu/bjmlocapsaicin.html
2. Cayenne. In: Grieve M. *A Modern Herbal*. Botanical.com website. Available at: http://www.botanical.com/botanical/mgmh/c/cayenn40. html.

3. Chren M-M, Bickers DR. Dermatological pharmacology. In: Gilman AG, Rall TW, et al, eds. *Goodman and Gilman's The Pharmacological Basis of Therapeutics.* 8th ed. New York, NY: Pergamon Press; 1990:1572.
4. Archer VE, Jones DW. Capsaicin pepper, cancer and ethnicity. *Med Hypotheses* 2002;59:450.
5. Singh S, Asad SF, Ahmad A, Khan NU, Hadi SM. Oxidative DNA damage by capsaicin and dihydrocapsaicin in the presence of Cu(II). *Cancer Lett* 2001;169:139.

CAOWU

See ACONITE.

CARNITINE

See L-CARNITINE.

CASCARA

■ SOURCE, DESCRIPTION, USES

Cascara, also known as *cascara sagrada* (Spanish for sacred bark) is a cathartic herb that comes from the bark of a tree, *Rhamnus purshianus* (similar to buckthorn) native to the Pacific coast of North America. It was in use by Native Americans for constipation and upset stomach in pre-Columbian times. Extracts and fluid extracts are used in over-the-counter laxative preparations.[1]

■ PHARMACOLOGY

Fresh bark is too irritating to the gastrointestinal tract; therefore, bark is usually stored for 1 year before use. Cascara is a relatively safe cathartic when taken in a standard proprietary form, but capsules containing dried bark are unreliable and may be harsh. Cascara contains anthraquinone glycosides as the active principle.

■ ADVERSE EFFECTS AND INTERACTIONS

The toxicity, contraindications, and interactive potential are the same as those of aloe vera.[2] (See ALOE VERA for details.)

■ REFERENCES

1. Schulz V, Hansel R, Tyler VE. *Rational Phytotherapy: A Physician's Guide to Herbal Medicine.* New York, NY: Springer-Verlag; 1998:210.
2. Jafri S, Pasricha PJ. Agents used for diarrhea, constipation and inflammatory bowel disease; agents used for biliary and pancreatic disease. In Hardman JG, Limbird L, Gilman AG, eds. *Goodman and Gilman's The Pharmacological Basis of Therapeutics.* 10th ed. New York, NY: McGraw-Hill; 2001:1046.

CASCARA AMARGA

■ SOURCE, DESCRIPTION, USES

Another tree, *Picramnia antidesma*, native to the West Indies, yields a bark known as *cascara amarga*, meaning bitter bark (also mountain damson bark, simaruba, Honduras bark).

■ PHARMACOLOGY

Cascara amarga is used as a purgative, tonic, and diaphoretic.

■ ADVERSE EFFECTS, INTERACTIONS

These are the same as for cascara sagrada. See preceding entry for CASCARA.

CATNIP

■ SOURCE, DESCRIPTION, USES

Catnip (*Nepeta cataria*), family Labiatae, is well known for inducing bizarre behavior in cats, presumably because it resembles the odor of feline pheromones. It has no similar effect on humans but, nevertheless, it has been used as an herbal remedy for decades. This European native is now well established throughout North America. It has a single slim stalk growing to 0.5 m, with opposing jagged-toothed leaves and is topped by a tight cluster of white to violet, purple-spotted flowers that bloom in late summer.[1]

Traditionally, catnip has been, and continues to be, used as an aid to digestion, a diaphoretic and antipyretic, antispasmodic, expectorant, and mild stimulant (but also as an aid to sleep). Topically, it is used as a poultice for local inflammation and pain, sprains, and insect bites.[2] Currently, there is interest in its use as a mosquito repellant, and it seems to possess some significant activity in this regard. (No mention is made of possible complications for cat owners!) A tea usually is prepared from the dried leaves and flowering tops, when used as a sedative or for stomach problems.

■ PHARMACOLOGY

Catnip contains many of the active substances encountered in botanicals, such as essential oils (carvacrol, citronellal, geraniol, nepetol, nepetelactones, pulegone, and thymol), as well as iridoids and tannins.[3]

Antibacterial and antifungal activity has been demonstrated for various *Nepeta* species.[4] One study reported that 1/2-MIC levels of extract of *N. cataria* inhibited significantly coagulase, DNAase, thermonuclease, and lipase activity of both methicillin-resistant and methicillin-sensitive strains of *Staphylococcus aureus*.[4] These enzymes are believed to contribute to the pathogenicity of this organism. A related species, *N. ucrainica*, is used for similar purposes in Kazakhstan, and it was reported recently that a component, verbascoside, has immunomodulatory activity, promoting chemotaxis in neutrophils but appearing to have immunosuppressive activity at higher concentrations.[5]

■ ADVERSE EFFECTS AND INTERACTIONS

Despite the claims that catnip has sedative properties, clinical evidence for such activity has been scarce. There is a suggestion that it may have mind-altering properties if smoked.[6] Jackson and Reed[7] described four cases of young adults, two males and two females, who smoked catnip and described effects similar to those of marijuana, which two of the subjects had used previously. One review[8] attributes this claim to confusion of catnip with marijuana, but this impression probably arose from the fact that in Jackson and Reed's article, the captions for the illustrations for *N. cataria* and *Cannabis sativa* were accidentally interchanged. There is one case report of a toddler who consumed an excessive amount of catnip and subsequently developed marked central nervous system (CNS) depression that could not be attributed to any other cause.[9] It seems probable that under appropriate conditions, catnip may have some CNS activity. To date, no reports of drug interactions have appeared, but it is conceivable that potentiation of CNS depressants or interference with other CNS drugs could occur.

■ REFERENCES

1. Peterson RT, McKenny M. *Northeastern Wildflowers: Roger Tory Peterson Field Guides.* Norwalk, Conn: Easton Press; 1984:350.
2. Catmint. In: Grieve M. *A Modern Herbal.* Botanical.com website. Available at: http://www.botanical.com/botanical/mgmh/c/catmin36.html.
3. Catnip. Available at: http://www.viableherbal.com/singles/herbs/s826.htm.
4. Nostro A, Cannatelli MA, Crisafi G, Alonzo V. The effect of Nepeta cataria extract on adherence and enzyme production of Staphylococcus aureus. *Int J Antimicrobial Agents* 2001;18:583.
5. Akbay P, Calis I, Undeger U, Basaran N, Basaran AA. In vitro immunomodulatory activity of verbascoside from Nepeta ucrainica L. *Phytother Res* 2002;16:593..
6. Fisher CR, Veronneau SJH. Herbal preparations: A primer for the aeromedical physician. *Aviat Space Environ Med* 2000;71:45.
7. Jackson B, Reed A. Catnip and the alteration of consciousness. *JAMA* 1969;207:1349.
8. Cauffield JS, Forbes HJM. Dietary supplements used in the treatment of depression, anxiety, and sleep disorders. *Prim Care* 1999;3:290.
9. Osterhoudt KC, Lee SK, Callahan JM, Henretig FM. Catnip and the alteration of human consciousness. *Vet Human Toxicol* 1997;39:373.

CAT'S CLAW

■ SOURCE, DESCRIPTION, USES

Cat's claw, or *una de gato* in Spanish, is prepared from the inner bark of the vine *Uncaria tomentosa* or the closely related *Uncaria guianensis*. These are native to the Amazonian region of Peru and are considered to be sacred by certain aboriginal tribes. These vines can be several inches in diameter and grow to great heights. The inner bark is boiled and extracted to prepare the herbal medicine.[1] In native folk medicine, cat's claw has been used for a wide variety of purposes, including cancer, arthritis, gastritis, and infectious diseases.[2]

■ PHARMACOLOGY

Cat's claw has been shown to contain 29 different chemical constituents, including quinovic acid glycosides, sterols, at least 17 different alkaloids, tannins, flavonoids, and terpenes. Most of the pharmacological activity has been attributed to pentacyclic oxindole alkaloids.[1] These include antioxidant, anti-inflammatory, immunomodulatory, cytoprotective, antimutagenic, and antihypertensive activity, as well as possible protection against cerebral ischemia. Extracts have been shown to have antiproliferative and antimutagenic activity in a human breast cancer cell line, lending credence to the anticancer use in folk medicine.[2]

One study indicated that there are two chemotypes of *U. tomentosa*, the one having a predominance of pentacyclic oxindoles and the other containing primarily tetracyclic oxindoles.[3] The latter has central nervous system effects and may also antagonize the immunomodulatory activity of the former, so that they should not be given together.

In a 4-week, double-blind study of patients with osteoarthritis of the knee who were given a freeze-dried preparation of the related species *U. guiarensis*, also called cat's claw, a significant reduction in pain associated with activity was noted after 1 week. No significant change in nighttime pain was observed. There were no side effects of note, and no deleterious effects on blood or on liver function. Laboratory evidence of free radical scavenging and inhibition of tumor necrosis factor-α (TNFα) was seen.[4] Inhibition of the synthesis of TNFα has been reported by others[5] and this, plus increased phagocytosis and the ability to repair radiation-induced DNA strand breaks, have been cited as possible explanations for the nonspecific immunomodulatory activity of cat's claw.[1]

■ ADVERSE EFFECTS AND INTERACTIONS

Although cat's claw seems to be remarkably free of side effects, there is one case on record of a woman with systemic lupus erythematosus who suffered acute renal failure after taking it.[6] The patient had first been diagnosed in 1984 and had renal insufficiency with nephrotic-range proteinuria and hematuria. The patient had responded well to immunosuppressive therapy. In 1996, her serum creatinine had increased from 2.0 mg/dL to 3.6 mg/dL. She had started taking cat's claw, four capsules daily, for her arthritic problems. Her renal function improved when the herb was withdrawn.

There is also experimental evidence that cat's claw is a fairly potent inhibitor of cytochrome P450 3A4, raising the possibility that it could potentiate many drugs that are metabolized by this oxidative enzyme system.[7] This herbal preparation is too recent an addition to western usage for all of the pitfalls to have been identified. Long-term systemic use should be avoided, especially in patients with autoimmune disorders, as should use in pregnant women and young children until more is known about the effects of the herb and its active principles.

■ REFERENCES

1. Williams JL. Review of antiviral and immunomodulating properties of plants of the Peruvian rain forest with a particular emphasis on una de gato and sangre de grado. *Altern Med Rev* 2001;6:567.
2. Riva L, Coradini D, Di Fronzo G, et al. The antiproliferative effects of Uncaria tomentosa extracts and fractions on the growth of breast cancer cell line. *Anticancer Res* 2001;21:2457.
3. Reinhard KH. Uncaria tomentosa (Willd.) D.C.: Cat's claw, una de gato, or saventaro. *J Altern Compliment Med* 1999;5:143.
4. Piscoya J, Rodriguez Z, Bustamante SA, Okuhama NN, Miller MJ, Sandoval M. Efficacy and safety of freeze-dried cat's claw in osteoarthritis of the knee: Mechanisms of action of the species Uncaria guianensis. *Inflamm Res* 2001;50:442.
5. Sandoval M, Okuhama NN, Zhang XJ, et al. Anti-inflammatory and antioxidant activities of cat's claw (Uncaria tomentosa and Uncaria guianensis) are independent of their alkaloid content. *Phytomedicine* 2002;9:325.
6. Hilepo JN, Bellucci AG, Mossey RT. Acute renal failure caused by cat's claw herbal remedy in a patient with systemic lupus erythematosus. *Nephron* 1997;77:361.
7. Budzinski JW, Foster BC, Vandenhoek S, Arnason JT. An in vitro evaluation of human cytochrome P450 3A4 inhibition by selected commercial herbal extracts and tinctures. *Phytomedicine* 2000;7:273.

CELANDINE (GREATER)

■ SOURCE, DESCRIPTION, USES

Herbal celandine comes from the plant greater celandine (*Chelidonium majus*), a member of the poppy (Papaveraceae) family. Greater celandine, also known as common or garden celandine, is a perennial having a yellow flower with four petals and grows up to 1 m in height. The yellow juice is acrid, nauseating, and an irritant.[1] It is a native of Europe and Asia and a garden escapee in North America.[2] Traditionally, it has been used for jaundice, as a diuretic and purgative, and topically for skin conditions.

Currently, it is often taken for gastric and biliary conditions. The aerial or whole herb is dried and is used as an infusion. Fluid extracts also are prepared, and the fresh juice may be used.[1] In Russia, it is used for cancer, and in Suffolk, in the United Kingdom, for toothache. It is more popular in Europe than in North America, and it has been tested in a double-blind controlled study for treating dyspepsia (see later discussion).

■ PHARMACOLOGY

Much of the literature concerning celandine is from Europe, and only the abstracts are available in English. More than 30 isoquinoline alkaloids have been identified, the root being the primary source, and their biological effects may be antagonistic.[3] A thiophosphoric acid derivative of celandine is marketed as Ukrain in Europe and is being investigated extensively for the treatment of cancer. Ukrain has been shown to protect animals against whole-body gamma radiation, increase survival time, and enhance hematopoiesis. It affects stem cell pool size and cell kinetics to enhance hematopoiesis and immunopoiesis.[4] Ukrain enhanced radiotoxicty of ionizing radiation in some, but not all, human tumor cell lines, but appeared to be radioprotective to lung and skin normal human fibroblasts.[5] Cytotoxicity (without radiation) was dose-dependent. In another study using the Guerin carcinoma cell line, Ukrain continued to be cytotoxic by acting on thiol groups even in cells that had become resistant to cisplatin.[6]

Celandine has been combined with numerous other herbs for the treatment of functional dyspepsia, where the mixture has shown promise.[7] There is some experimental evidence that it promoted bile flow in rats.[8]

■ ADVERSE EFFECTS AND INTERACTIONS

Overdose, usually associated with use as a tea, may result in stomach pain, intestinal colic, urinary urgency, hematuria, dizziness, and stupor.[8] It may be more difficult to control dosage when a tea is used. Commercial preparations are standardized to a specific alkaloid and dosage is more easily controlled.[8]

Acute cholestatic hepatitis is by far the most serious adverse effect associated with greater celandine. Numerous cases are on record, mostly from Germany. Benninger and colleagues[9] reviewed ten cases of mild to severe, acute, cholestatic hepatitis in which the herb had been taken for gastric or biliary disorders. Other potential causes were eliminated. All patients recovered quickly when the herb was discontinued.

Other reports document cases in several women aged 39 to 42 years who took celandine for a variety of purposes, sometimes in conjunction with other herbs.[10,11] All recovered quickly after the herb preparation was withdrawn, but liver function tests required up to 2 months to become normal. Contact dermatitis has been reported following exposure to celandine.[12]

To date, no serious problems have been reported resulting from use of the Ukrain product, possibly because its use occurs in a much better controlled environment. This is a new and emerging area, however, and caution is advised until more data are accumulated. The usual caveats regarding use during pregnancy, in young children, and for protracted periods pertain. Any herbal preparation with the potential to cause liver damage should be avoided in patients taking prescription or over-the-counter drugs.

■ REFERENCES

1. Celandine, greater. In: Grieve M. *A Modern Herbal.* Botanical.com website. Available at: http://www.botanical.com/botanical/mgmh/c/cel-gre43.html.
2. Peterson RT, McKenny M. *Northeastern Wildflowers: Roger Tory Peterson Field Guides.* Norwalk, Conn: Easton Press; 1984:130.
3. Taboeska E, Bochorakova H, Dostal J, Paulova H. The greater celandine (Chelidonium majus L.)—review of present knowledge. *Ceska Slov Farm* 1995;44:71.
4. Boyko VN, Balskiy SN. The influence of a novel drug ukrain on hemo- and immunopoiesis at the time of maximum radioprotective effect. *Drugs Exp Clin Res* 1998;24:335.
5. Cordes N, Plasswilm L, Bamberg M, Rodemann HP. Ukrain, an alkaloid thiophosphoric acid derivative of Chelidonium majus L, protects human fibroblasts but not human tumour cells against ionizing radiation. *Int J Radiat Biol* 2002;78:17.
6. Kulik GI. Comparative in vitro study of the effects of the new antitumor drug ukrain and several cytostatic agents on the thiol groups in the tissue of Guerin carcinoma and its resistance to cisplatin variant. *Drugs Exp Clin Res* 1998;24:277.
7. Madisch A, Melderis H, Mayr G, Sassin I, Hotz J. A plant extract and its modified preparation in functional dyspepsia. Results of a double-blind placebo controlled comparative study [in German]. *Z Gastroenterol* 2001;39:511.
8. Schulz V, Hansel R, Tyler VE. *Rational Phytotherapy: A Physician's Guide to Herbal Medicine.* New York, NY: Springer-Verlag; 1998:176.
9. Benninger J, Schneider HT, Schuppan D, Kirchner T, Hahn EG. Acute hepatitis induced by greater celandine (Chelidonium majus). *Gastroenterology* 1999;117:1234.
10. Strahl S, Ehret V, Dahm HH, Maier KP. Necrotizing hepatitis after taking herbal remedies [in German]. *Dtsch Med Wochenschr* 1998;123:1410.
11. Crijns AP, de Smet PA, van den Heuvel M, Schot BW, Haagsma EG. Acute hepatitis after use of an herbal preparation with celandine (Chelidonium majus). *Ned Tijdschr Geneeskd* 2002;146:124.
12. Etxenagusia MA, Anda M, et al. Contact dermatitis from Chelidonium majus. *Contact Dermatitis* 2000;43:47.

CELANDINE (LESSER)

■ SOURCE, DESCRIPTION, USES

Lesser celandine, also known as small celandine, figwort, smallwart, and pile-wort, is prepared from the dried, whole plant of *Ranunculus ficaria* of the family Ranunculaceae.[1] Other than having yellow flowers, it bears no relationship to greater celandine, being more closely related to the buttercup.[2] Its principal use appears to be as an astringent for the treatment of hemorrhoids ("piles"), which is an ancient application; hence, the old English name *pilewort*.[1]

■ PHARMACOLOGY

When used topically in an ointment for hemorrhoids, there does not appear to be associated risk of adverse effects. Lesser celandine also has been taken internally as an infusion, but no reports of adverse effects could be found. Nor could any information be found regarding its active principles or pharmacology. It would seem to make sense to restrict the use of lesser celandine to topical applications.

■ REFERENCES

1. Celandine, lesser. In: Grieve M. *A Modern Herbal.* Botanical.com website. Available at: http://www.botanical.com/botanical/mgmh/c/celles44.html.
2. Peterson RT, McKenny M. *Northeastern Wildflowers: Roger Tory Peterson Field Guides.* Boston, Mass: Houghton Mifflin; 1984:130.

CHAMOMILE

■ SOURCE, DESCRIPTION, USES

Chamomile comes from the plants *Matricaria recutita* (German chamomile) and *Anthemis nobilis* (Roman chamomile). German chamomile is most commonly used. Related species, introduced to North America from Europe, are *M. chamomilla* and *M. maritima.*[1]

Traditionally considered a "cure-all," chamomile tea has been recommended for a host of afflictions involving the central nervous system, the respiratory system, the digestive system, the urogenital system, the musculoskeletal system, and topical preparations for various skin conditions.[2] It is currently used for nausea, irritable bowel syndrome, peptic ulcer and colic, as well as disorders of the nervous system and dysmenorrhea.

■ PHARMACOLOGY

Bioactive ingredients in German chamomile include terpenoids (bisabolol, chamazulene, and matricin, which is converted to chamazulene) and flavonoids (apigenin, luteolin, and quercetin).[2,3] Roman chamomile also includes coumarins and angelic and tiglic acid esters.[2] In laboratory studies, apigenin has been shown to possess anti-inflammatory and anxiolytic properties and to act as a ligand for benzodiazepine receptors.[3] It also has been shown to inhibit the hepatic tumor-promoting action (mitogenic and anti-apoptotic) of peroxisome proliferators.[4] Numerous other pharmacological actions have been demonstrated for compounds from chamomile.[2]

■ ADVERSE EFFECTS AND INTERACTIONS

Side effects appear to be rare. Cross-allergenicity with other members of the Compositae family (ragweed, daisy) have been reported.[2] Because of the possible presence of coumarins, especially in Roman chamomile, co-administration with oral anticoagulants should be avoided. Tannin-containing herbs, such as chamomile, may interfere with iron absorption.[5] This may not be a serious problem clinically but should be considered in anemic patients, and it is advisable to avoid taking iron and the herbal preparation together.

See also Appendices I and IX.

■ REFERENCES

1. Peterson RT, McKenny M. *Northeastern Wildflowers: Roger Tory Peterson Field Guides.* Norwalk, Conn: Easton Press; 1984:92.
2. Gardner P. Chamomile: Complete monograph. The Longwood Herbal Task Force, and the Center for Holistic Pediatric Education and Research. Available at: http://www.mcp.edu/herbal//chamomile/chamomile.pdf.
3. Hadley SK, Petry JJ. Medicinal herbs: A primer for primary care. *Hosp Pract* 1999;34:105.
4. Mounho BJ, Thrall BD. The extracellular signal-regulated kinase pathway contributes to mitogenic and antiapoptotic effects of peroxisome proliferators in vitro. *Toxicol Appl Pharmacol* 1999;159:125.
5. Miller LG. Herbal medicinals: Selected considerations focusing on known or potential drug-herb interactions. *Arch Intern Med* 1998;158:2200.

CHAPARRAL

■ SOURCE, DESCRIPTION, USES

A thorny scrub brush (*Larrea tridentata*), chaparral grows in the arid southwest of the United States.

■ PHARMACOLOGY

See PHYTOESTROGENS AND PHYTOPROGESTINS.

■ ADVERSE, EFFECTS AND INTERACTIONS.

Chaparral has been associated with cases of toxic hepatitis,[1] attributed to the presence of nordihydroguaiaretic acid[2]; otherwise adverse effects are the same as for phytoestrogens.

■ REFERENCES

1. Haller CA, Dyer JE, Ko RJ, et al. Making a diagnosis of herbal related toxic hepatitis. *Western J Med* 2002;176:39.
2. Sheehan D. Herbal medicines, phytoestrogens and toxicity: Risk:benefit considerations. *Proc Soc Exp Biol Med* 1998;217:379.

CHASTEBERRY

■ SOURCE, DESCRIPTION, USES

In medieval times, the dried berries of the chasteberry tree (*Vitex agnus-castus*) were chewed by monks in the belief that they suppressed their libido; hence the name.[1] This tree is a native of southern Europe, and whether or not the berries worked for the monks, it is now clear that chasteberries possess estrogenic activity. Since ancient times, this herb has been used for treating menstrual complaints, and its current use remains the treatment of premenstrual symptoms (PMS) and those of the menopause.

■ PHARMACOLOGY

Vacuum-dried methanol extracts of chasteberry have been shown to have a high affinity for both α- and β-estrogen receptors.[2] The extract was also shown to stimulate estradiol-mediated expression of progestin receptor mRNA.[2] Animal studies have shown that chasteberry inhibits prolactin through stimulation of D_2 dopamine receptors.[3] A small, placebo-controlled, double-blind trial in men taking three different doses of chasteberry extract (120, 240, and 480 mg) did not, however, show a significant change in 24-hour serum prolactin levels.[3] In contrast, in women with mastodynia, a placebo-controlled, double-blind study indicated a significant reduction in serum prolactin levels.[3]

In one open-label, uncontrolled, clinical trial, 1634 women with PMS took a commercial preparation of chasteberry (Femicur) for three menstrual cycles and were assessed clinically as well as completing a self-assessment questionnaire. Both assessments indicated a significant reduction in a number of symptoms of PMS.[4] This study confirms similar findings from a multicenter, controlled (pyridoxine), double-blind study in women with PMS.[3] Another placebo-controlled, randomized study in women with PMS also found significant benefits of treatment with chasteberry extract.[5]

■ ADVERSE EFFECTS AND INTERACTIONS

These clinical studies did not reveal any serious side effects, the preparations being well tolerated. In the previously described open-label study,[2] the overall incidence of undesirable side effects was 2%, and none was serious. They included skin rashes (allergic reactions, acne, hair loss, etc.), gastrointestinal symptoms (nausea, vomiting, bloating), vertigo (one case), nosebleed (one case), and vaginal spotting (one case). As is usual for estrogen-containing products, chasteberry should not be taken by pregnant women or nursing mothers.

See also PHYTOESTROGENS AND PHYTOPROGESTINS and Appendix IV.

■ REFERENCES

1. Chasteberry at: WholeHealthmd.com website. Available at: http://www.wholehealthmd.com.
2. Liu J, Burdette JE, Xu H, et al. Evaluation of estrogenic activity of plant extracts for the potential treatment of menopausal symptoms. *J Agric Food Chem* 2001;49:2472.
3. Schulz V, Hansel R, Tyler VE. *Rational Phytotherapy: A Physician's Guide to Herbal Medicine.* New York, NY: Springer-Verlag; 1998:240.

4. Loch E-G, Selle H, Boblitz N. Treatment of premenstrual syndrome with a phytopharmaceutical formulation containing Vitex agnus castus. *J Womens Health Gender Med* 2000;9:315.

5. Schellenberg R. Treatment for the premenstrual syndrome with agnus castus fruit extract: Prospective, randomized, placebo controlled study. *BMJ* 2001;322:134.

CHICKWEED

■ SOURCE, DESCRIPTION, USES

Common chickweed (*Stellaria media*, family Caryophyllaceae) is a native of Europe that has spread widely throughout North America. This fairly short (to 35 cm) plant has short, opposed ovate leaves on long stalks and flowers with pink, deeply cleft petals, often on branches at the head of the plant.[1] Many species of plant have been commonly called chickweed, but *S. media* is widely regarded as having first call on the name and is the one meant in the context of herbal remedies. The dried, whole plant is generally used and traditional uses were as a topical demulcent and refrigerant for inflammatory conditions and ulcers of the skin, usually in the form of an ointment.[2] A decoction of the fresh plant has also been used for constipation, and a fluid extract is used for hoarseness and cough.[2] Historically, the plant also has been employed as a food source (e.g., in salads) in many cultures.

■ PHARMACOLOGY

Chickweed contains many nutritional elements as well as potential medicinal ones. It is high in carotenoids,[3] contains ascorbic acid and dehydroascorbic acid,[3] and has potential as an antioxidant by virtue of being a strong inhibitor of xanthine oxidase.[4] Inhibition of growth of several cell lines of hepatoma has also been demonstrated.[5]

■ ADVERSE EFFECTS AND INTERACTIONS

No evidence of adverse effects was revealed from the literature. This may in part be due to the fact that the use of chickweed has been largely restricted to topical applications. In light of current research findings, internal use may become more common and may be accompanied by an increase in adverse reactions.

■ REFERENCES

1. Peterson RT, McKenny M. *Northeastern Wildflowers: Roger Tory Peterson Field Guides.* Norwalk, Conn: Easton Press; 1984:130.
2. Chickweed. In: Grieve M. *A Modern Herbal.* Botanical.com website. Available at: http://www.botanical.com/botanical/mgmh/c/chickw60.html.
3. Guil JL, Rodriguez-Garcia I, Torija E. Nutritional and toxic factors in selected wild edible plants. *Plant Foods Hum Nutr* 1997;51:99.
4. Pieroni A, Janiak V, Durr CM, Ludeke S, Trachsel E, Heinrich M. In vitro antioxidant activity of non-cultivated vegetables of ethnic Albanians in southern Italy. *Phytother Res* 2002;16:467.
5. Lin LT, Liu LT, Chiang LC, Lin CC. In vitro anti-hepatoma activity of fifteen natural medicines from Canada. *Phytother Res* 2002;16:440.

CHINESE KUDZU

The uses and activities of Chinese kudzu (*Pueraria pseudohirsuta*) are virtually identical to those of kudzu (*P. lobata*). See KUDZU.

CHOLESTIN

■ SOURCE, DESCRIPTION, USES

Cholestin is a component of red yeast rice. The red yeast, *Monascus purpureus,* has been used for millennia in China to ferment rice for rice wine, as a food coloring and flavoring agent, and as a medicine. In a Chinese text from AD 800, it was recommended to improve circulation of the blood.[1] More recently, it was recognized to lower circulating lipids and later entered western herbal medicine for that purpose.

The status of Cholestin, apparently a registered trademark of Pharmanex Inc., is currently in a state of flux. On May 20, 1998, the U.S. Food and Drug Administration (FDA) concluded that it was not a dietary supplement as defined by the Federal Food Drug and Cosmetic Act, but rather an unapproved drug.[2] This decision was challenged in court by Pharmanex, and a preliminary decision favored their challenge. At time of writing, however, the product Cholestin is described as containing polycosanol, en extract of beeswax, as the active principle (Pharmanex website). Polycosanol also has been shown to possess antilipidemic properties.[3] For purposes of this monograph, the term *Cholestin* shall be replaced by red yeast rice (RYR).

■ PHARMACOLOGY

RYR contains a large number of monocolins, a class of compound to which the "statin" group of antilipidemic agents belongs.[2] Statins work by inhibiting cholesterol synthesis through a mechanism that involves inhibition of β-hydroxy-β-methylglutaryl coenzyme A (HMG-CoA).[4] Not surprisingly, the same mechanism has been demonstrated for RYR.[4] One of the statins in RYR is monacolin-K (lovastatin), marketed by Merck & Co. as Mevacor. Merck has become another player in the litigious proceedings. Also present in RYR are the sterols B-sitosterol, campesterol, stigmasterol, and sapogenin, as well as isoflavones and monounsaturated fatty acids.[5] Clinical trials have confirmed that RYR lowers serum cholesterol and triglycerides by about 15% to 25%.[1,5] A pilot study found that in patients with human immunodeficiency virus (HIV)–related dyslipidemia, RYR lowered total and low-density lipoprotein cholesterol.[6]

■ ADVERSE EFFECTS AND INTERACTIONS

Side effects in human trials appear to have been limited to gastrointestinal discomfort and headache.[5] The general contraindications for statins include pregnancy, nursing mothers, a history of liver or kidney disease, or co-administration of niacin, gemfibrozil, cyclosporin, azole antifungals, erythromycin and related macrolide antibiotics, and protease inhibitor antiviral agents.[5]

In patients who have undergone organ transplantation, statin therapy for posttransplant hyperlipidemia sometimes results in rhabdomyolysis as a complication. There is one report of this complication developing in a stable renal transplant patient taking an RYR supplement. The condition resolved when the supplement was discontinued.[7] An anaphylactic reaction also has been reported after exposure to RYR.[8]

In summary, it may be that RYR has a somewhat lower incidence of side effects than the pure prescription statins, but there is a need for further study of RYR supplement in comparison with its proprietary derivatives.

■ REFERENCES

1. Heber D, Yip, I, Ashley JM, Elashoff DA, Elashoff RM, Go VL. Cholesterol-lowering effects of a proprietary Chinese red-rice dietary supplement. *Am J Clin Nutr* 1999;69:231.
2. Havel RJ. Dietary supplement or drug? The case of cholestin. *Am J Clin Nutr* 1999;69:175.

3. Nikitin IuP, Slepchenko NV, Gratsianskii NA, et al. Results of the multicenter controlled study of polycosanol in Russia [in Russian]. *Ter Arkh* 2000;72:7.

4. Man RY, Lynn EG, Cheung F, Tsang PS, O K. Cholestin inhibits cholesterol synthesis and secretion in hepatic cells (HepG2). *Mol Cell Biochem* 2002;233:153.

5. Patrick L, Uzick M. Cardiovascular disease: C-reactive protein and the inflammatory disease paradigm: HMG-CoA reductase inhibitors, alpha-tocopherol, red yeast rice, and olive oil polyphenols. A review of the literature. *Altern Med Rev* 2001;6:248.

6. Keithley JK, Swanson B, Sha BZ, Zeller JM, Kessler HA, Smith KY. A pilot study on the safety and efficacy of cholestin in treating HIV-related dyslipidemia. *Nutrition* 2002;18:201.

7. Prasad GV, Wong T, Meliton G, Bhaloo S. Rhabdomyolysis due to red yeast rice (Monascus purpureus) in renal transplant recipient. *Transplantation* 2002;74:1200.

8. Wigger-Alberti W, Bauer A, Hipler UC, Elsner P. Anaphylaxis due to Monascus purpureus-fermented rice (red yeast rice). *Allergy* 1999;54:1330.

CHONDROITIN SULFATE

■ SOURCE, DESCRIPTION, USES

Chondroitin sulfates (CSs) are glycosaminoglycans that are structural components of joint cartilage. Their polysaccharide chains are composed of similar but unique disaccharides. CS is employed in the same manner as, and often in combination with, glucosamine sulfate (GAS) as a so-called chondroprotective agent[1] (see also GLUCOSAMINE). Commercial preparations are frequently prepared from bovine cartilage.

■ PHARMACOLOGY

The most abundant CSs are CS-A (chondroitin-4-sulfate) and CS-C (chondroitin-6-sulfate).[1] CSs function as components of proteoglycans. The metabolic fate of CS is unclear. There is little evidence that orally administered CS changes plasma CS levels. Although studies with radiolabeled CS indicated 70% of the label was absorbed, only 8.5% of the label was associated with intact CS. Biochemical studies suggest that any benefit must result from the incorporation of subunits of CS, or from some effect at the level of the gastrointestinal wall.[1] Studies with cultured chondrocytes demonstrated that CS stimulates the synthesis of proteoglycans and, therefore, could assist in the repair of damaged cartilage.[1,2] In rabbits with experimentally damaged joint cartilage, CS has shown a protective effect.[2] CS has been shown to increase mRNA synthesis by chondrocytes.[3] It also has been shown, in cultured chondrocytes from osteoarthritic cartilage, to neutralize the catabolism induced by interleukin-1.[4]

The clinical efficacy of CS is virtually identical to that for GAS. Numerous clinical trials have been conducted, and most have shown evidence of efficacy in treating osteoarthritis (OA). Seven studies of CS were reviewed, and all were considered positive (treatment group ≥ 25% better than the placebo group).[5] A meta-analysis was conducted on four, suitable, randomized, double-blind, placebo- or nonsteroidal anti-inflammatory drug–controlled trials involving 227 subjects.[5] Study endpoints were 150 to 180 days. All four studies found CS to be superior to placebo, with at least 50% improvement in the study variables.

Criticisms of clinical trials of CS have been similar to those of GAS regarding small sample size, lack of standardization of selection criteria, and so on (see GLUCOSAMINE). In both cases there has been a concern over publication bias (i.e., that only positive trials are likely to be submitted for publication and that the manufacturer of the product being tested funded many studies). Another concern is that, whereas agents such as CS and GAS are treated as drugs in Europe, they are considered to be nutritional supplements in Great Britain and North America and, therefore, less rigorously controlled with respect to standardization. Some preparations in the United States have been found to contain little or no active ingredient.[5]

Trials have also been conducted using intramuscular and intra-articular injections with generally positive findings.[1] This route of administration, however, is outside the realm of herbal remedies and, therefore, of this text.

Although the results of studies of CS in OA of the knee have been generally positive, trials of its usefulness in relieving OA in other joints, such as finger joints, have been disappointing.[6] When used in conjunction with naproxen, however, it tended to slow the erosion of finger joints after 24 months and to reduce the number of new joints involved after 2 years.[7]

■ ADVERSE EFFECTS AND INTERACTIONS

Side effects in the clinical trials were uncommon and minor and usually related to the gastrointestinal tract.[2] There is one as yet theoretical hazard of using CS, especially by an injectable route, for treating OA. Wang and Roehrl[8] gave intradermal injections of glycosaminoglycans (GAGs), including CSs, to mice on days 1, 16, 43, 80, and 100 and found that after two injections, signs of inflammation and swelling in the paws appeared by day 31. The authors propose, on the basis of immunological and histological findings, that GAGs provoke autoimmune dysfunction, resulting in inflammation and pathology similar to those of rheumatoid arthritis (RA).

Although this was proposed as a possible factor in the development of RA, it raises the question of RA as a possible consequence of CS treatment of OA, especially by the intra-articular and intramuscular routes in which the biotransformation that occurs in the gut is absent.

In summary, CS appears to hold promise for the treatment of OA of the knee, but unequivocal endorsement must await the results of additional, well-designed clinical trials. Currently a National Institutes of Health–sponsored multicenter, double-blind, placebo-controlled trial of CS and GAS, alone and in combination, is under way. The results are expected in 2004.[3] It is hoped they will provide a definitive answer regarding the efficacy of these compounds.

■ REFERENCES

1. Kelly GS. The role of glucosamine and chondroitin sulfates in the treatment of degenerative joint disease. *Altern Med Rev* 1998;3:27.

2. Hauselmann HJ. Nutripharmaceuticals for arthritis. *Best Pract Res Clin Rheum* 2001;15:595.

3. Felson DT, Lawrence RC, Hochberg, MC, et al. Osteoarthritis: New insights. Part 2: Treatment approaches. *Ann Intern Med* 2000;133:726.

4. Mathieu P. A new mechanism of action of chondroitin sulfates ACS4, ACS6 in osteoarthritic cartilage. *Presse Med* 2002;31:1383.

5. Deal CL, Moskowitz RW. Nutriceuticals as therapeutic agents in osteoarthritis. The role of glucosamine, chondroitin sulfate, and collagen hydrolysate. *Rheum Dis Clin North Am* 1999;25:379.

6. Verbruggen G, Goemaere S, Veys EM. Systems to assess the progression of finger joint osteoarthritis and the effects of disease modifying osteoarthritis drugs. *Clin Rheumatol* 2002;21:231.

7. Rovetta G, Monteforte P, Molfetta G, Balestra V. Chondroitin sulfate in erosive osteoarthritis of the hands. *Int J Tissue React* 2002;24:29.

8. Wang JY, Roehrl H. Glycosaminoglycans are a potential cause of rheumatoid arthritis. *Proc Natl Acad Sci U S A* 2002;99:14362.

CHONDROITIN SULFATE/GLUCOSAMINE SULFATE COMBINATION

To date there is no convincing evidence that the combination of chondroitin sulfate and glucosamine sulfate is more efficacious than either alone,[1,2] although on theoretical grounds this would appear to be probable. Currently a National Institutes of Health–sponsored multicenter, double-blind, placebo-controlled trial of CS and GAS, alone and in combination, is under way. The results are expected in 2004,[3] and it is hoped they will provide a definitive answer regarding the efficacy of these compounds. See also individual monographs for CHONDROITIN SULFATE and GLUCOSAMINE.

■ REFERENCES

1. Kelly GS. The role of glucosamine and chondroitin sulfates in the treatment of degenerative joint disease. *Altern Med Rev* 1998;3:27.
2. Hauselmann HJ. Nutripharmaceuticals for arthritis. *Best Pract Res Clin Rheum* 2001;15:595.
3. Felson DT, Lawrence RC, Hochberg MC, et al. Osteoarthritis: New insights. Part 2: Treatment approaches. *Ann Intern Med* 2000;133:726.

CHUANWU

See ACONITE.

CINEOLE

See EUCALYPTUS OIL.

COENZYME Q10

■ SOURCE, DESCRIPTION, USES

Coenzyme Q10, also known as ubiquinone, ubidecarenone, and vitamin Q10, is, as the names suggest, a group of similar quinones that is present in most living cells, including those of animals, plants, and microorganisms. It is intimately involved in cell respiration processes and seems to be essential for normal cell function. Because of its widespread distribution in mammalian tissues and its importance to cell function, it has been touted to be effective for a host of medical problems and for nonmedical applications, such as to reverse the aging process and improve athletic and sexual performance.[1] It is now available in pure form and can be prepared from a variety of sources.

■ PHARMACOLOGY

Ubiquinone (CoQ10) is chemically related to water-soluble vitamin K_2 and to certain derivatives of vitamin E. It is essential to mitochondrial function, being involved in electron transport, cell respiration, and free-radical scavenging.[2,3] Supplements claim to be able to counter heart failure, prevent and treat cancer, improve exercise ability and physical stamina, and aid in weight loss.[1] There is evidence that some, but not all, of these claims are valid.

It has been known for some time that levels of CoQ10 are significantly lower in patients with congestive heart failure (CHF) than in normal subjects.[2] Several controlled clinical trials have shown that patients with milder forms of CHF benefit from treatment with CoQ10 in having improved quality of life and increased exercise tolerance and heart function.[3–5] More severely affected individuals do not appear to benefit as much. Not all studies support these findings,[3,4] and it would appear that the benefit of CoQ10 in CHF is modest and restricted to milder forms of the condition. Some recent studies suggest that a supplement containing CoQ10, taurine, and L-carnitine improves left ventricular end-diastolic volume in patients with left ventricular dysfunction and that this approach may be useful prior to surgery for revascularization. See L-CARNITINE for details.

There is some evidence of efficacy of CoQ10 in essential hypertension. One study in 26 patients found that 50 mg twice daily resulted in a drop in systolic pressure from 164.5 ± 3.1 to 146.7 ± 4.1 after 10 weeks.[6]

There are numerous anecdotal reports in the literature suggesting that CoQ10 is beneficial for patients with muscular dystrophy, chronic fatigue syndrome, breast cancer, and primary biliary cirrhosis.[7] Indeed, double-blind studies have provided evidence that CoQ10 is useful for patients with muscular dystrophy.[8] There is some experimental evidence that multiple effects of CoQ10 could be mediated through an effect on gene expression, because it resulted in upregulation of 47 genes while downregulating 68 others.[7] A rare congenital disorder associated with a deficiency in CoQ10 has been shown to respond positively to supplementation with the enzyme.[9]

There is as yet no convincing evidence for the usefulness of CoQ10 in the numerous other conditions for which it has been recommended. Further studies must be conducted before firm conclusions can be reached.

■ ADVERSE EFFECTS AND INTERACTIONS

Although CoQ10 itself appears to be well tolerated, there are some areas of concern. There are reports that patients with CHF who have been placed on CoQ10 supplements suffer a clinical relapse if the enzyme is withdrawn suddenly, and improvement on reinstatement of the therapy.[10]

The anticholesterolemic statins, such as lovastatin (Mevacor) and cerivastatin (Lipobay), work by inhibiting the enzyme β-hydroxy-β-methylglutaryl coenzyme A (HMG-CoA) reductase, a key enzyme in cholesterol biosynthesis. They also, however, increase the free radical oxidation of low-density lipoproteins (LDLs), increasing their atherogenic potential. It appears that this is the result of a reduction in circulating levels of CoQ10, which is normally reduced to ubiphenol Q10, a potent antioxidant that protects LDLs from oxidation.[11,12] This action may provide a rationale for supplementation with CoQ10 in patients who take statins.

Finally, several cases are on record of patients undergoing anticoagulant therapy with warfarin whose anticoagulant response fell below the therapeutic range after taking CoQ10.[5] The similarity of the enzyme to vitamin K_2 appears to impart some procoagulant properties, and its use in patients receiving warfarin should be undertaken only with the realization that warfarin dosage will need to be adjusted and clotting activity monitored closely. There is also a danger of an excessive anticoagulant effect if CoQ10 is discontinued abruptly.

In summary, CoQ10 may have a place in adjunctive therapy of CHF, but its use requires recognition of the potential problems. Its application in other conditions must await further data. See also Appendix II.

■ REFERENCES

1. Anti-aging products, part I: Can supplements rewind our body clocks? *Harv Womens Health Watch* 2001;9:2.
2. Mortensen SA. Perspectives on therapy of cardiovascular diseases with coenzyme Q10 (ubiquinone). *Clin Invest* 1993;71(suppl):S116.
3. Massey PB. Dietary supplements. *Med Clin North Am* 2002;86:127.
4. Morrelli V, Zoorob RJ. Alternative therapies: Part II, congestive heart failure and hypercholesterolemia. *Am Fam Physician* 2000;62:1325.
5. Heck AM, DeWitt BA, Lukes A. Potential interactions between alternative therapies and warfarin. *Am J Health Syst Pharm* 2000;57:1221.
6. Mancini F, Littarru GP. Coenzyme Q10 in essential hypertension. *Mol Aspects Med* 1994;15(suppl):S257.
7. Linnane AW, Zhang C, Yarovaya N, et al. Human aging and global function of coenzyme Q10. *Ann N Y Acad Sci* 2002;959:396.
8. Folkers K, Simonsen R. Two successful double-blind trials with coenzyme Q10 (vitamin Q10) on muscular dystrophies and neurogenic atrophies. *Biochim Biophys Acta* 1995;1271:281.
9. Rotig A, Appelkvist EL, Geromel V, et al. Quinone-responsive multiple respiratory-chain dysfunction due to widespread coenzyme Q10 deficiency. *Lancet* 2000;356:391.
10. Mortensen SA, Vadhanavikit S, Baandrup U, Folkers K. Long-term coenzyme Q10 therapy: A major advance in the management of resistant myocardial failure. *Drugs Exp Clin Res* 1985;11:581.
11. Folkers K, Langsjoen P, Willis R, et al. Lovastatin decreases coenzyme Q levels in humans. *Med Sci* 1990;87:8931.

12. Lankin VZ, Tikhaze AK, Konovalova GG, et al. Intensification of free radical oxidation of low-density lipoproteins in the plasma of patients with ischemic heart disease receiving β-hydroxy-β-methylglutaryl-coenzyme A reductase inhibitor cerivastatin and inhibition of low-density lipoprotein peroxidation with antioxidant probucol. *Bull Exp Biol Med* 2002;134:48.

COLCHICUM

■ SOURCE, DESCRIPTION, USES

Colchicum herb is the dried root of the autumn crocus (*Colchicum autumnale,* family Liliaceae) known also as meadow saffron, naked lady, naked boy, and father-before-the-son. These last three names derive from the fact that the plant flowers in the fall after the leaves have withered and fallen off. It has long, narrow, lanceolate leaves with parallel veins and light purple or white crocus-like flowers. The plant grows widely throughout the northern hemisphere.[1] It has a medicinal history going back 1500 years, and its toxic properties were known to the 1st century Greek physician Dioscorides.[2] It was used for arthritic conditions, including gout. Colchicum remains the 22nd most commonly prescribed single herb preparation in Germany.[3]

■ PHARMACOLOGY

The active principle in colchicum is the alkaloid colchicine. Its chemical structure is well known, and it provides dramatic relief from acute attacks of gouty arthritis. This antirheumatic effect is highly specific for gout, and colchicum has little effect on nongouty arthritis and no analgesic property. The mechanism involves binding to microtubule protein (tubulin) and preventing mitosis. It also causes depolymerization and disappearance of fibrillar microtubules in granulocytes, preventing release of lactic acid and proinflammatory enzymes in joints, including a glycoprotein thought to be the initiating agent in acute gouty arthritis.

Colchicine has a number of other pharmacological actions, including lowering body temperature, depressing the respiratory center, and enhancing the action of central depressants. It has also been shown to activate T lymphocytes.[4]

■ ADVERSE EFFECTS AND INTERACTIONS

Nausea, vomiting, diarrhea, and abdominal pain result from the antimitotic effect of colchicine on the rapidly proliferating intestinal epithelial cells. Several hours may elapse between the ingestion of the plant and the onset of signs and symptoms.[1] Leukopenia also may occur. Because of the antimitotic effect, the signs and symptoms of colchicum poisoning are similar to those of radiation sickness. Aplastic anemia and other blood dyscrasias have been reported.[5]

There are numerous reports of poisonings with colchicum, both accidental and deliberate, many of them fatal. Jaspersen-Schib and colleagues[6] reported on 152 cases of severe plant poisoning in Switzerland between 1966 and 1994. Ten were the result of ingesting *Colchicum autumnale*. All ten had severe diarrhea, nine developed liver necrosis, and two died of multiple organ failure. In severe cases of poisoning, hemorrhagic gastroenteritis, vascular damage, nephrotoxicity, muscle paralysis, and ascending central nervous system paralysis occur.[7] Hypersensitivity reactions also may occur.[5] All parts of the plant are poisonous.

Debilitated patients, elderly patients, and those with organ disease (heart, kidney, liver, etc.) are not appropriate candidates for treatment with colchicum, nor are children and pregnant women. The drug colchicine has been reported to enhance the action of central depressants, enhance the response to sympathomimetic agents, depress the respiratory center (and, hence, may increase depression caused by narcotic analgesics), and act as a vasoconstrictor (and, thus, may increase the effect of other vasoconstrictors).[2] Similar effects could be expected from high doses of the herbal preparation. Alkalinizing agents may increase the toxicity of colchicum and acidifying agents may decrease it.[5]

Sannohe and colleagues[8] described a fatal case of colchicum poisoning resulting from accidental ingestion. A 48-year-old man in northern Japan mistook *Colchicum autumnale* for *Allium victorialis platyphyllum*, a species of wild onion. Gastrointestinal symptoms commenced about 3 hours after ingestion, and he initially was misdiagnosed as having acute hepatitis or food poisoning. He was admitted to hospital on day 3 and collapsed on day 5, expiring despite 50 minutes of intensive resuscitation.

Given that the pure active principle of this herb is available as a prescription drug, it is difficult to see any justification for using the herbal form, in which dosage regulation and medical supervision are much more likely to be deficient.

■ REFERENCES

1. Saffron, meadow. In: Grieve M. *A Modern Herbal*. Botanical.com website. Available at: http://www.botanical.com/botanical/mgmh/s/safmea04.html.

2. Roberts LJ, Morrow JD. Analgesic-antipyretic and antiinflammatory agents and drugs employed in the treatment of gout. In: Hardman JG, Limbird L, Gilman AG, eds. *Goodman and Gilman's The Pharmacological Basis of Therapeutics.* 10th ed. New York, NY: McGraw-Hill; 2001:719.

3. Schulz V, Hansel R, Tyler VE. *Rational Phytotherapy: A Physician's Guide to Herbal Medicine.* New York, NY: Springer-Verlag; 1998:288.

4. Bemer V, Van Damme EJ, Peumans WJ, Perret R, Truffa-Bachi P. Colchicum autumnale agglutinin activates all murine T-lymphocytes but does not induce the proliferation of all activated cells. *Cell Immunol* 1996;172:60.

5. Ehrenpreis S, Ehrenpreis ED, eds. *Clinician's Handbook of Prescription Drugs.* New York, NY: McGraw-Hill; 2001:244.

6. Jaspersen-Schib R, Theus L, Guirguis-Oeschger M, Gossweiler B, Meier-Abt PJ. Serious plant poisonings in Switzerland 1966-1994 [in German]. Case analysis from the Swiss Toxicology Information Center. *Schweiz Med Wochenschr* 1996;126:1085.

7. Hood RL. Selected topics in toxicology: Colchicine poisoning. *J Emerg Med* 1994;12:171.

8. Sannohe S, Makino Y, Kita T, Kuroda N, Shinozuka T. Colchicine poisoning resulting from accidental ingestion of meadow saffron (Colchicum autumnale). *J Forensic* 2002;Sci 47:1391.

COLTSFOOT

■ SOURCE, DESCRIPTION, USES

Coltsfoot (*Tussilago farfara*) is a native of Europe and member of the Compositae (daisy) family that has spread throughout eastern North America. It grows 20 to 40 cm in height, with a stalk topped by a yellow, dandelion-like flower and broad, hoof-shaped, toothed leaves that give the plant its name.[1] The aerial plant is dried and used as the herb. Traditional uses include as a decoction or tea, with honey or licorice, as an expectorant and cough suppressant. The Latin word *tussilago* means "cough dispeller." Coltsfoot also has been used as a poultice for inflamed skin.[2]

■ PHARMACOLOGY

The plant contains mucilaginous elements, tannins, glucosides, phytosterols, and faradiol, a dihydride alcohol.[2] The mucilages (polysaccharide hydrophilic colloids) coat and soothe mucous membranes and contribute to the antitussive action.

■ ADVERSE EFFECTS AND INTERACTIONS

Coltsfoot contains hepatotoxic (hepatic venoocclusive disease) and carcinogenic pyrrolizidine alkaloids (PAs).[3,4] Hepatotoxic PAs are those containing an unsaturated nucleus, whereas those with a saturated nucleus are not hepatotoxic.[4] Some countries (e.g., Austria) have banned the sale of coltsfoot entirely, and Germany has limited the amount of PAs that can be consumed in 1 day to 1 µg, but whether this level is safe for chronic, long-term use has not been established beyond question.

As a member of the Compositae family, coltsfoot has the potential to elicit contact dermatitis in sensitive persons, and cross-reactivity may occur with other Compositae. One study examined the sensitizing properties of ether extracts of 20 Compositae using the guinea pig maximization test and found that coltsfoot was only weakly sensitizing.[5] Sensitizing capacity depends on the presence of specific sesquiterpene lactones.[5]

In summary, because there are other, safer mucilage-containing herbs, such as marshmallow leaves and mallow leaves,[3] that are equally effective as antitussives, there seems little justification for using coltsfoot. See also Appendices III and IX.

■ REFERENCES

1. Peterson RT, McKenny M. *Northeastern Wildflowers: Roger Tory Peterson Field Guides.* Norwalk, Conn: Easton Press; 1984:130.
2. Coltsfoot. In: Grieve M. *A Modern Herbal.* Botanical.com website. Available at: http://www.botanical.com/botanical/mgmh/c/coltsf88.html.
3. Schulz V, Hansel R, Tyler VE. *Rational Phytotherapy: A Physician's Guide to Herbal Medicine.* New York, NY: Springer-Verlag; 1998:34.
4. Miller LG, Murray WJ. *Herbal Medicines: A Clinician's Guide.* New York, NY: Pharmaceuticals Products Press; 1998:66.
5. Zeller W, de Gols M, Hausen BM. The sensitizing capacity of Compositae plants. VI. Guinea pig sensitization experiments with ornamental plants and weeds using different methods. *Arch Dermatol Res* 1985;277:28.

COMFREY

■ SOURCE, DESCRIPTION, USES

The herb comfrey is derived from *Symphytum officinale*, an introduced plant that grows along roadsides and in waste places throughout the northeast of

North America. It has pale, bell-like flowers—white, yellow, blue, or pink—and grows up to 1 m in height.[1] It should not be confused with wild comfrey, which belongs to a different genus and species (*Cynoglossum virginianum*) and is native to North America.[1] Both plants are members of the forget-me-not family. Comfrey has been used for numerous conditions, including as a poultice for varicose ulcers, as an infusion of the leaves for "intestinal troubles" and arthritic pain, as a preparation of the root for cough, and as an expectorant.

■ PHARMACOLOGY

Little is known about the pharmacology of comfrey. More is known about its toxicology.

■ ADVERSE EFFECTS AND INTERACTIONS

The main concern regarding use of comfrey is the presence of hepatotoxic pyrrolizidine alkaloids (PAs) in the plant. Although moderate, occasional use of comfrey does not appear to constitute a significant health hazard, there are several cases on record of hepatic veno-occlusive disease associated with excessive use of comfrey. Haller and colleagues[2] identified five such cases in the older literature and others more recently have been reported.[3,4] Accidental exposure to PAs can occur also through contaminated foodstuffs.[5] PAs are converted in the liver to reactive metabolites capable of forming adducts with macromolecules. These macromolecules, in turn, can lead both to acute and chronic toxicity.[5] Studies in rats have confirmed the hepatotoxicity of comfrey at relatively low doses.[6] Vascular congestion, necrosis, and damage to hepatocytes were observed. Some PAs have been shown to persist for a long time in animal tissues and may be re-released much later after a prolonged period of ingestion.[4] Mutagenicity and carcinogenicity have also been demonstrated experimentally.[4] After reviewing the existing evidence, Abbott[7] concluded that there is a small but significant health risk associated with prolonged, low levels of comfrey ingestion and that its intake should be limited. Studies in rats have indicated that PAs can be absorbed transdermally.[8] In cases where the skin has been damaged, as in burns or ulcers, there is a potential for percutaneous absorption to cause systemic PA to reach toxic levels. The use of poultices on damaged skin is ill advised.

It should be evident that consumption during pregnancy or in the presence of existing liver disease is contraindicated. Long-term use even at low levels is ill advised. Although no reports of herb-drug interactions were found in the literature, it should be evident that even minor impairment of liver function could have serious consequences for the biotransformation of many drugs. Nothing is known about long-term effects on growth and reproduction.

Because of its toxicity, comfrey has been banned by both the United States and Canada for internal consumption, but it may still appear in topical preparations such as poultices and lotions. In some parts of Europe and elsewhere, it is sometimes used in salads.[5] See also Appendix VIII.

■ REFERENCES

1. Peterson RT, McKenny M. *Northeastern Wildflowers: Roger Tory Peterson Field Guides.* Norwalk, Conn: Easton Press; 1984:144.
2. Haller CA, Dyer JE, Ko RJ, et al. Making a diagnosis of herbal-related toxic hepatitis. *West J Med* 2002;176:39.
3. Yeong ML, Swinburn B, Kennedy M, et al. Hepatic veno-occlusive disease associated with comfrey ingestion. *J Gastroenterol Hepatol* 1990;5:211.
4. McDermott WV, Ridker PM. The Budd-Chiari syndrome and hepatic veno-occlusive disease. Recognition and treatment. *Arch Surg* 1990;125:525.
5. Prakash AS, Pereira TN, Reilly PE, et al. Pyrrolizidine alkaloids in human diet. *Mutat Res* 1999;443:53.
6. Yeong ML, Wakefield SJ, Ford HC. Hepatocyte membrane injury and bleb formation following low dose comfrey toxicity in rats. *Int J Exp Path* 1993;74:211.
7. Abbott PJ. Comfrey: Assessing the low-dose health risk. *Med J Aust* 1988;149:678.
8. Brauchli J, Luthy J, Zweifel U, Schlatter C. Pyyolizidine alkaloids from Symphytum officinale L. and their percutaneous absorption in rats. *Experientia* 1982;38:1085.

COPTIS

See GOLDTHREAD.

COTTON ROOT

■ SOURCE, DESCRIPTION, USES

Gossypium herbaceum is a species of cotton indigenous to India. It also grows in southern Europe and around the Mediterranean. The root of the bark is rich in mucilaginous polysaccharides and has been used as a demul-cent.[1] Cottonseeds have been used in the southern United States to treat fever. The bark also contains sugars, oils, tannins, and chlorophyll. The herbal preparation has been used as an abortifacient, a practice employed by slaves in the south.[1]

■ PHARMACOLOGY

One of the most important constituents of all *Gossypia* species is gossypol, a polyphenolic aldehyde that has been used as a male contraceptive and antineoplastic agent.

■ ADVERSE EFFECTS AND INTERACTIONS

The use of gossypol may be associated with significant side effects and drug interactions. See GOSSYPOL.

■ REFERENCE

1. Cotton root. Available at: http://www.botanical.com/botanical/mgmh/c/cotto109.htm.

COWITCH

■ SOURCE, DESCRIPTION, USES

Cowitch (English name) is the herb prepared from the *Mucuna pruriens* (family Pappillonaceae), a plant native to India where it is known as *kawaanch* or *kavach* in Hindi.[1] It has been used in traditional Indian medi-cine for treating diabetes mellitus.

■ PHARMACOLOGY

Cowitch has been shown to possess hypoglycemic activity in alloxan dia-betic rabbits[2] and streptozotocin diabetic mice.[3] It also was shown to atten-uate renal damage in these mice. Cowitch increased glycogen content in the liver in a partially insulin-independent manner but was partially dependent on the existence functional insulin-secreting β cells.

■ ADVERSE EFFECTS AND INTERACTIONS

No adverse effects on hematological parameters were found in the study with streptozotocin diabetic mice.[3] The possibility of interactions with other antidiabetic medications cannot be dismissed. This interaction has been shown for other hypoglycemic herbs (see KARELA). More data are required to determine the safety and efficacy of this herb and whether adverse reactions and interactions with drugs are a problem. See also Appendix X.

■ REFERENCES

1. Rathi SS, Grover JK, Vats V. The effect of Momordica charantia and Mucuna pruriens in experimental diabetes and their effect on key metabolic enzymes involved in carbohydrate metabolism. *Phytother Res* 2002:16:236.
2. Akhtar MS, Qureshi AQ, Iqbal J. Antidiabetic evaluation of Mucuna pruriens, Linn seed. *J Pak Med Assoc* 1990;40:147.
3. Grover JK, Vats V, Rathi SS, Dawar R. Traditional Indian anti-diabetic plants attenuate progression of renal damage in streptozotocin induced diabetic mice. *J Ethnopharmacol* 2001;76:233.

CRANBERRY

■ SOURCE, DESCRIPTION, USES

Several species of cranberries (*Vaccinium*) are native to North America and grow in many locales from southern Canada to Illinois and the mountains of New England.[1] The juice of the so-called large cranberry (*V. macrocarpon,* bog cranberry), which is grown commercially, has been reported to assist in the prevention of urinary tract infections in a controlled study of elderly individuals who received 300 mL daily, and in another study involving young women.[2] It also is felt to be useful for people with spinal cord injuries.[2,3]

■ PHARMACOLOGY

Initially, it was thought that cranberry's beneficial action was the result of acidifying the urine, owing to the fairly high concentration of hippuric acid in cranberry juice. It is now felt that the presence of compounds called proanthocyanidins, also found in blueberries, prevent the adhesion of *Escherichia coli* bacteria to the bladder wall.[2]

■ ADVERSE EFFECTS AND INTERACTIONS

None has been reported to date.

■ REFERENCES

1. Peterson LA. *Edible Wild Plants: Roger Tory Peterson Field Guides.* Norwalk, Conn: Easton Press; 1985:102.
2. Rodblatt MD. Cranberry, feverfew, horse chestnut and kava. *West J Med* 1999;171:195.
3. Riering-Sorensen F. Urinary tract infections in individuals with spinal cord lesion. *Curr Opin Urol* 2002;12:45.

DAMIANA

■ SOURCE, DESCRIPTION, USES

Turnera diffusa var. (family Turneraceae), also known as *Damiana aphrodisiaca* or damiana, is a small shrub native to Texas, Mexico, South America, and the West Indies. It has pale green, ovolanceolate leaves and an aromatic odor.[1] Traditional uses includes as a laxative, diuretic, tonic, stimulant, and, as the name suggests, aphrodisiac. A greenish volatile oil is made from the leaves.[1] *T. diffusa* is widely reputed throughout Latin America to possess aphrodisiac properties and is used by men to stimulate libido and improve performance.[2]

■ PHARMACOLOGY

Studies have been conducted on alcohol-water extracts, but not much appears to be known about the active principles. *A Modern Herbal* by Mrs. M. Grieve,[1] dating to the 1930s, refers to an amorphous bitter principle, damianin, resins, and tannin. Certainly, damiana contains many ingredients with the potential for pharmacological activity including β-sitosterol (see β-SITOSTEROL), 5-hydroxy-7,3'4'-trimethyloxyflavone, α- and β-pinene, 1,8-cineole, *p*-cymene, hydroquinone glycosides, and cyanogenic glycosides.[2]

Arletti and colleagues[2] conducted a study in which male rats were selected for poor sexual responsiveness when presented with a female rat in estrus (hormonally induced in ovariectomized animals). An ethanol-water extract of damiana was prepared from dried, crushed leaves and given by gastric lavage 1 hour before testing. There was a significant improvement in sexual performance as indicated by shortened mount and intromission latencies, postejaculatory intervals, and other measures. These changes were not observed in saline-treated controls.

One human double-blind, placebo-controlled study looked at the ability of a mixture of herbs and vitamins to improve female human sexual function.[3] The mixture, known as ArginMax for Women, contained extracts of ginkgo, ginseng, and damiana; L-arginine; multivitamins; and minerals. Seventy-seven women who were 21 years of age and had an interest in improving their sexual function were given either the mixture (34 subjects) or a placebo (43 subjects) daily for 4 weeks. At the end of the study, 73.4% of women in the treatment group reported greater satisfaction with their sex life compared with 37.2% of the placebo group. The treatment group reported improved lubrication, clitoral sensitivity, frequency of orgasm, and increased sexual desire. Not all of these differences were statistically significant, but significant differences were noted in improved sexual relationship with the partner, improved lubrication, and decreased discomfort during intercourse. As the authors note, the high placebo response frequency is indicative of a significant psychological component to sexual dysfunction in young women. These authors also reviewed a study using a similar product that improved men's ability to maintain an erection.

T. diffusa has demonstrated hypoglycemic activity in diabetic mice and rabbits.[4,5]

A mixture of the herbs, guarana, damiana, and yerba maté was studied as a weight loss aid in overweight patients.[6] Body weight and gastric emptying time were measured after 10 days of treatment with either the mixture in capsule form or a placebo capsule containing apple juice. Gastric emptying was delayed and significant weight loss occurred in the treated subjects.

■ ADVERSE EFFECTS AND INTERACTIONS

Given the paucity of clinical studies on single herb effects of damiana, not much can be said with certainty regarding adverse reactions and interactions. There is a theoretical possibility of an interaction with oral hypoglycemic agents or insulin, and close monitoring of blood glucose obviously should be instituted in anyone who elects to combine herbal therapy with prescription medications. In the previously mentioned study using ArginMax, the authors stated that no adverse effects were reported, specifically listing headache, nausea, vomiting, visual disturbances, blood pressure alterations, dizziness, and hypersensitivity.[3]

In summary, although there have been some promising findings with herb mixtures incorporating damiana, it is difficult to evaluate the efficacy and safety of this herb on the basis of existing evidence. See also the individual monographs for GINKGO, GINSENG, and GUARANA, and Appendix X.

■ REFERENCES

1. Damiana. In: Grieve M. *A Modern Herbal.* Botanical.com website. Available at: http://www.botanical.com/botanical/mgmh/d/damian05.html.
2. Arletti R, Benelli A, Cavazutti E, Scarpetta G, Bertolini A. Stimulating property of Turnera diffusa and Pfaffia paniculata extracts on the sexual behavior of male rats. *Psychopharmacol* 1999;143:15.
3. Ito TY, Trant AS, Polan ML. A double-blind placebo-controlled study of ArginMax, a nutritional supplement for enhancement of female sexual dysfunction. *J Sex Marital Ther* 2001;27:541.
4. Alarcon-Aguilara FJ, Roman-Ramos R, Perez-Gutierrez S, Aguilar-Contreras A, Contreras-Weber CC, Flores-Saenz JL. Study of the anthyperglycemic effect of plants used as antidiabetics. *J Ethnopharmacol* 1998;61:101.
5. Alarcon-Aguilar FJ, Roman-Ramos R, Flores-Saenz L, Aguirre-Garcia F. Investigation of the hypoglycaemic effects of extracts of four Mexican plants in normal and alloxan-diabetic mice. *Phytother Res* 2002;16:383.
6. Anderson T, Fogh J. Weight loss and delayed gastric emptying following a South American herbal preparation in overweight patients. *J Hum Nutr Diet* 2001;14:243.

DANDELION

■ SOURCE, DESCRIPTION, USES

Many species of plants are called dandelion. All are members of the Compositae family.[1] The common dandelion (*Taraxacum officinale*) is unhappily familiar to all gardeners and lawn care specialists and grows widely throughout the northern hemisphere. It is also familiar to traditional herbalists wherever it grows. Traditionally, all parts of the plant have been used medicinally, but the dried root is used most commonly.[2] It was taken as a diuretic, tonic, "general stimulant," and especially for kidney and liver disorders.[1] The plant has a long, hollow stem topped by a bright yellow composite flower; long, narrow toothed leaves with the teeth pointing toward the stem; and bitter, milky latex. The Rocky Mountain dandelion (*T. eriophorum*) has strap-like leaves without teeth.

■ PHARMACOLOGY

The dandelion is known to contain several flavonoids, including caffeic acid, chlorogenic acid, luteolin, and luteolin-7-glucoside.[3] Both water and ethyl acetate extracts of dandelion flowers demonstrate free-radical scavenging activity that appears to be associated with their content of luteolin and luteolin-7-glucoside.[3] Studies with rats found that dandelion herbal tea significantly inhibited hepatic cytochrome P450 (CYP)1A2 and CYP2E1, raising the possibility that it could potentiate the effects of drugs metabolized by these enzymes.[4] Other studies with rats showed that a water extract of dandelion leaves increased antioxidant activity by increasing superoxide dismutase and catalase activities in both normal and streptozotocin-induced diabetic mice, and the authors of these studies suggested that this property could be useful to improve lipid metabolism and free radical scavenging in diabetics.[5]

Current herbal medicinal use for dandelion includes as a diuretic, laxative, and digestive aid; as a protectant for liver and gallbladder; and to prevent iron-deficiency anemia, premenstrual syndrome, and breast tenderness.[6]

■ ADVERSE EFFECTS AND INTERACTIONS

As a member of the Compositae family, dandelion has the potential to cause allergic contact dermatitis as well as cross-reactivity with other members of this large botanical family.[7] See also Appendix IX. Because of the diuretic action of dandelion, interaction with other diuretics is a possibility and concomitant use should likely be avoided.[6]

Dandelions growing in urban lawns and waste ground may accumulate toxic materials, such as heavy metals and pesticides. Frequent use of plants from such sites, whether as an herb or a foodstuff (as in dandelion wine or salad), is unwise. Studies have shown that lead content rises in the leaves in the autumn as compared with the spring,[8] and the insecticide chlordane has been detected in the leaves in areas where it has been used.[9] There has been a suggestion that dandelion is toxic for young children, resulting in gastrointestinal distress, vomiting, and diarrhea,[10] and it has been recommended that it not be used in cases of biliary obstruction or infection.[10]

Apart from these considerations, dandelion appears to be a relatively innocuous remedy or food source. See also Appendices V, IX, and XI.

■ REFERENCES

1. Peterson RT, McKenny M. *Northeastern Wildflowers: Roger Tory Peterson Field Guides.* Norwalk, Conn: Easton Press; 1984:218.

2. Dandelion. In: Grieve M. *A Modern Herbal*. Botanical.com website. Available at: http://www.botanical.com/botanical/mgmh/d/dandel08.html.

3. Hu C, Kitts DD. Antioxidant, prooxidant, and cytotoxic activities of solvent-fractionated dandelion (Taraxacum officinale) flower extracts in vitro. *J Agric Food Chem* 2003;51:301.

4. Maliakal PP, Wanwimolruk S. Effect of herbal teas on hepatic drug metabolizing enzymes in rats. *J Pharm Pharmacol* 2001;53:1323.

5. Cho SY, Park JY, Park EM, et al. Alteration of hepatic activities and lipid profile in streptozotocin-induced diabetic rats by supplementation of dandelion water extract. *Clin Chim Acta* 2002;317:109.

6. Fisher CR, Veronneau SJH. Herbal preparations: A primer for the aeromedical physician. *Aviat Space Environ Med* 2000;71:45.

7. Paulsen E, Andersen KE, Hausen BM. Sensitization and cross-reaction patterns in Danish Compositae-allergic patients. *Contact Dermatitis* 2001;45:197.

8. Keane B, Collier MH, Shann JR, Rogstad SH. Metal content of dandelion (Taraxacum officinale) leaves in relation to soil contamination and airborne particulate matter. *Sci Total Environ* 2001;281:63.

9. Mattina MJ, Iannucci-Berger W, Dykas L. Chlordane uptake and its translocation in food crops. *J Agric Food Chem* 2000;48:1909.

10. Miller LG, Murray WJ. *Herbal Medicinals: A Clinician's Guide*. New York, NY: Pharmaceutical Products Press; 1998:127.

DANSHEN

■ SOURCE, DESCRIPTION, USES

Danshen is the root of *Salvia miltiorrhiza*. It also is known as red sage root and tan seng. It is a Chinese herbal remedy and it is grown commercially in China and elsewhere in Asia. Related *Salvia* species are native to North America (see SAGE). Danshen is used primarily as an herbal remedy for cardiovascular problems, including angina pectoris and high blood pressure. It also is used for menstrual discomfort.[1,2]

■ PHARMACOLOGY

A wide range of pharmacological actions have been claimed for danshen, including hypotensive effect, positive inotropism and negative chronotropism, inhibition of platelet function, and prolongation of the prothrombin time and the international normalized ratio (INR).[1,2] Animal studies indicate that the hypotensive action of danshen is mediated through inhibition of angiotensin-converting enzyme.[3] Inhibition of thromboxane synthesis also has been reported.[4] An investigation of diterpene quinones isolated from ether extracts of danshen root found several with partial agonist activity for benzodiazepine receptors.[5] One in particular, militrone, had significant potency and displayed tranquilizing properties when given orally to mice.

■ ADVERSE EFFECTS AND INTERACTIONS

Given the pharmacological activity of danshen, it is not surprising that it can increase the risk of bleeding when given concomitantly with oral anticoagulants, such as warfarin, or platelet-inhibiting drugs, such as acetylsalicylic acid and clopidogrel (Plavix), and a number of such cases have been recorded.[1,2,6–8] In addition to being effective orally, danshen is active when inhaled, and some Chinese cigarettes actually contain danshen.[9]

It is clear from these findings that danshen should not be taken by anyone undergoing medical treatment with anticoagulants or platelet-inhibiting drugs. The partial agonist activity of danshen for benzodiazepine receptors[5] creates the theoretical possibility of additive effects with tranquilizers and sedatives. It should be used cautiously, if at all, with these medications until more information regarding its safety is available. Its use in pregnant women and nursing mothers is not advisable. The safety of long-term use has not been established, and use could entail risks even when no other medications are involved. See also Appendix VII.

■ REFERENCES

1. Izzat MB, Yim APC, El-Zufari H. A taste of Chinese medicine. *Ann Thorac Surg* 1998;66:941.
2. Lambrecht JE, Hamilton W, Rabinovich A. A review of herb-drug interactions: Documented and theoretical. *US Pharmacist* 25:8. Available at: http:/www.uspharmacist.com/NewLook/DisplayArticle.cfm?item_num=566.
3. Kang DG, Yun YG, Ryoo JH, Lee HS. Anti-hypertensive effect of water extract of danshen on renovascular hypertension through inhibition of the renin angiotensin system. *Am J Chinese Med* 2002;30:87.
4. Cheng TO. *The International Textbook of Cardiology.* New York, NY: Pergamon Press; 1987:1067.
5. Chang HM, Chui KY, Tan FW, et al. Structure-activity relationship of miltirone, an active central benzodiazepine receptor ligand isolated from Salvia miltiorrhiza Bunge (Danshen). *J Med Chem* 1991;34:1675.
6. Miller LG. Herbal medicines: Selected clinical considerations focusing on known or potential herb-drug interactions. *Arch Intern Med* 1998;158:2200.

7. Fugh-Berman A. Herb-drug interactions. *Lancet* 2000;355:134.

8. Yu CM, Chan JC, Sanderson JE. Chinese herbs and warfarin potentiation by "danshen". *J Intern Med* 1997;241:337.

9. Cheng TO. Warfarin danshen interaction. *Ann Thorac Surg* 1999;67:894.

DEVIL'S CLAW

■ SOURCE, DESCRIPTION, USES

The seedpods of *Harpagophytum procumbens* resemble a desiccated bird's foot, with many hooked protuberances. The plant is native to the Kalahari and Madagascar and has been used traditionally in those areas for arthritic pain, probably because of the seedpod's resemblance to an arthritic hand. A standardized root extract is currently used for rheumatic pain. It also has been used as a carminative ("bitters") because of its ability to stimulate gastric acid secretion.

■ PHARMACOLOGY

Active ingredients include iridoid glycosides, harpagoside being of main interest, flavonoids, and sterols.[1] Several clinical studies have now confirmed that devil's claw has antirheumatic properties and may be associated with fewer adverse reactions than conventional, nonsteroidal, anti-inflammatory drugs (NSAIDs).[1–4] The mechanism of action appears to differ from that of NSAIDs, however, because no inhibition of prostaglandin synthesis and no anti-inflammatory activity could be shown in an animal model of inflammation.[5] A number of other pharmacological effects involving the cardiovascular system and the central nervous system have been reported both in animal studies and in humans.[6,7] Not all of these effects could be attributed to harpagoside.

■ ADVERSE EFFECTS AND INTERACTIONS

Although this herb has been recommended for dyspepsia, its ability to promote gastric acid secretion makes it a poor choice for anyone with acid reflux disorder or peptic ulcer. Diarrhea was reported as the most frequent side effect in one clinical study, involving 8.1 % of patients treated with powdered herb.[4]

Specific drug interactions do not appear to be associated with devil's claw, but the complex nature of its pharmacology makes these a possibility. Flavonoids, in particular, have been associated with inhibition of cytochrome P450 3A4, with resulting potentiation of several drugs, including felodipine, midazolam, and quinidine.[8,9] This interaction has been reported for naringenin in grapefruit juice[8] and for quercetin and kaemferol.[9] Given the presence of flavonoids in devil's claw, the possibility of a similar interaction cannot be discounted. Easy bruising as a result of an interaction with warfarin has been reported,[10] apparently as a result of inhibition of cyclooxygenase enzyme.

There are no reliable data regarding the effects of long-term use, use in pregnancy, or effects on growth and development. See also Appendices VII and VIII.

■ REFERENCES

1. Purvis G. Nature's pharmacy. *The Guardian* Nov 1, 2001. Available at: http://www.education.guardian.co.uk/Print/0,3858,4289474.00.html.

2. Schulz V, Hansel R, Tyler VE. *Rational Phytotherapy: A Physician's Guide to Phytotherapy.* New York, NY: Springer-Verlag; 1998:263.

3. Leblan D, Chantre P, Fournie B. Harpagophytum procumbens in the treatment of knee and hip osteoarthritis. Four-month results of a prospective multicenter, double-blind trial versus diacerhein. *Joint Bone Spine* 2000;67:462.

4. Chantre P, Cappelaere A, Leblan D, Guerdon D, Vandermander J, Fournie B. Efficacy and tolerance of Harpagophytum procumbens versus diacerhein in treatment of osteoarthritis. *Phytomedicine* 2000;7:177.

5. Whitehouse LW, Znamirowska M, Paul CJ. Devil's claw (Harpagophytum procumbens): No evidence for anti-inflammatory activity in the treatment of arthritic disease. *Can Med Assoc J* 1983;128:249.

6. Circosta C, Occhiuto F, Raguse S, et al. A drug used in traditional medicine: Harpagophytum procumbens DC. II. Cardiovascular activity. *J Ethnopharmacol* 1984;11:259.

7. Gobel H, Heinze A, Ingwersen M, Niederberger U, Gerber D. Effects of Harpagophytum procumbens LI 174 (devil's claw) on sensory, motor and vascular muscle reagibility in the treatment of unspecific back pain [in German]. *Schmerz* 2001;15:10.

8. Bailey DC, Kreeft JH, Munoz C, et al. Grapefruit juice-felodipine interaction: Effect of naringin and 6,7-dihydroxybergamottin in humans. *Clin Pharmacol Ther* 1998;64:248.

9. Ha HR, Chen J, Leuenberger PM, Frieburghaus AU, Follath F. In vitro inhibition of midazolam and quinidine metabolism by flavonoids. *Eur J Clin Pharmacol* 1995;48:367.

10. Fugh-Berman A, Ernst E. Herb-drug interactions: Review and assessment of report reliability. *Br J Clin Pharmacol* 2001;52:587.

DHEA

■ SOURCE, DESCRIPTION, USES

Dehydroepiandrosterone (DHEA) and its sulfated form (DHEAs) are the main steroid hormones synthesized and secreted by the adrenal cortex and are precursors in both androgen and estrogen synthesis. They also are the most prominent circulating steroids.[1,2] Because DHEA has a wide range of physiological effects, and because studies indicate that levels in the body decline with age, many health food advocates have embraced it as the elixir of youth. In the mid 1990s, studies in France provided some evidence that DHEA could counteract some of the effects of aging, lending support to this belief.[3] Animal studies have shown that caloric restriction, which is known to prolong longevity, also retards the decline in serum DHEAs associated with aging in animals and people.[4] Competitive athletes also began to use the drug in the belief that it would improve stamina and energy.[2] It is widely available in health food stores in the United States and elsewhere. Most DHEA is synthesized pharmaceutically from diosgenin, a precursor found in Mexican wild yam (see also PHYTOESTROGENS AND PHYTOPROGESTINS and WILD YAM).

■ PHARMACOLOGY

The pharmacology of DHEA is the same as that of androgens and estrogens. Its effects depend on the age and sex of the recipient and, if female, on pre- or postmenopausal state. Although animal studies have indicated a plethora of activities, clinical studies are largely inconclusive if not controversial. An extensive literature has developed in the past few years regarding DHEA. The following is a brief summary compiled from some recent review articles.[1,2,5]

AGING

Circulating DHEA levels decline with age in both animals and humans. Clinical studies in elderly subjects reported that DHEA supplementation was associated with an improved sense of well being, sleep patterns, and energy levels. Evidence showing that these subjective changes are paralleled by improved physiological parameters, including improved cognition, is controversial. Larger and better-designed studies are required.

CARDIOVASCULAR DISEASE

Some epidemiological studies have suggested that men with low DHEA levels are at a slightly increased risk of cerebrovascular disease, but not all studies support this finding.

OBESITY

Treatment with DHEA has been shown to reduce body fat mass in obese, but not nonobese, young men. However, in postmenopausal women, a positive association was found between DHEA levels and central obesity. No firm conclusion can be reached regarding the usefulness of DHEA for obesity.

CANCER

Endogenous levels of DHEA could obviously play a role in the development of hormone-dependent cancers, such as breast and prostate cancers, but the effect appears to be dependent on the prevailing hormonal milieu. In premenopausal women, DHEA seems to be protective against breast cancer, possibly acting as an estrogen antagonist by virtue of being weakly estrogenic itself. In postmenopausal women, this activity could promote the development of estrogen-dependent breast cancer. High levels of DHEA have been associated with an increased risk of ovarian cancer.

MOOD

Several studies have reported improvement in cognition and mood in depressed patients and in those with systemic lupus erythematosus (SLE). Mania in men taking high doses has been reported.

ATHLETIC PERFORMANCE

DHEA has been taken by athletes to increase androgen levels and, hence, strength. Increases in testosterone levels are transient, however, and there are no data to indicate that performance is enhanced by DHEA.

IMMUNE FUNCTION

There is an association between low levels of DHEA and diseases in which immune function is impaired, including acquired immunodeficiency syndrome and SLE. Although animal studies have suggested that supplementation with DHEA improves antibody response, human studies have failed to confirm this finding. Clinically, there is substantial evidence that DHEA may benefit women with SLE.[6] Double-blind, placebo-controlled studies showed that DHEA (200 mg/day for 3 months) decreased the required dose of prednisolone, the frequency of flare-ups, and the activity of the disease. In another study, DHEA was shown to reduce bone density loss associated with corticosteroid therapy.

DHEA has been examined in numerous other disease states or for age-related problems with inconclusive results.

■ ADVERSE EFFECTS AND INTERACTIONS

There have been several reports of mania in men resulting from taking high doses of DHEA.[3,7] In one case,[7] the 68-year-old man had suffered from bipolar disorder in the past. There is no information regarding the effects of long-term consumption of DHEA. Excessive use could result in signs and symptoms of excessive androgen or estrogen levels, such as oily skin, pimples, fine facial hair in women (some women in the SLE studies showed these effects[6]), mood changes, irritability, and, in men, aggressiveness. DHEA could interfere with estrogen replacement therapy, oral contraceptives, and therapies for breast and prostate cancers.

In summary, much more information is needed before firm conclusions can be reached regarding the usefulness of DHEA as a supplement or a drug.

■ REFERENCES

1. Johnson MD, Bebb RA, Sirrs SM. Uses of DHEA in aging and other disease states. *Ageing Res Rev* 2002;1:29.
2. Corigan B. DHEA and sport. *Clin J Sport Med* 2002;12:236.
3. Holden C. Interest grows in anti-aging drug. *Science* 1995;269:33.
4. Roth GS, Lane MA, Ingram DK, et al. Biomarkers of caloric restriction may predict longevity in humans. *Science* 2002;297:811.
5. Allolio B, Arlt W. DHEA treatment: Myth or reality? *Trends Endocrinol Metab* 2002;13:288.
6. Patavino T, Brady DM. Natural medicine and nutritional therapy as an alternative treatment in systemic lupus erythematosus. *Altern Med Rev* 2001;6:460.
7. Vacheron-Trystram MN, Cheref S, Gauillard J, Plas J. A case report of mania precipitated by use of DHEA [in French]. *Encephale* 2002;28:563.

DONG QUAI

■ SOURCE, DESCRIPTION, USES

The Chinese herb dong quai or dang gui (various spellings) is prepared from the root of *Angelica sinensis* (in the parsley family, Umbelliferae), a perennial that grows to a height of about 1 m throughout Southeast Asia. It is commonly referred to an angelica in the West and will be referred to as angelica here. Traditionally, it has been used for a variety of conditions, most especially as a phytoestrogen for treating dysmenorrhea and menopausal symptoms. It also is claimed to have analgesic, anticholesterolemic, anti-inflammatory, antispasmodic, and hepatoprotective properties. Dong quai also is used for bone and tendon injuries.[1] North American members of the Umbelliferae family include cow parsnip, snakeroot, Alexander's angelica (*Angelica atropurpurea*), and honeywort.[2]

■ PHARMACOLOGY

The USDA medicinal plant database[3] lists dozens of chemical components of angelica, including many vitamins and many agents with pharmacological activity. Whether they are all present in sufficient quantity to have clinical significance is questionable. Earlier attention focused on the estrogenic activity of angelica. Several members of the Umbelliferae family have been shown to be only weakly estrogenic.[4,5] Dong quai showed only weak estrogen-receptor binding activity and ability to induce progestin receptors.[6]

Other pharmacological activities have been ascribed to angelica. It has been shown to stimulate, dose dependently, proliferation and several biochemical functions (e.g., collagen synthesis) of human bone (osteoprecursor) cells, supporting its traditional use for bone and tendon injuries.[7] A crude extract of the plant also has been shown to stimulate proliferation of gastric epithelial cells,[8,9] and a polysaccharide-rich fraction was shown to protect mouse livers from acetaminophen-induced damage.[10]

■ ADVERSE EFFECTS AND INTERACTIONS

Despite the apparent lack of significant estrogenic activity, estrogen-related adverse effects have been reported. There is a report of a man in Singapore who developed gynecomastia after taking dong quai pills as a tonic; a traditional use recommended for both men and women.[11] There is an obvious risk associated with men taking excessive doses of herbal preparations with estrogenic activity. The possibility of interference with estrogen replacement therapy and oral contraceptives cannot be ignored.

Easy bruising as a result of an interaction with warfarin has been reported,[12] apparently as a result of inhibition of cyclooxygenase enzyme. Interactions with digoxin and furosemide also have been reported.[12]

Several allergens have been identified in angelica[3]; thus, allergic reactions are possible, and cross-sensitivity with other Umbelliferae could occur. See also PHYTOESTROGENS AND PHYTOPROGESTINS and Appendix IV.

■ REFERENCES

1. Introduction to Angelica sinensis (Dong quai, Dang Gui). DreamPharm.com website. Available at: http://dreampharm.com/garlic/angelica.asp.
2. Peterson RT, McKenny M. *Northeastern Wildflowers: Roger Tory Peterson Field Guides*. Norwalk, Conn: Easton Press; 1984:50.
3. Dr. Duke's phytochemical and ethnobotanical databases. Available at: http://www.ars-grin.gov/duke.
4. Golden RJ, Noller KL, Titus-Ernstoff L, et al. Environmental endocrine modulators and human health: An assessment of the biological evidence. *Crit Rev Toxicol* 1998;28:109.
5. Zava DT, Dollbaum CM, Blen M. Estrogen and progestin bioactivity of foods, herbs and spices. *Proc Soc Exp Biol Med* 1998;217:369.
6. Liu J, Burdette JE, Xu H, et al. Evaluation of estrogenic activity of plant extracts for the potential treatment of menopausal symptoms. *J Agric Food Chem* 2001;49:2472.
7. Yang Q, Populo S, Zhang J, Yang G, Kodama H. Effect of Angelica sinensis on the proliferation of human bone cells. *Clin Chim Acta* 2002;324:89.
8. Ye YN, Koo MW, Li Y, Matsui H, Cho CH. Angelica sinensis modulates migration and proliferation of gastric epithelial cells. *Life Sci* 2001;68:961.
9. Ye YN, Liu ES, Shin VY, et al. A mechanistic study of proliferation induced by Angelica sinensis in the normal gastric epithelial cell line. *Biochem Pharmacol* 2001;61:1439.
10. Ye YN, Liu ES, Li Y, et al. Protective effect of polysaccharide-enriched fraction from Angelica sinensis on hepatic injury. *Life Sci* 2001;69:637.
11. Goh SY, Loh KC. Gynaecomastia and the herbal tonic "dong quai". *Singapore Med J* 2001;42:115.
12. Fugh-Berman A, Ernst E. Herb-drug interactions: Review and assessment of report reliability. *Br J Clin Pharmacol* 2001;52:587.

ECHINACEA

■ SOURCE, DESCRIPTION, USES

Echinacea is derived from the coneflower *Echinacea purpurea L.* and related species *E. pallida* and *E. augustifolia* and is available in numerous forms, including teas, capsules, prepared beverages, and chewing gum marketed under various trade names by many companies. It also is combined frequently with conventional over-the-counter medications such as dextromethorphan (Benylin).

■ PHARMACOLOGY

It is claimed that this botanical improves immune function and shortens the duration of the common cold if taken at the onset of symptoms. Both laboratory studies and clinical trials lend some credence to this claim. In one Swedish study of 119 cold sufferers, those who took an echinacea supplement (two Echinoforce tablets three times daily for 1 week) reported slightly less severe symptoms than those who took a matching placebo.[1] In a similar randomized, double-blind, controlled study, 80 patients were assigned to placebo treatment or echinacea (Echinacin, EC312J0). The treated group had symptoms for an average of 6 days compared with 9 days for the placebo group, and the difference was statistically significant.[2] In another study, a polysaccharide extract of E. purpurea was given to 15 patients with advanced gastric cancer undergoing palliative chemotherapy. Two mg of the polysaccharide were given intravenously daily. Two weeks after treatment, the leukocyte count was 3630/uL compared to 2370/uL for a historical control group. This difference was statistically significant ($p = .015$). No clinically relevant effects on phagocytic activity of granulocytes were observed, nor were effects on lymphocyte subpopulations noted.[3]. Yet another study showed that dietary administration of E. purpurea extract to aging mice stimulated the activity of natural killer cells.[4]

Other pharmacological properties have been reported. Alkamides extracted from echinacea have been shown to have anti-inflammatory activity, attributed to their ability to inhibit both cyclooxygenase (COX)-1 and COX-2 enzymes.[5]

■ ADVERSE EFFECTS AND INTERACTIONS

Coneflowers are related to ragweed, daisies, sunflowers, chrysanthemums, and asters. The possibility for cross-allergenicity exists, although reported reactions are rare. Underreporting may be a problem, because of failure to recognize the connection. An Australian study reviewed reports to the Australian Adverse Drug Reaction Committee and found 51 cases implicating an allergic reaction to echinacea. Twenty-six cases were suggestive of immunoglobulin E–mediated hypersensitivity. Two patients suffered anaphylaxis and another had an asthma attack within 10 minutes of first exposure. Milder reactions occurred in other patients on first exposure, suggesting cross-allergenicity with other environmental agents.[6]

The greatest concern relates to the potential for interference with immunosuppressive therapy, exacerbation of autoimmune disorders such as systemic lupus erythematosus, and the unknown effects in immunocompromised individuals such as those with human immunodeficiency virus infection or acquired immunodeficiency syndrome.

Additive effects with nonsteroidal anti-inflammatory agents, including gastrointestinal hemorrhage, have not been reported but are a theoretical possibility as are interactions with low-dose acetylsalicylic acid therapy for thromboembolic disorders.

As is the case with most herbal agents, no long-term animal or human studies have been undertaken; thus, the chronic, long-term toxicity of echinacea is unknown. Only one study has looked at pregnant women taking echinacea, and it found no untoward effects. Effects in nursing mothers or in women trying to conceive are unknown.[1]

■ REFERENCES

1. Echinacea. *Nutrition Action Newsletter* 2002;29:4.
2. Schulten SB, Bulitta M, Ballering-Bruhl B, et al. Efficacy of Echinacea purpurea in patients with a common cold. A placebo-controlled, randomized, double-blind clinical trial. *Arzneimittelforschung* 2001;51:563.
3. Kim LS, Walters RF, Burkholder PM. Immunological activity of larch arabinogalactan and echinacea: A preliminary, randomized, double-blind, placebo-controlled trial. *Altern Med Rev* 2002;7:138.
4. Currier NL, Miller SC. Natural killer cells from aging mice treated with extracts from Echinacea purpurea are quantitatively and functionally rejuvenated. *Exp Gerontol* 2000;35:627.
5. Clifford LJ, Nair MG, Rana J, Dewitt DL. Bioactivity of alkamides isolated from Echinacea purpurea (L.) Moench. *Phytomedicine* 2002;9:249.
6. Mullins RJ, Heddle R. Adverse reactions associated with echinacea: The Australian experience. *Ann Allergy Asthma Immunol* 2002;88:7.

EPHEDRA

■ SOURCE, DESCRIPTION, USES

Known as *ma huang* in Chinese herbal medicine, ephedra comes from a group of evergreen shrubs native to central Asia. These include *Ephedra sinica, E. equisetina,* and *E. intermedia.* The crude herb is prepared from the dried, young stems. Ephedra is used to promote weight loss, to increase energy levels, as a bronchodilator for asthmatics, as a vasoconstrictor for nasal congestion, to enhance athletic performance, and even to induce a euphoric state and improve sexual enjoyment.[1,2]

■ PHARMACOLOGY

Ephedrine constitutes 30% to 90% of the active alkaloids in ephedra, but pseudoephedrine, norephedrine, methylephedrine, and norpseudoephedrine also may be present.[3] Ephedrine and related alkaloids are both α- and β-adrenergic agonists. They may thus increase heart rate and cardiac output, increase peripheral resistance, and, hence, increase blood pressure. Stimulation of β receptors in the lungs accounts for the bronchodilatory action. Action on α receptors of the smooth muscle of the bladder increases resistance to urine flow, especially in men with benign prostatic hypertrophy (BPH) (4).

■ ADVERSE EFFECTS AND INTERACTIONS

These effects result from the adrenergic agonist activity of the ephedra alkaloids. The U.S. Food and Drug Administration has investigated more than 1000 incidents of untoward reactions in which ephedra-containing products were suspected.[1,2] Reported adverse effects include insomnia, nervousness, tremor, headaches, hypertension, seizures, kidney stones, arrhythmia, heart attack, stroke, and death.[1,2,5] At least one case of hepatitis has been associated with ephedra use.[6]

The oral use of ephedra for any purpose is questionable at best. It is absolutely contraindicated in individuals with a history of cardiovascular disease (e.g., heart attack, stroke) and ill advised in persons with risk factors for cardiovascular conditions. Ephedra also is contraindicated in patients with hyperthyroidism, diabetes mellitus, BPH, prostatic cancer, pheochromocytoma, and glaucoma.[2] Because adverse reactions have been reported at the low end of recommended doses, and because the actual content of active agents can never be guaranteed (standardization is generally adjusted to ephedrine content, only), it is not possible to identify a safe dose.

Numerous interactions between ephedra and prescription and over-the-counter medications are possible. Ephedra should not be taken with other stimulants, including caffeine and pseudoephedrine, or other vasoconstrictors (often present in nasal decongestants). Ephedra also has been reported to raise blood glucose levels, to reduce the effectiveness of dexamethasone, and to interfere with the actions of the following medications: digoxin and other cardiac glycosides, antihypertensives, oxytocin, theophylline, and diabetes medications.[7,8] In one case of hypersensitivity myocarditis, ephedra (ma huang) was the suspected causative agent.[9] Given the number and serious nature of the adverse reactions associated with ephedra, this product should be avoided at all costs. See also Appendix VII.

■ REFERENCES

1. Ang-Lee MK, Moss J, Yuan C-S. Herbal medicines and perioperative care. *JAMA* 2001;286:208.
2. Cupp MJ. Herbal remedies: Adverse effects and drug interactions. *Am Fam Physician* 1999;69:1239.
3. Gurley BJ, Gardner FS, Hubbard MA. Content versus label claims in ephedrine-containing dietary supplements. *Am J Health Syst Pharm* 2000;57:963.
4. Hoffman BB, Lefkowitz RJ. Catecholamine and sympathomimetic drugs. In Gilman AG, Rall TW, Neis AS, Taylor P, eds. *Goodman and Gilman's The Pharmacological Basis of Medical Practice.* 8th ed. New York, NY: Pergamon Press; 1990:213.
5. Haller CA, Benowitz NL. Adverse cardiovascular and central nervous system events associated with dietary supplements containing ephedra alkaloids. *N Eng J Med* 2000;343:1833.
6. Haller CA, Dyer JE, Ko R, Olson KR. Making a diagnosis of herbal related toxic hepatitis. *West J Med* 2002;176:39.
7. Angell D. Herb and drug interactions. Ohio State University extension fact sheet. Available at: http://ohioline.osu.edu/hyg-fact/5000/5406.html.
8. Herb/drug interactions. Space Coast Medical Associates website. Available at: http://spacecoastalmedicalassociates.com/herbalsupplements/interactions.htm.
9. Zaacks SM, Klein L, Tan CD, Rodriguez ER, Leikin JB. Hypersensitivity myocarditis associated with ephedra use. *J Toxicol Clin Toxicol* 1999;37:485.

EUCALYPTUS OIL

■ SOURCE, DESCRIPTION, USES

Eucalyptus oil is distilled from the leaves of *Eucalyptus globulus* (family Myrtaceae), one of several species of eucalyptus that are native to Australia, where they are called gum trees, but which have become established in many parts of the world including Africa, India, southern Europe, and even California.[1] About 25 of some 500 species are used to prepare commercial eucalyptus oil. Traditional use includes as a general stimulant, aromatic, antiseptic, disinfectant, and cardiac stimulant.

Current uses for eucalyptus oil include for coughs and colds, in aromatherapy[2] and in soaps and bath products. In addition, it frequently is used as a flavor enhancer in baked goods, dairy products, beverages, and other foodstuffs.[3]

■ PHARMACOLOGY

Synonyms for oil of eucalyptus are eucalyptol, cineole, and cajeputol.[3] Similar to cold air, eucalyptol stimulates cold receptors in the nasal passages and promotes increased secretion of watery mucus to cause a flushing effect without actually having a decongestant action.[2] The active principles in the oil are monoterpene oxides 1,4-cineole and 1,8-cineole. They are present in a wide variety of unrelated botanicals and their essential oils. Many of these botanicals are used as herbal remedies[3] and included in this text (see PEPPERMINT, ROSEMARY, SAGE, and WORMWOOD). The cineoles are metabolized to 2-hydroxylated products by cytochrome P450 3A enzymes in both rat and human hepatic microsomes. The biological activity of these metabolites is not presently known.[4] These agents have additional pharmacological properties associated with the autonomic nervous system. In one study, intravenous administration of 1,8-cineole to normotensive rats caused a reduction in mean arterial pressure and heart rate and caused relaxation of isolated strips of rat aorta[5]. The researchers felt that the hypotensive effect resulted from a direct relaxation of vascular smooth muscle. In another study, skin conductance and heart rate were measured in subjects exposed to a variety of essential oils and components, including 1,8-cineole. Other researchers found that autonomic variations in response to olfactory stimuli were affected by subjective impressions of pleasantness and arousal.[6]

■ ADVERSE EFFECTS AND INTERACTIONS

Eucalyptol was given "generally regarded as safe" (GRAS) status by the Flavor and Extract Manufacturer's Association in 1965 and is approved by the U.S. Food and Drug Administration for use as a food.[3] Deaths have been reported after ingestion of a few milliliters of the essential oil. Larger doses have been associated with severe gastrointestinal distress, central nervous system depression and collapse, generally followed by recovery.[3] Eucalyptol has been shown to cross the placental barrier in rats and reach concentrations sufficient to stimulate hepatic enzymes.[3] There was no evidence of teratogenicity.

At the concentrations that are encountered in foodstuffs, cough remedies or inhalation therapy there does not seem to be any appreciable risk of adverse reactions. The internal use of concentrated essential oil is ill advised and could well be the cause of serious effects.

■ REFERENCES

1. Eucalyptus. In: Grieve M. *A Modern Herbal*. Botanical.com website. Available at: http://www.botanical.com/botanical/mgmh/e/eucaly14.html.

2. Schulz V, Hansel R, Tyler VE. *Rational Phytotherapy: A Physician's Guide to Herbal Medicine.* New York, NY: Springer-Verlag; 1998:146.

3. De Vincenzi M, Silano M, De Vincenzi A, Maialetti F, Scazzocchio B. Constituents of aromatic plants: Eucalytptol. *Fitoterapia* 2002;73:269.

4. Miyazawa M, Shindo M, ShinadaT. Roles of cytochrome P4503A enzymes in the 2-hydroxylation of 1,4-cineole, a monoterpene cyclic ether by rat and human liver microsomes. *Xenobiotica* 2001;31:713.

5. Lahlou S, Figueiredo AF, Magalhaes PJ, Leal-Cardoso JH. Cardiovascular effects of 1,8-cineole, a terpenoid oxide present in many plant essential oils, in normotensive rats. *Can J Physiol Pharmacol* 2002;80:1125.

6. Bensafi M, Rouby C, Farget V, Bertrand B, Vigouroux M, Holley A. Autonomic nervous system responses to odours: The role of pleasantness and arousal. *Chem Senses* 2002;27:703.

EVENING PRIMROSE

■ SOURCE, DESCRIPTION, USES

The common evening primrose (*Oenothera biennis*) is a tall, biennial plant that produces clusters of yellow flowers with four petals in a cross-like form. It grows throughout northeastern North America in open areas and ditches.[1] It also is known as evening star. It has been promoted for a wide variety of conditions, including menstrual discomfort, menopausal symptoms, to promote weight loss, for hypertension, rheumatoid arthritis, multiple sclerosis (MS), cardiovascular disease, and some skin conditions.[2] The seeds contain up to 25% of a fatty oil that is extracted with hexane. The extract contains 60% to 80% linoleic acid and 8% to 14% linolenic acid.[3]

■ PHARMACOLOGY

It is widely held that the benefits, real or purported, of evening primrose oil are the result of the presence of these fatty acids. Linoleic acid is an essential fatty acid. It is converted in the body to γ-linolenic acid (GLA, also known as gamolenic acid), an omega-6 fatty acid synthesized in the body from linoleic acid via an enzyme, Δ-6-desaturase.[3] This is a precursor for dihomo-γ-linolenic acid and arachidonic acid and, hence, for prostaglandin synthesis.[4] The multiplicity of actions of prostaglandins forms the theoretical basis for using evening primrose oil in such conditions as cardiovascular disease (prostacyclin inhibits platelet aggregation)[5] and MS (prostaglandin E_1 may play a role in regulating T-lymphocyte function).[4] Clinical evidence that dietary supplementation with primrose oil is beneficial in these conditions is scanty. Horrobin[4] reviewed three studies involving patients with MS. One reported significant benefits, one some slight benefit and one found no benefit. Another study looked at the effect of evening primrose oil on several tests of platelet function in MS patients and controls and found that the tests were not significantly affected in either group by the oil.[6] More positive results have been reported for patients with certain types of dermatitis. Neurodermatitis, which appears to involve a deficiency in the Δ–6-desaturase enzyme, has been reported to respond well to the oil,[3] and Morse and colleagues[7] conducted a meta-analysis of several studies of atopic eczema and found that both patient and physician evaluations reported significant improvement.

■ ADVERSE EFFECTS AND INTERACTIONS

Research in many areas related to essential fatty acid intake is continuing. Not all the findings are positive. Renaud[8] reviewed data from the Framingham study and other evidence and concluded that these data suggest that a high intake of linoleic acid, the main polyunsaturated acid prescribed for coronary heart disease, could be a significant risk factor for stroke. There is one report[9] of a possible interaction between evening primrose oil and anesthetics, resulting in seizures; however, no details were provided. Oil of primrose has been used in schizophrenia to differentiate it from temporal lobe epilepsy.[10] Three patients became worse when given the oil and responded to carbamazepine. Primrose oil also has been suggested as a treatment for schizophrenia and tardive dyskinesia.[11]

Side effects of evening primrose oil are generally mild and include nausea, gastric upset, and headache.[2,3] There is a theoretical possibility that consuming large amounts could affect the absorption of fat-soluble vitamins (A, K, E). In the case of vitamin K, this could compromise normal hemostasis. Because of the effect of GLA on prostaglandin synthesis, there is a potential for interaction with oral anticoagulants[12] and platelet-inhibiting drugs if large amounts are taken. Similarly, it has been reported that GLA lowers the convulsant threshold, which may necessitate an adjustment in the dosage of anticonvulsant.[13] The use of evening primrose oil in pregnant women is unwise. Consumption of large amounts, or consumption over an extended period, should probably be avoided.

■ REFERENCES

1. Peterson RT, McKenny M. *Northeastern Wildflowers. Roger Tory Peterson Field Guides.* Norwalk, Conn: Easton Press; 1984:156.

2. Coleman E, Taylor M. Evening primrose oil. HCRC FAQ Sheet. Healthcare Reality Check website. Available at: http://www.hcrc.org/faqs/eveprim.html.

3. Schulz V, Hansel R, Tyler VE. *Rational Phytotherapy: A Physician's Guide to Herbal Medicine*. New York, NY: Springer-Verlag; 1998:258.

4. Horrobin DF. Multiple sclerosis: The rational basis for treatment with colchicine and evening primrose oil. *Med Hypotheses* 1979;5:365.

5. Philp RB. *Methods of Testing Proposed Antithrombotic Drugs*. Boca Raton, Fla: CRC Press; 1981:44.

6. Mcgregor L, Smith AD, Sidey M, Belin J, Zilka KJ, McGregor JL. Effects of dietary linoleic acid and gamma linolenic acid on platelets of patients with multiple sclerosis. *Acta Neurol Scand* 1989;80:23.

7. Morse PF, Horrobin DF, Manku MS, et al. Meta-analysis of placebo-controlled studies of the efficacy of Epogam in the treatment of atopic eczema. Relationship between plasma essential fatty acid changes and clinical response. *Br J Dermatol* 1989;121:75.

8. Renaud SC. Diet and stroke. *J Nutr Health Aging* 2001;5:167.

9. Fugh-Berman A, Ernst E. Herb-drug interactions: Review and assessment of report reliability. *Br J Clin Pharmacol* 2001;52:587.

10. Vaddadi KS. The use of gamma-linolenic acid and linoleic acid to differentiate between temporal lobe epilepsy and schizophrenia. *Prostaglandins Med* 1981;6:375.

11. Vaddadi KS. Use of gamma-linolenic acid in the treatment of schizophrenia and tardive dyskinesia. *Prostaglandins Leukot Essent Fatty Acids* 1992;46:67.

12. Heck AM, Dewitt BA, Lukes AL. Potential interactions between alternative therapies and warfarin. *Am J Health Syst Pharm* 2000;57:1221.

13. Miller LG. Herbal medicines: Selected clinical considerations focusing on known or potential drug-herb interactions. *Arch Intern Med* 1998;158:2200.

EVENING STAR

See EVENING PRIMROSE.

FANGCHI

The Chinese herbal remedy fangchi, or hanfangchi, is *Stephania tetranda*. *Aristolochia fangchi* is extremely toxic.

See ARISTOLOCHIA for more details..

FENNEL

■ SOURCE, DESCRIPTION, USES

Fennel or sweet fennel (*Foeniculum vulgare*, family Umbelliferae) has been used for centuries as a flavoring agent and an herbal remedy. It is a perennial herb with yellow flowers and feathery leaves that is native to temperate Europe, the Mediterranean region, and east to India.[1] It also is cultivated in many parts of the world. Both seeds and fresh leaves are used as a flavoring, and the essential oil is often employed as an herbal remedy.[1] It has been used as a carminative, with purgatives to moderate their griping action, and as an ingredient in "gripe water" for treating infant colic.[1] Modern use includes as a carminative, an expectorant, and a tea to treat dyspepsia and diarrhea in infants.[2] It also is used in throat lozenges and cough remedies.

■ PHARMACOLOGY

The main active principle in fennel is anethole, which also is present in anise oil.[3] The two, in fact, have a similar taste and odor. Anethole is believed to stimulate ciliary activity in the bronchi. Anethole is rapidly absorbed from the gastrointestinal tract and rapidly eliminated in urine and, to some extent, in expired air. Some metabolites have been identified, such as 4-methoxyhippuric acid and 4-methoxybenzoic acid.[4] Anethole has been shown to possess anti-inflammatory and anticancer properties in laboratory rodents, possibly by blocking tumor necrosis factor–mediated responses.[4] See ANISE for details.

Extracts of fennel have been shown to possess free radical–scavenging and antioxidant activity,[5] and antimicrobial action.[6] It has been claimed that fennel essential oil (FEO) relieves the pain of dysmenorrhea.[7] FEO was shown to reduce both oxytocin and prostaglandin E_2 (PGE_2)–stimulated contractions of rat uterine strips.[7] It also reduced the frequency of PGE_2-induced contractions, but not those induced by oxytocin.

■ ADVERSE EFFECTS AND INTERACTIONS

Studies in rats found that fennel could interfere with the absorption of ciprofloxacin from the gastrointestinal tract.[8] Distribution and elimination also were affected. Total bioavailability was reduced by almost one half.

FEO contains an oxygenated monoterpene, fenchone, which has convulsant properties.[9] The concentrated oil poses a significant risk to children, in particular.

Cross-allergic reactivity has been demonstrated among anise, coriander, fennel, and cumin (all Umbelliferae) and allergens include Bet v 1- and pro-filin-related ones and higher molecular weight allergens causing type I allergy (see ANISE). See also Appendix V.

Similar to other members of the Umbelliferae family, fennel may contain psoralens and cause phytophotodermatitis, mostly on contact with the skin. This is a photochemical reaction and not a true antibody-based allergic reaction. For more details on phytophotodermatitis, see AMMI; see also Appendix XIII.

In summary, the use of fennel as a flavoring agent or in cough medicines and lozenges does not appear to constitute a significant risk. Children should not be exposed to the high concentrations present in the essential oil, which could pose a convulsant risk, as they might for epileptics, as well. Dermal contact could elicit an allergic dermatitis or phytophotodermatitis. Experimental evidence suggests the possibility of interference with the pharmacokinetic profile of some drugs.

■ REFERENCES

1. Fennel. In: Grieve M. *A Modern Herbal.* Botanical.com website. Available at: http://www.botanical.com/botanical/mgmh/f/fennel01.html.
2. Schulz V, Hansel R, Tyler VE. *Rational Phytotherapy: A Physician's Guide to Herbal Medicine.* New York, NY: Springer-Verlag; 1998:180.
3. Schulz V, Hansel R, Tyler VE. *Rational Phytotherapy: A Physician's Guide to Herbal Medicine.* New York, NY: Springer-Verlag; 1998:159.
4. Chainy GB, Manna SK, Chaturvedi MM, Aggarwal BB. Anethole blocks both early and late cellular responses transduced by tumor necrosis factor: Effect on NF-kappaB, AP-1, JNK, MAPKK and apoptosis. *Oncogene* 2000;19:2943.
5. Parejo I, Viladomat F, Bastida J, et al. Comparison between the radical scavenging activity and antioxidant activity of six distilled and nondistilled Mediterranean herbs and aromatic plants. *J Agric Food Chem* 2002;50:6882.
6. Kwon YS, Choi WG, Kim WJ, et al. Antimicrobial constituents of Foeniculum vulgare. *Arch Pharm Res* 2002;25:154.
7. Ostad SN, Soodi M, Shariffzadeh M, Khorshidi N, Marzban H. The effect of fennel oil on uterine contraction as a model for dysmenorrhea, pharmacology and toxicology study. *J Ethnopharmacol*; 76:299,304.
8. Zhu M, Wong PY, Li RC. Effect of oral administration of fennel (Foeniculum vulgare) on ciprofloxacin absorption and disposition in the rat. *J Pharm Pharmacol* 1999;51:1391.
9. Burkhard PR, Burkhardt K, Haenggeli CA, Landis T. Plant-induced seizures: Reappearance of an old problem. *J Neurol* 1999;246:667.

FENUGREEK

■ SOURCE, DESCRIPTION, USES

From *Trigonella foenum-graecum*, fenugreek (the dried plant) is used primarily as a cooking and pickling spice in the Middle East and India. The plant is a member of the bean family.

■ PHARMACOLOGY

Fenugreek has been shown to possess hypoglycemic activity. Shapiro and Gong[1] reviewed the experimental and clinical evidence. In one crossover, placebo-controlled trial involving 60 patients having type 2 diabetes, use of 12.5 mg of fenugreek powder twice daily in the food for 24 weeks resulted in a 40.6% reduction in the area under the blood glucose curve. Fasting blood glucose levels also were reduced in a small, controlled study with patients with type 1 diabetes.[1] Fenugreek also reduces total cholesterol and triglycerides.[1] Fenugreek contains phytoestrogens. See PHYTOESTROGENS AND PHYTOPROGESTINS.

■ ADVERSE EFFECTS AND INTERACTIONS

Adverse effects are the same as those for phytoestrogens. In addition, fenugreek seeds have been shown to adsorb oral medications because of the high soluble fiber content of the crushed seeds. Oral medications should not be taken within 2 hours of consuming fenugreek. Significant hypoglycemia can occur if high doses are taken without titration. If other antidiabetic medications are being used, fenugreek could promote a hypoglycemic crisis. See also Appendices IV and X.

■ REFERENCE

1. Shapiro K, Gong WC. Natural products used in diabetes. *J Am Pharmaceut Assoc* 2002;42:217.

FEVERFEW

■ SOURCE, DESCRIPTION, USES

Feverfew (*Chrysanthemum parthenium, Pyrethrum parthenium, Tanacetum parthenium*) is a member of the Compositae family. It is described as a bushy plant with broad, toothed leaves and a pungent aromatic odor.[1] It is a roadside escapee from gardens and has numerous, small, daisy-like white or yellow flowers.[1,2] The name is thought to be a corruption of febrifuge, one of its early uses. Synonyms include featherfew, fetherfoil, flirtwort, and bachelor's button.[2] Teas and fluid extracts of the leaves and stems are used. Current uses are primarily for arthritic pain and migraine headache.[3,4] Feverfew also may be used for menstrual discomfort.[5]

■ PHARMACOLOGY

Feverfew may inhibit prostaglandin synthesis, inhibit release of histamine from mast cells, inhibit platelet aggregation, and inhibit vascular smooth muscle contractility.[5] Its effect on prostaglandin synthesis does not involve inhibition of cyclooxygenase enzyme. Clinical studies suggest moderate efficacy in treating migraine but perhaps less for arthritic pain.[4,5] Parthenolide (parthenocide) has been suggested as the active ingredient, but content in preparations may vary widely[4] and some clinical studies do not indicate that this component is the active agent.[6]

■ ADVERSE EFFECTS AND INTERACTIONS

Feverfew may be cross-allergenic with other Compositae (Asteraceae), including chamomile, yarrow, and ragweed.[4] Rapid withdrawal has been associated with a syndrome that involves nervousness, tension headaches, insomnia, stiffness, joint pain, and fatigue.[7] Ulcers and inflammation of the mouth have been reported infrequently.[5] Contact dermatitis also has been reported.[3] Feverfew is known to cause abortion in cattle and, therefore, is contraindicated in pregnancy.[5] Effects of long-term consumption are not known, but in view of the withdrawal syndrome such a practice is unwise.

Because of the inhibitory effect of feverfew on PG synthesis, there is an increased risk of bleeding when it is given concomitantly with warfarin and other oral anticoagulants or platelet-inhibiting drugs (e.g., acetylsalicylic acid, clopidogrel [Plavix]). Nonsteroidal anti-inflammatory drugs and feverfew may be mutually antagonistic.[3,4] Tannin-containing herbs such as feverfew may interfere with iron absorption.[8] This may not be a serious problem clinically but should be considered in anemic patients. It is advisable to avoid taking iron and the herbal preparation together.

See also Appendices I and IX.

■ REFERENCES

1. Peterson RT, McKenny M. *Northeastern Wildflowers. Roger Tory Peterson Field Guides.* Norwalk, Conn: Easton Press; 1984:92.
2. Feverfew. In: Grieve M. *A Modern Herbal.* Botanical.com website. Available at: http://www.botanical.com/botanical/mgmh/f/feverf10.html.
3. Ko R. Adverse reactions to watch for in patients using herbal remedies. *West J Med* 1999;171:181.
4. Miller LG. Herbal medicines; selected clinical considerations focusing on known or potential drug-herb interactions. *Arch Intern Med* 1998;158;2200.
5. Rodblatt MD. Cranberry, feverfew, horse chestnut, and kava. *West J Med* 1999;171:196.
6. Goldman P. Herbal medicines today and the roots of modern pharmacology. *Ann Intern Med* 2001;135:594.
7. Pribitkin E deA, Boger G. Herbal therapy: What every facial plastic surgeon must know. *Arch Facial Plast Surg* 2001;3:127.
8. Miller LG. Herbal medicinals: Selected clinical considerations focusing on known or potential herb-drug interactions. *Arch Intern Med* 1998;158:2200.

FEVERWORT

See BONESET.

FRENCH MARITIME PINE BARK EXTRACT

■ SOURCE, DESCRIPTION, USES

Pycnogenol and PYC are registered trade names for the standardized extract of the bark of the French maritime pine (*Pinus maritima* or *P. pinaster*),[1,2] henceforth referred to as PBE (pine bark extract). PBE is used for a wide variety of conditions, including chronic venous insufficiency (CVI), retinal microhemorrhages, and premenstrual symptoms, among others.[1,2]

■ PHARMACOLOGY

PBE is a mixture of bioflavonoids that includes procyanidins and phenolic acids.[2] Procyanidins are bipolymers consisting of units of catechin or epicatechin. These are potent antioxidants, free radical scavengers, and inhibitors of lipid peroxidation.[1] As such, they preserve capillary integrity and are antiatherosclerotic and anti-inflammatory.

PBE has been shown to inhibit the increase in platelet aggregation induced by smoking.[3] In a study of CVI, PBE was shown to decrease lower limb circumference, improve subjective symptoms (leg pain, cramps, feeling of heaviness), and significantly decrease blood cholesterol and low-density lipoprotein values.[4] Rohdewald[2] reviewed other studies with similar findings. Inhibition of gene expression of proinflammatory cytokines has been demonstrated and may account for the anti-inflammatory activity of PBE.[5]

Because of anecdotal reports of improved concentration in adults with attention-deficit/hyperactivity disorder (ADHD), a placebo-controlled study was conducted with PBE and methylphenidate in adults with ADHD.[6] According to self-reported rating scales, all three groups showed improvement after 3 weeks, but there were no significant differences among the groups.

■ ADVERSE EFFECTS AND INTERACTIONS

According to Rohdewald the incidence of untoward side effects with PBE is 1.5%, and these consist mainly of gastrointestinal disturbances, dizziness, nausea, and headache.[2] Because of the platelet-inhibiting properties of PBE, there is a theoretical possibility of an increased risk of bruising or bleeding if it is given in conjunction with oral anticoagulants and platelet-inhibiting drugs. Interactions with anti-inflammatory drugs (e.g., nonsteroidal anti-inflammatory drugs) are undocumented but theoretically possible. Effects of long-term administration and use during pregnancy are unknown. See also Appendix VII.

■ REFERENCES

1. Schulz V, Hansel R, Tyler VE. *Rational Phytotherapy: A Physician's Guide to Herbal Medicine.* New York, NY: Springer-Verlag; 1998:283.
2. Rohdewald P. A review of the French maritime pine bark extract (Pycnogenol®), a herbal medication with a diverse clinical pharmacology. *Int J Clin Pharmacol Ther* 2002;40:158.
3. Putter M, Grotemeyer KH, Wurthwein G, et al. Inhibition of smoking-induced platelet aggregation by aspirin and pycnogenol. *Thromb Res* 1999;95:155.

4. Koch R. Comparative study of Venostatin and Pycnogenol in chronic venous insufficiency. *Phytother Res* 2002;16(suppl 1):S1.

5. Cho KJ, Yun CH, Packer L, Chung AS. Inhibition mechanisms of bioflavonoids extracted from the bark of Pinus maritima on the expression of proinflammatory cytokines. *Ann N Y Acad Sci* 2001;928:141.

6. Tenenbaum S, Paull J, Sparrow EP, Dodd DK, Green L. An experimental comparison of pycnogenol and methylphenidate in adults with attention deficit/hyperactivity disorder (ADHD). *J Atten Disord* 2002;6:49.

FRANKINCENSE (INDIAN)

See SALAI GUGGAL.

GARLIC

■ SOURCE, DESCRIPTION, USES

Garlic, from the perennial *Allium sativum*, is related to the onion and both are of the lily family (Liliaceae). Garlic was known as a vegetable and herb to the ancient Egyptians, and the use of garlic was documented in Sanskrit documents dating back 5000 years. Louis Pasteur noted its antibiotic properties.[2] Garlic is used as a cholesterol-lowering agent.

■ PHARMACOLOGY

Garlic is believed to inhibit cholesterol biosynthesis at several enzymatic steps. It has been shown to lower the levels of free and esterified cholesterol in cultured human cells and to decrease fatty streak development in rabbits. Clinical studies have confirmed a moderate cholesterol-lowering effect in patients with hypercholesterolemia.[1,2] Low-density lipoproteins were lowered less than 25%.[3] Garlic also has been shown to lower blood pressure,[2] but the effect seems to be marginal in humans.[2] These effects have been attributed to sulfur-containing allicin and related compounds. Commercial preparations are standardized to these compounds (allicin and alliin).[2] Inhibition of platelet aggregation is attributed to ajoene, and the effect is irreversible. Dried garlic preparations seem to be more effective than the oil.[4] Some moderate inhibition of tumor promotion also has been shown for garlic (and onion) oil.[5] Antibacterial, antiviral, and antifungal activity of allicin has been shown experimentally.

■ ADVERSE EFFECTS AND INTERACTIONS

The main medical concern with garlic is its potential to increase the risk of bleeding by potentiating oral anticoagulants and platelet-inhibiting agents. Although this does not seem to be a common problem, one case of an epidural hematoma in an elderly man was attributed to heavy use of garlic, and two cases of prolonged coagulation times (international normalized ratio) were reported in patients taking warfarin and garlic.[6]

A more recent concern stems from studies in human volunteers that demonstrated that garlic reduces by half the area under the curve of a protease inhibitor antiviral agent, saquinavir (Fortovase), commonly used to treat acquired immunodeficiency syndrome (AIDS) and human immunodeficiency virus infection.[7] Thus, garlic has significant potential to interfere with AIDS therapy. Patients taking anticoagulants, platelet-inhibiting drugs, anticholesterolemic drugs, antiviral protease inhibitors, and antihypertensives are not good candidates for garlic supplementation.

Based on some experimental evidence that garlic has antidiabetic properties,[8] not confirmed in human studies,[9] concomitant use of garlic and antidiabetic medication should be monitored closely, if not discouraged. Little is known about the long-term effects of garlic supplementation.

Some individuals may be allergic to garlic.[10] See also Appendix VII.

■ REFERENCES

1. Hadley SK, Petry JJ. Medicinal herbs: A primer for primary care. *Hosp Pract* 1999;34:105.
2. Ang-Lee MK, Moss J, Yuan C-S. Herbal medicines and perioperative care. *JAMA* 2001;286:208.
3. Caron MF, White CM. Evaluation of the antihyperlipidemic properties of dietary supplements. *Pharmacotherapy* 2001;21:481.
4. Fugh-Berman A. Herbs and dietary supplements in the prevention and treatment of cardiovascular disease. *Prev Cardiol* 2000;3:24.
5. Belman S. Onion and garlic oils inhibit tumor promotion. *Carcinogenesis* 1983;4:1063.
6. Izzo AA, Ernst E. Interactions between herbal medicines and prescribed drugs. *Drugs* 2001;61:2163.
7. Piscitelli SC, Burstein AH, Welden N, Gallicano KD, Falloon J. The effect of garlic supplement on the pharmacokinetics of saquinavir. *Clin Infect Dis* 2002;34:234.
8. Swanston-Flatt SK, Day C, Bailey CJ, Flatt PR. Traditional plant treatments for diabetes. Studies in normal and streptozotocin diabetic mice. *Diabetologia* 1990;33:462.

9. Ackermann RT, Mulrow CD, Rameriz G, Gardner CD, Morbidoni L, Lawrence VA. Garlic shows promise for improving some cardiovascular risk factors. *Arch Intern Med* 2001;161:813.

10. Papageorgiou C, Corbet JP, Menezes-Brandao F, Peceguiero M, Benezra C. Allergic contact dermatitis to garlic (Allium sativum L.). Identification of the allergens: The role of mono-, di-, and trisulfides present in garlic. A comparative study in man and animal (guinea-pig). *Arch Dermatol Res* 1983;275:229.

GERMANDER

■ SOURCE, DESCRIPTION, USES

Germander is the name applied to a number of species of *Teucrium*, which are low, shrubby plants with felt-like leaves, members of the Labiatae family.[1] The species most commonly associated with herbal use is *T. chamaedrys,* but *T. polium* (golden germander) may also be used. *T. chamaedrys* is a native of Europe. *T. canadense*, also known as wood sage, is the North American native species of germander.[1] The name germander is thought to be a corruption of the Latin *chamaedrys,* meaning "dwarf oak" (the leaves were thought to bear some resemblance to those of oaks). The leaves and other parts of the above-ground plant are dried and used in capsules or as a tea or infusion. Traditionally, germander was recommended as a tonic, an appetizer, a choleretic, for snakebite, and for a number of vaguely defined conditions. Current use is largely for obesity and weight loss.[2]

■ PHARMACOLOGY

Germander contains numerous potentially active principles, but which, if any, are responsible for weight loss is unclear. Saponins, glycosides, flavonoids, and furanoterpenoids have been identified.[3]

Little attention was paid to germander until it was claimed to promote weight loss. This was followed by a marked increase in usage in France, followed by an outbreak, bordering on an epidemic, of hepatotoxicity. After 27 cases with 1 death from acute, nonviral hepatitis, the French Ministry of Health banned the sale of products containing germander on May 12, 1992.[3]

■ ADVERSE EFFECTS AND INTERACTIONS

Considerably more is known about the toxicology of germander. Use of the herb has been associated with cytolytic hepatitis, fulminant hepatitis, chronic hepatitis, and cirrhosis. The onset of hepatitis can be delayed for several weeks and does not appear to be dose related.

Attention has focused on one of the furanoterpenoids, teucrin A, as the hepatotoxic ingredient. It has been shown to bind covalently to hepatocytes, causing membrane blebbing and cell death. It also leads to depletion of glutathione through induction of cytochrome P450 3A (CYP 3A). Inhibition of CYP 3A reduced toxicity and glutathione depletion, whereas induction of CYP 3A had the opposite effect.[3] A teucrin A metabolite formed by CYP 3A4 binds and inhibits human epoxide hydrolase, which would further contribute to hepatotoxicity.[4]

One might have expected the use of germander to decline after it was banned in France, but in 1996 two cases were reported in Canada. Both patients were women. One, 55 years of age, had been taking the herb for months, possibly years, for hypercholesterolemia. The other, 45, had been taking it for weight loss for 6 months. Both were jaundiced, with abnormal liver function tests, and a liver biopsy of the first patient revealed necrosis and other pathology. Both patients recovered over a period of 2 months after discontinuing the herb.[5]

Although no drug interactions have been reported, disturbed liver function has obvious implications for drug biotransformations. Germander should not be taken for any reason. In the past it has been mislabeled as skullcap,[6] and there is no guarantee that it will not cause problems in the future.

■ REFERENCES

1. Peterson RT, McKenny M. *Northeastern Wildflowers: Roger Tory Peterson Field Guides.* Norwalk, Conn: Easton Press; 1984:278.

2. Larrey D, Vial T, Pauwels A, et al. Hepatitis after germander (Teucrium chamaedrys) administration: Another instance of herbal medicine toxicity. *Ann Intern Med* 1992;117:129.

3. Lekehal M, Pessayre D, Lereau JM, Moulis C, Fouraste I, Fau D. Hepatotoxicity of the herbal medicine germander: Metabolic activation of its furano diterpenoids by cytochrome P450 3A depletes cytoskeleton-associated protein thiols and forms plasma membrane blebs in rat hepatocytes. *Hepatology* 1996;24:212.

4. Loeper J, De Berardinis V, Moulis C, Beaune P, Pessayre D, Pompton D. Human epoxide hydrolase is the target of germander autoantibodies on the surface of human hepatocytes: Enzymatic implications. *Adv Exp Med Biol* 2001;500:121.

5. Laliberte L, Villeneuve JP. Hepatitis after the use of germander, a herbal remedy. *Can Med Assoc J* 1996;154:1689.

6. Huxtable RA. The myth of beneficent nature: The risks of herbal preparations. *Ann Intern Med* 1992;117:165.

GINKGO BILOBA

■ SOURCE, DESCRIPTION, USES

Leaves from the tree of the same name (*Ginkgo biloba*) have been used for 4000 years to improve mentation and respiratory function. This tree is the only surviving member of an ancient family, the Ginkoaceae. It is claimed to improve cerebral and peripheral blood flow and to combat geriatric depression when given as the standardized extract EGb 761.

■ PHARMACOLOGY

The leaves contain flavone glycosides (quercetin, kaempherol, isohamnetin) that have antioxidant and platelet aggregation-inhibiting properties. Terpene lactones (ginkolides A, B, C and bilobalide) may have neuroprotective properties through several mechanisms, including improved blood flow and inhibition of platelet-activating factor. Animal and clinical studies, including double-blind trials, support the claims for ginkgo's usefulness in peripheral vascular disease and geriatric depression.[1,2]

Recently, a number of placebo-controlled clinical studies have shown benefit of a standardized extract of ginkgo leaf in patients with Alzheimer's disease. There was a significant improvement in cognitive function, memory, and social functioning compared with placebo. These beneficial effects were attributed to antioxidant components of ginkgo.[3–5] A recent study, however, casts doubt on ginkgo's ability to improve memory. In a controlled, double-blind study, healthy men and women over 60 years of age received 40 mg of an over-the-counter ginkgo preparation three times daily for 6 weeks. There was no difference in their performance on objective memory tests compared with the control group.[6] The study did not address the effects of longer-term administration.

■ ADVERSE EFFECTS AND INTERACTIONS

Reported adverse reactions and interactions relate to the platelet-inhibiting properties of ginkgo and involve bleeding episodes and interactions with anticoagulants and drugs that inhibit platelet function. Spontaneous bleeding has been reported in patients taking aspirin, warfarin, and acetaminophen with caffeine-ergotamine, as well as with ginkgo alone.[7,8] This herbal should not be taken with oral anticoagulants, preparations containing acetylsalicylic acid, or other platelet-inhibiting drugs such as ticlopidine (Ticlid), clopidogrel (Plavix), and dipyridamole (Persantine). Caution also should be used when ginkgo is taken in conjunction with other agents that could compromise hemostasis, such as vitamin E or oils containing omega 3 fatty acids. It also is recommended that patients be taken off ginkgo at least 36 hours before surgery.[8] Convulsions have been reported in children following consumption of large numbers of seeds.[9,10] There is at least one report of a 36-year-old woman with no past personal or family history of epilepsy, who developed frequent vomiting and convulsions after consuming 70 to 80 ginkgo seeds 4 hours earlier as an aid to memory.[11] Ginkgo seeds (nuts) appear to be considerably more toxic than the extract of the leaves, but patients with controlled, preexisting epilepsy developed recurrent seizures within 2 weeks of beginning to take commercial extract. The seizures stopped when the herb was discontinued.[12]

Ginkgo biloba contains potent pharmacological agents that may well play a useful part in the treatment of some forms of dementia[13] and peripheral vascular disorders. As with all potent drugs, there may serious side effects and drug interactions. Long-term effects and effects in pregnant women and on conception are unknown.

■ REFERENCES

1. Hadley SK, Petry JJ. Medicinal herbs: A primer for primary care. *Hosp Pract* 1999;34:105.

2. Curtis-Prior P, Vere D, Fray P. Therapeutic value of *Ginkgo biloba* in reducing symptoms of decline in mental function. *J Pharm Pharmacol* 1999;51:535.

3. Kanowski S, Herrmann WM, Stephan K, Wierich W, Horr R. Proof of efficacy of the ginkgo biloba special extract EGb 761 in outpatients suffering from mild to moderate primary degenerative dementia of the Alzheimer type or multi-infarct dementia. *Phytomedicine* 1997;4:3.

4. Le Bars PL, Katz MM, Berman N, Itil TM, Freedman AM, Schatzberg AF. A placebo-controlled, double-blind, randomized trial of an extract of ginkgo biloba for dementia. *JAMA* 1997;278:1327.

5. Brautigam MRH, Blommant FA, Verleye G, et al. Treatment of age-related memory complaints using Ginkgo biloba extract: A randomized double blind placebo-controlled clinical study. *Phytomedicine* 1998;5: 425.

6. Solomon PR, Adams F, Silver A, Zimmer J, DeVeaux R. Ginkgo for memory enhancement: A randomized controlled trial. *JAMA* 2002;288:835.

7. Cupp MJ. Herbal remedies: Adverse effects and drug interactions. *Am Fam Physician* 1999;69:1239.

8. Ang-Lee MK, Moss J, Yuan C-S. Herbal medicines and perioperative care. *JAMA* 2001;286:208.

9. Ernst E. The risk-benefit profile of commonly used herbal therapies: Ginkgo, St. John's wort, ginseng, echinacea, saw palmetto and kava. *Ann Intern Med* 2002;136:42.

10. Kajiyama Y, Fujii K, Takeuchi H, Manabe Y. Ginkgo seed poisoning. *Pediatrics* 2002;109:325.

11. Miwa H, Iijima M, Tanaka S, Mizuno Y. Generalized convulsions after consuming a large amount of ginkgo nuts. *Epilepsia* 2001;42:280.

12. Granger AS. Ginkgo biloba precipitating epileptic seizures. *Age Aging* 2001;30:523.

13. Beaubrun G, Gray GE. A review of herbal medicines for psychiatric disorders. *Psychiatr Serv* 2000;51:1130.

GINGER

■ SOURCE, DESCRIPTION, USES

Common ginger, used as a cooking spice, is the root of *Zingiberis rhizoma* (*Zingiber officinale*). It has been used for centuries for dyspepsia, nausea and vomiting, motion sickness, and as an aid to digestion (a carminative). More recently, it has been recommended for thrombosis, for relief of pain of musculoskeletal disorders, and rheumatism.[1] It is grown commercially in many locales.

■ PHARMACOLOGY

Several clinical trials indicate that ginger is as effective as, or more effective than, many prescription and over-the-counter drugs for controlling motion sickness, postoperative nausea and vomiting, and hyperemesis gravidarum (morning sickness).[2] Its mechanism of action does not appear to be central; rather, it appears to act locally in the stomach.[2] Ginger also has been found to inhibit thromboxane synthetase and to prolong bleeding time.[2,3] In studies on rats, a standardized extract of ginger, EV.EXT 33, did not significantly affect blood glucose, coagulation parameters, or warfarin-induced changes; it neither decreased systolic blood pressure nor increased heart rate.[4]

■ ADVERSE EFFECTS AND INTERACTIONS

The finding that ginger is positive in the *E. coli* bacteria test for mutagenesis raises concerns about its use in pregnant women.[2] More information is required before such use can be recommended without reservation. Because it is a potent inhibitor of thromboxane synthetase, there is a possibility that ginger could increase the risk of bleeding or bruising if given concomitantly with anticoagulants or platelet-inhibiting drugs. Studies of one component of ginger, 6-shogaol, in anesthetized rats have shown pressor activity.[5] The significance of this finding for patients with hypertension is not known at present. See also Appendices VII and VIII.

■ REFERENCES

1. Ko R. Adverse reactions to watch for in patients taking herbal remedies. *West J Med* 1999;171:181.
2. Miller L. Herbal medicines: Selected clinical considerations focusing on known or potential drug-herb interactions. *Arch Intern Med* 1998;158:2211.
3. Probitkin E deA, Boger G. Herbal therapy: What every facial plastic surgeon must know. *Arch Facial Plast Surg* 2001;3:127.
4. Weidner MS, Sigwart K. The safety of ginger extract in the rat. *J Ethnopharmacol* 2000;73:513.
5. Suekawa M, Aburada M, Hosoya E. Pharmacological studies on ginger. II. Pressor action of (6)-shogaol in anesthetized rats, or hindquarters, tail and mesenteric vascular beds of rats. *J Pharmacobiodyn* 1986;9:842.

GINSENG

■ SOURCE, DESCRIPTION, USES

This herb has been a staple in Chinese medicine for over 2000 years, but the name *ginseng* is applied to herbs prepared from the root of several different species. Asian ginseng is from *Panax ginseng,* Siberian (Russian) ginseng comes from *Eleutherococcus senticosus,* American ginseng from *P. quinquefolius,* and Japanese ginseng from *P. japonicus.*[1] The roots frequently take a bifurcated form resembling the human body, and this is thought to have promoted belief in their mystical properties. Asian and American ginsengs are most commonly used in North America.[2] This herb has been taken to improve vitality, immune function, cognitive and physical performance, and sexual function. It has been described as an "adaptogen"[2] because it is reputed to restore homeostasis.

■ PHARMACOLOGY

A review of randomized clinical trials failed to reveal convincing evidence of efficacy for the previously mentioned indications.[1,3] Nonetheless, ginseng contains numerous pharmacologically complex active agents called ginsenosides. Attele and colleagues[4] reviewed the pharmacology of ginseng. More than 20 ginsenosides have been isolated, and new ones are being found in *P. quinquefolius* and *P. japonicus*. Many ginsenosides bear structural similarity to the steroid hormones. Both inhibitory and excitatory effects on the central nervous system have been reported, as has protection of neurons from ischemic damage and, possibly, enhancement of learning. The uptake of neurotransmitters into rat brain synaptosomes has been reported. There also is experimental evidence for antineoplastic and immunomodulatory effects. The steroid nature of the ginsenosides imparts high lipid solubility and the ability to pass through cell membranes, possibly interacting with cytosolic steroid receptors and nuclear receptors, including those for glucocorticoids with downstream genomic consequences. Interactions with cell membrane components also have been cited as a possible cause for some of ginseng's pharmacological effects.[5] Recent clinical studies[6] showed that American ginseng attenuated postprandial hyperglycemia in both ten normal and nine diabetic (type 2) subjects. Subjects were given 3 g of ginseng in capsule form or matching placebo before a glucose challenge. Ginseng also has been reported to exert cardioprotective effects through the release of nitric oxide.[7,8] Given that ginseng has more than two dozen active components with multiple sites of action and sometimes opposing actions, its pharmacology is too complex to review in detail here, and its in vivo effects are likely too variable and unpredictable to be useful. The herb may, however, provide a source of new drugs in the future.

■ ADVERSE EFFECTS AND INTERACTIONS

Although the frequency of interactions and adverse effects has been reported as low,[1] their nature is varied as one might expect, and some are potentially serious. Reported adverse effects include insomnia, diarrhea, vaginal bleeding, mastalgia and headache, schizophrenia, and Stevens-Johnson syndrome.[1] Inhibition of platelet aggregation and interference with the coagulation cascade have been reported.[2] The antiplatelet effect has been attributed to the ginsenoside panaxynol, and it may, like that of aspirin, be irreversible.[2] Use in nondiabetic individuals may prevent postprandial glycemia that could be a hazard for patients undergoing surgery.[2,6]

There is one widely quoted case report of a man with a mechanical heart valve who was taking warfarin (and several other medications) and whose clotting tests fell to subtherapeutic levels after self-medicating with ginseng.[9,10] Based on the multiplicity of active agents, the potential for interactions with many drugs has been noted.[11] These include interference with antipsychotic drugs by affecting neurotransmitter transport; interference with monoamine oxidase inhibitors; increasing the stimulant effect of caffeine, with possible hypertension as a result; interference with steroidal hormone therapy; and interference with hypoglycemic medication. There is one report of Siberian ginseng elevating serum digoxin levels, although no toxic effects were noted. The mechanism for the elevation was not identified.[12]

It should be evident that the use of ginseng in the presence of prescription medications is unwise, and that its use should be discontinued some days before surgery.[2]

■ REFERENCES

1. Ernst E. The risk-benefit profile of commonly used herbal therapies: Ginkgo, St. John's wort, ginseng, echinacea, saw palmetto and kava. *Ann Intern Med* 2002;136:42.

2. Ang-Lee MK, Moss J, Yuan C-S. Herbal medicines and perioperative care. *JAMA* 2001;286:208.

3. Vogler BK, Pittler MH, Ernst E. The efficacy of ginseng: A systematic review of randomized clinical trials. *Eur J Clin Pharmacol* 1999;55:567.

4. Attele AS, Wu JA, Yuan C-S. Ginseng pharmacology: Multiple constituents and multiple actions. *Biochem Pharmacol* 1999;58:1685.

5. Coon JT, Ernst E. Panax ginseng: A systematic review of adverse effects and drug interactions. *Drug Saf* 2002;25:323.

6. Vuksan V, Sievenpiper JL, Koo VY, et al. American ginseng (*Panax quinquefolius L.*) reduces postprandial glycemia in nondiabetic subjects and subjects with type 2 diabetes mellitus. *Arch Intern Med* 2000;160:1009.

7. Chen X. Cardiovascular protection by ginsenosides and their nitric oxide releasing action. *Clin Exp Pharmacol Physiol* 1996;23:738.

8. Gillis CN. *Panax ginseng* pharmacology: A nitric oxide link? *Biochem Pharmacol* 1998;54:1.

9. Janetzky K, Morreale AP. Probable interaction between warfarin and ginseng. *Am J Health Syst Pharm* 1997;54:692.

10. Cupp MJ. Herbal remedies: Adverse effects and drug interactions. *Am Fam Physician* 1999;69:1239.

11. Angell D. Herb and drug interactions. Ohio State University extension fact sheet. Available at: http://ohioline.osu.edu/hygfact/5000/5406.html.

12. McRae S. Elevated serum digoxin levels in a patient taking digoxin and Siberian ginseng. *Can Med Assoc J* 1996;155:293.

GLUCOSAMINE

■ SOURCE, DESCRIPTION, USES

Glucosamine is an amino-monosaccharide that is a normal component of cartilage. Because of this, it was theorized that glucosamine supplementation might assist in the rebuilding of cartilage in people with osteoarthritis. Glucosamine is synthesized or extracted from the chitin of seashells and is usually provided as the sulfate. It has become one of the most popular alternative remedies for osteoarthritis on the market.

■ PHARMACOLOGY

Chemically, glucosamine is 2-amino-2-deoxyglucose. It has a molecular weight of 179 and is well absorbed from the gastrointestinal tract and selectively taken up by cartilage and other joint tissues to form glycosaminoglycans, the main structural element of cartilage.[1,2] Osteoarthritis affects 10% of all persons over age 65. Chondrocytes, the cells involved in cartilage synthesis and repair, disappear with age, so that cartilage lost through wear and tear is not replaced. Exposed joint bone then becomes damaged, causing pain. Bony protrusions called osteophytes form, and the joint space becomes narrower. So-called chondroprotective agents, such as glucosamine sulfate (GAS) and chondroitin sulfate, are thought to accelerate the repair process and retard cartilage degeneration.[1]

There is evidence from laboratory studies to support this hypothesis. Studies with human and animal chondrocytes have shown that GAS can promote the synthesis of glycosaminoglycan and retard its breakdown.[2] The proposed mechanism is inhibition of proinflammatory cytokines such as interleukin-1β and other pain and inflammation mediators such as prostaglandin E_2.[2] GAS has been shown to inhibit inducible nitric oxide synthase and, thus, the formation of nitrite, another proinflammatory mediator.[3] Neutrophils have been implicated as effector cells in the inflammatory process. In response to local chemical stimuli, they migrate to the inflamed site and release superoxide anion. Although this has an antibacterial effect, it may also contribute to the breakdown of cartilage.[4] Studies with human neutrophils have shown that GAS inhibited the formation of superoxide anion generated in response to experimental stimuli and inhibited phagocytosis and granule lysozyme release.[4] The GAS analog N-acetyl-glucosamine did not possess these anti-inflammatory effects on neutrophils.

The debate over the clinical efficacy of GAS has been ongoing for some years. Numerous reviews of clinical trials and editorials on the subject have been written.[1–2,5–7] By 2001, some 15 clinical trials had been conducted on the use of GAS for treating osteoarthritis, mostly involving the knee. The great majority of these demonstrated at least modest efficacy in the form of reduced pain and improved flexibility but were also criticized for a number of flaws, best summarized by an editorial in the *Medical Journal of Australia*.[7] These included:

- Lack of standardized selection criteria
- Small sample size
- Short duration of follow-up
- Inadequate radiographic evidence
- Heterogeneous patient population
- Lack of standardized patient outcome measures such as Western Ontario and McMaster Universities (WOMAC) or Lequesne indices

In addition, criticism has been frequently leveled at some studies for being funded by a manufacturer of GAS. Given that many clinical trials units in academic hospitals could not function without at least some funding from the pharmaceutical industry, this criticism seems mildly sanctimonious.

Two clinical studies of note were published in 2002, one negative[8] and one positive.[9] A comparison of them is useful. Both were randomized, placebo-controlled, double-blind studies, involving patients with osteoarthritis (OA) of at least one knee. Both studies were funded by proprietary companies (the negative one by Health Perceptions UK, and the positive one by Rottapharm). Both used accepted evaluation techniques such as WOMAC and visual analog scale (negative study) or WOMAC and Lequesne index (positive study), and both employed a daily dose of 1500 mg GAS. They differed in some substantial ways, as outlined in the accompanying table.

The negative study found that GAS was no better than placebo in modifying symptoms in patients with a wide range of pain severity. Conversely, the positive study found that GAS retarded the progression of OA of the knee, including largely preventing further joint narrowing, as well as improving symptoms by 20% to 25%. The placebo produced only a modest improvement.

The results of these studies appear to confirm the impressions from previous studies that GAS is of significant benefit in the treatment of mild to moderate OA but not likely of much help in more severe forms. Currently a National Institutes of Health–sponsored multicenter, double-blind, placebo-controlled trial of condroitin sulfate and GAS, alone and in combination, is under way. The results are expected in 2004.[4] It is hoped they will provide a definitive answer regarding the efficacy of these compounds. Trials also have been conducted with intramuscular and intra-articular injections with generally positive results.[9] This route of administration, however, is outside the realm of herbal remedies and therefore of this text.

■ ADVERSE EFFECTS AND INTERACTIONS

In the positive study,[8] 64% of patients receiving placebo and 66% of those given GAS reported at least one side effect, mostly related to gastrointestinal symptoms. There were no significant differences between the groups. Similar results were reported for the negative study.[7]

There are some reports of adverse effects involving patients taking GAS, usually in combination with chondroitin sulfate. In one report,[10] one patient had photosensitization that was reproducible on rechallenge, three had moderate systolic hypertension, there were four episodes of 1+ to 2+ proteinuria, and three patients had elevated creatine phosphokinase levels. In all cases, the patients were taking the combination of GAS and chondroitin sulfate so it was not possible to assign responsibility to a particular agent. In another report, a 79-year-old woman who began taking GAS developed evidence of renal dysfunction 4 months later in the form of elevated blood urea nitrogen and creatinine levels that returned slowly to nor-

COMPARISON OF ONE NEGATIVE AND ONE POSITIVE STUDY OF GLUCOSAMINE SULFATE (1500 MG/DAY)

PARAMETER	NEGATIVE STUDY[8]	POSITIVE STUDY[9]
Subjects completing study	78	202
Dosage regimen	3 divided doses	Single dose
Duration of study	24 wk	3 yr
Age range of subjects	> 40 yr	45–70 yr
Exclusion criteria	Protheses in both knees Received arthroscopic washout within 3 mo	Lequesne index > 12 Presence of rheumatic disease other than OA, including trauma and inflammation
	Previous use of GAS	Body mass index > 27 Clinically significant alterations in hematology, renal, hepatic, or metabolic function, including diabetes mellitus
	Any intra-articular injection to knee	Systemic or intra-articular corticosteroid therapy in previous 3 mo

GAS, glucosamine sulfate; OA, osteoarthritis.

mal after discontinuing GAS.[11] This patient was also taking low doses of methylprednisolone and cyclosporine for myasthenia gravis. It was, therefore, not possible to determine whether the renal dysfunction was the result of a drug interaction, a side effect of GAS, or a coincidence.

In conclusion, it would appear the GAS could offer a safer alternative to NSAIDs for the treatment of mild to moderate OA.

■ REFERENCES

1. Sutton L, Rapport L, Lockwood B. Glucosamine: Con or cure? *Nutrition* 2002;18:534.
2. Hauselmann HJ. Nutripharmaceuticals for arthritis. *Best Pract Res Clin Rheum* 2001;15:595.
3. Meninger CJ, Kelly KA, Li H, Haynes TE, Wu G.: Glucosamine inhibits inducible nitric oxide synthase. *Biochem Biophys Res Commun* 2000;279:234.
4. Hua J, Sakamoto K, Nagaoka I. Inhibitory actions of glucosamine, a therapeutic agent for osteoarthritis, on the functions of neutrophils. *J Leukocyte Biol* 2002;71:632.
5. Felson DT, Lawrence RC, Hochberg MC, et al. Osteoarthritis: new insights. Part 2: Treatment approaches. *Ann Intern Med* 2000;133:726.
6. Chard J, Dieppe P. Glucosamine for osteoarthritis: Magic, hype, or confusion? [editorial.] *BMJ* 2001;322:1439.
7. Bellamy N, Lybrand SG. Glucosamine therapy: Does it work? *Med J Aust* 2001;175:399.
8. Hughes R, Carr A. A randomized, double-blind, placebo-controlled trial of glucosamine sulfate as an analgesic in osteoarthritis of the knee. *Rheumatology* 2002;41:279.
9. Pavelka K, Gatterova J, Olejarova M, Machacek S, Giacovelli G, Rovati LC. Glucosamine sulfate use and delay of progression of knee osteoarthritis: A 3-year, randomized, placebo-controlled, double-blind study. *Arch Intern Med* 2002;162:2113.
10. Kelly GS. The role of glucosamine and chondroitin sulfates in the treatment of degenerative joint disease. *Alt Med Rev* 1998;3:27.
11. Danao-Camara T. Potential side effects of treatment with glucosamine and chondroitin. *Arthritis Rheum* 2000;43:2853.
12. Guillaume M-P, Peretz A. Possible association between glucosamine treatment and renal toxicity: Comment on the letter by Danao-Camara. *Arthritis Rheum* 2001;44:2943.

GOLDENSEAL

■ SOURCE, DESCRIPTION, USES

Goldenseal (*Hydrastis canadensis*) is native to northeastern North America and is variously called eyebalm, eyeroot, goldenroot, tumeric root, yellow paint, and yellow root. An extract of the root has been used for a variety of conditions, including malaria, diarrhea, and ventricular tachyarrhythmias,[1] as an eyewash, and as a skin lotion. Other uses include as a bitter tonic; an aid to digestion; for genitourinary conditions, menorrhagia, and atrophic vaginitis; and as an oral antiseptic. It is among the ten most commonly used herbs in the United States.[2] Goldenseal tea was one of the most common herbs used by patients presenting at a New York hospital emergency department.[3]

■ PHARMACOLOGY

There are several pharmacologically active substances in goldenseal.[4,5] Among the activities that have been identified are various cardiovascular effects believed to be associated with berberine and hydrastinine. Berberine has been shown to generate free radicals when exposed to ultraviolet light.[5]

■ ADVERSE EFFECTS AND INTERACTIONS

High doses and prolonged use may cause diarrhea, hypertension, and vaso-constriction.[2] In infants with glucose-6-phosphate dehydrogenase deficiency, goldenseal may induce hemolysis.[1] Decreased anticoagulant effect has been reported when goldenseal is given with anticoagulants, including heparin, and platelet-inhibiting drugs.[4] Increased sedative effect has been reported when it is given with sedatives or tranquilizers.[4] Interference with the action of digoxin and with antihypertensive drugs is a possibility based on case reports.[4] Goldenseal is contraindicated in pregnant women and in infants with jaundice.[1] Photosensitivity reaction when goldenseal is used topically is a theoretical possibility.[5]

■ REFERENCES

1. Ko R. Adverse reactions to watch for in patients taking herbal remedies. *West J Med* 1999;171:181.
2. Mar C, Bent S. An evidence-based review of the ten most commonly used herbs. *West J Med* 1999;171:168.

3. Hung OL, Shih RD, Chiang WK, Nelson LS, Hoffman RS, Goldfrank LR. Herbal preparation use among urban emergency department patients. *Acad Emerg Med* 1997;4:209.

4. Lambrecht JE, Hamilton W, Rabinovich A. A review of herb-drug interactions: Documented and theoretical. *US Pharmacist* 25:8. Available at: http://www.uspharmacist.com/NewLook/DisplayArticle.cfm?/item_num=566.

5. Inbaraj JJ, Kukielczak BM, Bilski P, Sandvik SL, Chignell CF. Photochemistry and phytotoxicity of alkaloids from goldenseal (Hydrastis canadensis). 1. Berberine. *Chem Res Toxicol* 2001;14:1529.

GOLDTHREAD

■ SOURCE, DESCRIPTION, USES

Goldthread or gold-thread (*Coptis groenlandica, C. trifolia*) is a member of the buttercup (Ranunculaceae) family. A short (to 15 cm) plant with bright yellow roots (hence the name), it has white or pink buttercup-like flowers and shiny, dark evergreen, palmate leaves.[1] Goldthread favors dark woods and grows in eastern Canada, the northeastern United States, and further south in mountainous regions. Although goldthread is not commonly used today, traditional use (King's American Dispensatory, 1898) of the root and rootlets included as a bitter tonic, as a mouthwash for ulcers, and for dyspepsia and other stomach ills. It was generally taken as a powder or as a decoction of the dried root.[2]

■ PHARMACOLOGY

Two alkaloids, berberine and coptine, have been isolated from the root. The former is probably responsible for goldthread's traditional use.[2] Berberine is an isoquinoline alkaloid, present in many botanicals, that has been shown to possess anti-inflammatory, antinociceptive, and antipyretic actions,[3] as well as antimicrobial[4] and glucose-lowering properties.[5] Current interest in *C. groenlandica* centers on its potential antineoplastic properties. A crude extract has been shown to be the most potent of 15 natural medicines from Canada with respect to cytotoxicity in five human hepatoma cell lines.[6] This was true for cell lines containing hepatitis B (HB) virus genome and those not containing this genome.

■ ADVERSE EFFECTS AND INTERACTIONS

No information was revealed concerning adverse effects or interactions. In the absence of additional data, this herb probably should not be used in conjunction with anticancer drugs.

■ REFERENCES

1. Peterson RT, McKenny M. *Northeastern Wildflowers: Roger Tory Peterson Field Guides.* Norwalk, Conn: Easton Press; 1984:30.
2. Coptis—gold-thread. In: Felter HW, Lloyd JU. *King's American Dispensatory.* Available at: http://www.ibiblio.org/herbmed/eclectic/kings/coptis.html.
3. Kupeli E, Kosar M, Yesilada E, Husnu K, Baser C. A comparative study on the anti-inflammatory, antinociceptive and antipyretic effects of isoquinoline alkaloids from the roots of Turkish Berberis species. *Life Sci* 2002;72:645.
4. Cernakova M, Kostalova D. Antimicrobial activity of berberine—a constituent of Mahonia aquifolium. *Folia Microbiol (Praha)* 2002;47:375.
5. Yin J, Hu R, Chen M, et al. Effects of berberine on glucose metabolism in vitro. *Metabolism* 2002;51:1439.
6. Lin LT, Liu LT, Chiang LC, Lin CC. In vitro anti-hepatoma activity of fifteen natural medicines from Canada. *Phytother Res* 2002;16:440.

GOSSYPOL

■ SOURCE, DESCRIPTION, USES

Gossypol is a polyphenolic aldehyde extracted from cottonseed (*Gossypium hirsutum*) as a racemic mixture.[1] It has been researched extensively as a male contraceptive. It is not available for that purpose in North America but is so used in China,[2] and it is available from Internet sources.

■ PHARMACOLOGY

Gossypol in daily doses induces infertility in many mammalian species, including humans[3] Several clinical trials have shown that it can be an effective contraceptive for men when taken at doses of 10 to 15 mg/day.[3,4] In one trial,[4] it required 2 months of this loading dose before sperm counts began dropping to the generally accepted infertile level of less than 4 million/mL.

The maintenance dose was 10 to 15 mg every second day. Neither study reported any serious side effects, but one[3] reported a reversible reduction in testicular mass resulting from a decrease in mass of the germinal epithelium.

The mechanism of gossypol's antispermatogenic activity is not well understood, but it is known that this nutriceutical interferes with normal transmembrane movement of many ions, and it has been shown to inhibit a Ca^{2+} channel in mouse spermatogenic cell membranes, which could play a role in its mechanism of action.[5] It also has been shown to inhibit several intracellular dehydrogenases.[6]

Gossypol has shown some promise as an antineoplastic agent. In one study,[6] 27 patients with heavily pretreated gliomas and poor prognosis were given 10 mg of gossypol twice daily by mouth. Treatment was continued until the disease progressed. Six of the 27 showed a favorable, if modest, response in that progression of the disease was delayed. Only historical controls were used, and the authors concluded that gossypol was worth further study. Gossypol also has been shown to have an antiproliferative effect in a number of human carcinoma cell lines.[1]

■ ADVERSE EFFECTS AND INTERACTIONS

Early Chinese studies of gossypol as a male contraceptive used a higher dose than 10 to 15 mg/day and reported hypokalemia as a frequent side effect. Muscle weakness, fatigue, and malaise may occur as a consequence of higher doses.[3] In the study using gossypol as an antineoplastic agent, hypokalemia also was noted.[6] Another undesirable effect was irreversibility of the contraceptive action. Both side effects occurred in about 10% of treated subjects.[3] The mechanism involved appears to be inhibition of 11β-hydroxysteroid dehydrogenase (11β-OHSD). This enzyme normally oxidizes the active hormone cortisol to inactive cortisone. Inhibition of 11β-OHSD increases the amount of cortisol, enhancing mineralocorticoid action in the kidney. This in turn leads to Na^+ retention and K^+ loss, with resultant hypokalemia and hypertension.[7,8]

Although these effects do not appear to be associated with lower doses (10 to 15 mg/day), there is a potential for interaction of gossypol with many drugs, including corticosteroids, potassium-depleting thiazide diuretics, and high ceiling diuretics such as ethacrynic acid. Furosemide is also a potent inhibitor of 11β-OHSD, as is the flavonoid naringenin, which is present in grapefruit juice.[7] Interactions with these agents cannot be ruled out. Until more data regarding safety and efficacy are available gossypol, is not an agent to be recommended as a male contraceptive. The long loading period required and the potential for irreversibility of contraceptive effect also argue against its use. Tannin-containing preparations such as cottonseed oil may interfere with iron absorption.[9] This may not be a serious problem clinically but should be considered in anemic patients, and it is advisable to avoid taking iron and the herbal preparation together. Pure gossypol does not have this problem.

■ **REFERENCES**

1. Le Blanc ML, Russo J, Kudelka AP, Smith JA. An in vitro study of inhibitory activity of gossypol, a cottonseed extract, in human carcinoma cell lines. *Pharmacol Res* 2002;46:551.
2. Miller LG, Murray WJ, eds. *Herbal Medicinals: A Clinician's Guide.* New York, NY: Pharmaceutical Products Press; 1998:309.
3. Coutinho EM. Gossypol: A contraceptive for men. *Contraception* 2002;65:259.
4. Gu ZP, Mao BY, Wang YX, et al. Low dose gossypol for male contraception. *Asian J Androl* 2000;2:283.
5. Shi Y-L, Bai J-P, Wang W-P. Ion-channels in human sperm membrane and contraceptive mechanisms of male antifertility compounds derived from Chinese traditional medicine. *Acta Pharmacol Sin* 2003;24:22.
6. Bushunow P, Reidenberg MM, Wasenko J, et al. Gossypol treatment of recurrent adult malignant gliomas. *J Neuro-Oncol* 1999;43:79.
7. Reidenberg MM. Environmental inhibition of 11β-hydroxysteroid dehydrogenase. *Toxicology* 2000;144:107.
8. Song D, Lorenzo B, Reidenberg MM: Inhibition of 11β –hydroxysteroid dehydrogenase by gossypol and bioflavonoids. *J Lab Clin Med* 1992;120:792.
9. Miller LG. Herbal medicinals: Selected clinical considerations focusing on known or potential drug herb interactions. *Arch Intern Med* 1998;158:2200.

GROUNDSEL SPECIES (RAGWORTS)

■ **SOURCE, DESCRIPTION, USES**

The groundsels or ragworts (*Senecio* species) comprise some 900 members of the Compositae family and are distributed worldwide.[1] They are known mostly as troublesome weeds and frequently cause poisonings in livestock. Many, however, also are used around the world as herbal remedies and are being investigated as potential sources of pharmaceuticals. Several varieties that are of historical interest because of their traditional use as herbal remedies are described here.[1] Some of these varieties have established themselves in North America. Most can grow to nearly 1 m on a single stem, branching near the top.[2] The name *groundsel* derives from the Anglo-Saxon *groindeswelge*, meaning "ground-swallower," testimony to the rapidity with which these species can take over a site.

COMMON GROUNDSEL (*S. VULGARIS*)

Common throughout Europe and northern Asia, this annual plant is an alien in North America, growing throughout the northeast on waste ground.[2] It has dandelion-like leaves and flowers. The dried, whole herb has been used as a diaphoretic, antiscorbutic, purgative, diuretic, and anthelmintic. It also has been used for chapped hands and gout.[1]

GOLDEN GROUNDSEL (*S. AUREUS*)

Also known as life root and golden ragwort, this species is native to North America. It has yellow, daisy-like flowers. It has been used as an emetic, diuretic, and astringent. It is a perennial.

HOARY GROUNDSEL (*S. ERUCIFOLIUS*)

A native of Europe and northern Russia, hoary groundsel has been used in poultices, ointments, and plasters. It is a perennial.

VISCID OR STINKING GROUNDSEL (S. *VISCOSUS*)

A native of Europe, this species has become established in North America along the eastern seaboard. The leaves and flowers resemble those of the dandelion.[2] It is used as an emetic and carminative. This annual has an unpleasant odor, which gives rise to its name.

■ PHARMACOLOGY

Numerous pharmacologically active agents have been isolated from various *Senecio* species. β-Sitosterol has been isolated from a methanol extract of the aerial plant of *S. lyratus* and shown to have both antibacterial and antifungal activity.[3] β-Sitosterol is present in many botanicals and has been shown to be of benefit it treating benign prostatic hypertrophy.[4] See also β-SITOSTEROL. Perez and colleagues[5] identified a dozen constituents, including terpinoids, in the essential oil from *S. graveolens* from Argentina and found that the oil had antimicrobial activity. Antibacterial activity has been reported for *S. aegyptius* essential oil, and a sesquiterpene from the oil showed marked potency against gram-negative organisms.[6]

■ ADVERSE EFFECTS AND INTERACTIONS

Senecio species all contain pyrrolizidine alkaloids (PAs). These were originally identified in 1918 as the causative agents in a condition called bread poisoning associated with flour made from wheat contaminated with groundsel species.[7] PAs, which can be found in groundsels all over the world, cause veno-occlusive hepatitis. *S. latifolius,* a plant used in traditional medicine in South Africa, was shown to induce pathological changes in a human hepatoma cell line (HuH-7), including destruction of the cytoskeleton and necrosis.[8] The PA integerrimine, from *S. brasiliensis,* has been shown to be teratogenic for mice and mutagenic in several test systems and to induce micronuclei formation in bone marrow erythrocytes.[7]

As previously noted, livestock poisoning occurs frequently with groundsels. Tansy ragwort (*S. jacobaea*), an alien that has established itself widely in North America, has caused bizarre behavior, lameness, colic, and liver failure in horses that foraged on rough pasture.[9]

In addition to the toxicity of the PAs in groundsels, members of the Compositae family are noted for being a common cause of botanical contact dermatitis and for having a potential for cross-reactivity. It is possible that some of the antimicrobial effect noted earlier may simply be the result of the cytotoxicity of PAs. This class of botanicals is not a good candidate for use as herbal remedies. See also Appendices III and IX.

■ REFERENCES

1. Peterson RT, McKenny M. *Northeastern Wildflowers: Roger Tory Peterson Field Guides.* Norwalk, Conn: Easton Press; 1984:166,176.
2. Groundsel. In: Grieve M. *A Modern Herbal.* Botanical.com website. Available at: http://botanical.com/botanical//mgmh/g/grocom41.html.
3. Kiprono PC, Kaberia F, Keriko JM, Karanja JN. The in vitro antifungal and antibacterial activities of β-sitosterol from Senecio lyratus. *Z Naturforsch* 2000;55:485.
4. Klippel KF, Hiltl DM, Schipp B. A multicentric, placebo-controlled, double-blind clinical trial of beta-sitosterol (phytosterol) for the treatment of benign prostatic hyperplasia. German BPH-Phyto Study Group. *Br J Urol* 1997;80:427.
5. Perez C, Agnese AM, Cabrera JL. The essential oil of Senecio graveolens (Compositae): Chemical composition and antimicrobial activity tests. *J Ethnopharmacol* 1999;66:91.
6. El-Shazly A, Doral G, Wink M. Chemical composition and biological activity of the essential oils of Senecio aegyptius var. discoideus Boiss. *Z Naturforsch* 2002;57:434.
7. Santos-Mello R, Deimling LI, Almeida A. Induction of micronuclei by alkaloids extracted from Senecio brasiliensis and stored for 23 years. *Mutat Res* 2002;516:23.
8. Steenkamp V, Stewart MJ, van der Merwe S, Zuckerman M, Crowther NJ. The effect of Senecio latifolius a plant used as a South African traditional medicine, on a human hepatoma cell line. *J Ethnopharmacol* 2001;78:51.
9. de Lanux-Van Gorder V. Tansy ragwort poisoning in a horse in southern Ontario. *Can Vet J* 2000;41:409.

GUAR GUM

■ SOURCE, DESCRIPTION, USES

Guar gum is obtained from the seeds of *Cyamopsis tetragonolobus*, a plant native to India and Pakistan. It has numerous commercial uses as a thickening agent in foodstuffs, a binding agent for dying materials, and other applications. Guar gum has been marketed extensively as an alternative remedy to assist in weight loss.

■ PHARMACOLOGY

The theory underlying its use is that, by absorbing water and expanding in the stomach, guar gum creates a sensation of fullness that discourages overeating.[1] Guar gum has been used for gastrointestinal problems. It contains a hydroscopic, high polymer polysaccharide, galactomannan, as the principle active ingredient. One double-blind, controlled study examined the use of partially hydrolyzed guar gum to control chronic diarrhea in a group of critically ill, septic, tube-fed patients on life support. The treated group received 22 g/L of the guar preparation in addition to nutrient. Over a period of approximately 5 months, the treated group had significantly fewer days of diarrhea, on average, than the control group.[2]

Guar gum also has been used with some success in treating gastric and duodenal ulcers.[3] The nonabsorbable, mucilaginous substance offers physical protection to the mucosa and may have other useful properties.

Guar gum powder has been shown to reduce total and low-density lipoprotein cholesterol in patients with type 2 diabetes.[4]

■ ADVERSE EFFECTS AND INTERACTIONS

In the late 1980s, the introduction of guar tablets as a weight-loss aid was accompanied by an outbreak of cases of esophageal obstruction, some fatal. Unless they are taken with an adequate amount of water, the tablets may lodge in the esophagus where they can expand to many times their size, causing a physical blockade. Lewis[5] reported on 18 cases of esophageal obstruction, 7 of small bowel obstruction, and 1 death in individuals who had taken a guar-containing tablet called Cal-Ban. The tenacious, gel-like consistency of the substance made removal by endoscopy difficult. Two cases required the use of a rigid endoscope. One patient died of pulmonary embolism after the surgical repair of a mucosal tear in the esophagus.

The Food and Drug Administration subsequently banned such products, redefining them as "not being generally recognized as safe and effective."[5]

Such products also were banned in Australia. Pittler and Ernst[6] conducted a meta-analysis of 392 patients in 11 clinical trails and concluded that there was no significant effect from use of guar gum as a weight-loss aid compared with placebos. Many guar preparations are still available commercially.

Because it is bulky and not absorbed, guar gum can interfere with the absorption of many prescription drugs. Interference with the absorption of acetaminophen, nitrofurantoin, digoxin, bumetanide, metformin, phenoxymethylpenicillin, and some formulations of glibenclamide has been shown, and slowed absorption of oral contraceptives is possible.[7,8] Potentiation of insulin also has been demonstrated.

Although powdered guar preparations may be relatively safe when taken with adequate fluids, tablets should be avoided at all costs. This is not a substance that should be taken with prescription drugs. There may be an application for guar gum in treating some hyperlipidemias, but further study is required.

■ REFERENCES

1. Halama WH, Mauldin JL. Distal esophageal obstruction due to a guar gum preparation (Cal-Ban 3000). *South Med J* 1992;85:642.
2. Sappen H, Diltoer M, Van Malderen C, Opdenacker G, Suys E, Huyghens L. Soluble fiber reduces the incidence of diarrhea in septic patients receiving total enteral nutrition: A prospective, double-blind, randomized, and controlled trial. *Clin Nutrition* 2001;20:301.
3. Borrelli F, Izzo AA. The plant kingdom as a source of anti-ulcer remedies. *Phytother Res* 2000;14:581.
4. Bhardwaj PK, Dasgupta DJ, Prashar BS, Kaushal SS. Effective reduction of LDL cholesterol by indigenous plant product. *J Indian Med* 1994;92:80.
5. Lewis JH. Esophageal and small bowel obstruction from guar gum–containing "diet pills": Analysis of 26 cases reported to the Food and Drug Administration. *Am J Gastroenterol* 1992;87:1424.
6. Pittler MH, Ernst E. Guar gum for the reduction of body weight: A meta-analysis of randomized trials. *Am J Med* 2001;110:724.
7. Fugh-Berman A. Herb-drug interactions. *Lancet* 2000;355:134.
8. Ernst E, Pittler MH. Herbal medicine. *Med Clin North Am* 2002;86:149.

GUARANA

■ SOURCE, DESCRIPTION, USES

Guarana is prepared somewhat like coffee from the roasted, shelled seeds of a Brazilian climbing shrub, *Paullinia cupana*. It forms the basis of a popular drink in Brazil and contains significant levels of caffeine. The Guarinis, an Amazonian native tribe, originally prepared the herb.[1] It was used as a nerve tonic, stimulant, aphrodisiac, and febrifuge.[1] Several other drinks are prepared from *P. cupana*, and it has become a national beverage in Brazil. Miners there use it to stave off exhaustion.[1] In North America, guarana frequently shows up as an ingredient of multiherbal preparations for weight loss and as a so-called natural energy booster.

■ PHARMACOLOGY

The active principle of guarana is caffeine, which is present in a crystallized preparation called *guaranine*. Tannins also are present.[1] Guarana is exceptionally high in caffeine. Whereas the average cup of coffee might contain 100 mg of caffeine, the defined dose (30 mL) of one commercial product, Race 2005, may contain up to 570 mg.[2]

■ ADVERSE EFFECTS AND INTERACTIONS

The effects of excessive use of guarana are those of caffeine overdose. They include nervousness, restlessness, irritability, and insomnia; in more extreme cases, toxic effects may progress to mild delirium and emesis. Muscle tremors, tachycardia, extrasystole, and rapid respiration may occur. Toxic effects may occur with as little as 1 g of caffeine, and a dose of 10 g has been fatal.[3] Cannon and colleagues[2] describe a case of fatal ventricular fibrillation in a 25-year-old woman known to have mitral valve prolapse who had been advised to limit her intake of caffeine to one cup of tea daily. She worked in a bar where someone had given her a 55-mL squirt bottle of Race 2005 Energy Blast with Guarana and Ginseng, which she consumed almost completely. Her caffeine intake thus could have exceeded 1 g, the equivalent of 10 to 15 cups of coffee, in a relatively short time. Although this particular product was subsequently withdrawn from the Australian market, many others exist that contain guarana, as a search of the Internet will attest.

Guarana frequently is combined with other herbal ingredients that may increase the risk of an untoward event. Kaberi-Otarod and colleagues[4] describe a case of a 33-year-old man who was brought to an emergency department in California with left hemiparesis and slurred speech. He had no medical history of significance, smoked one pack of cigarettes a day, and was taking buproprion to assist him to cease smoking. The patient also was taking Thermadrene, an herbal product recommended for body building and energy boosting. He had taken his last dose 8 hours before the onset of symptoms. Although the patient improved gradually over several weeks, he still required physiotherapy after 5 months.

According to the product label, Thermadrene tablets contain ephedrine (24 mg), guarana (approximately 15 mg of caffeine), willow bark, caffeine (160 mg), and cayenne pepper. The dangers of ephedrine are well documented, and numerous reports of serious and even fatal consequences of its use are on record (see EPHEDRA). The possibility of an interaction with caffeine and guarana leading to the stroke in this patient cannot be discounted.

Guarana is one of several caffeine- and other methylxanthine-containing herbal products that include cola nuts, maté, cocoa beans, and, of course, coffee and tea.[5] The danger with many so-called nutritional supplements is that they can provide caffeine in a highly concentrated form, and they may be unpredictable with respect to the amount present. The risk of caffeine overdose is thus heightened. There is no information regarding safety during pregnancy of these preparations. Use in pregnant women should be discouraged, as should use in children.

Centrally acting agents, whether herbal remedies, prescription drugs, or over-the-counter (OTC) medications, carry a significant risk of adverse effects and interactions. Herbal products marketed for weight loss, body building, and to boost energy are especially risky because the user may not be aware of their caffeine content or the presence of other central nervous system stimulants such as ephedra. OTC nasal decongestants, sedating antihistamines, and antinausea agents may also interact with these herbal products (see also Appendix II).

■ REFERENCES

1. Guarana. In: Grieve M. *A Modern Herbal.* Botanical.com website. Available at: http://www.botanical.com/botanical/mgmh/g/guaran43.html.
2. Cannon ME, Cooke CT, McCarthy JS. Caffeine-induced cardiac arrhythmia: An unrecognized danger of healthfood products. *Med J Aust* 2001;174:520.
3. Rall TW. Drugs used in the treatment of asthma: The methylxanthines cromolyn sodium, and other agents. In: Gilman AG, Rall TW, Nies AS, Taylor P, eds. *Goodman and Gilman's The Pharmacological Basis of Therapeutics.* 8th ed. New York, NY: Pergamon Press; 1990:618.

4. Kaberi-Otarod J, Conetta R, Kundo KK, Farkash A. Ischemic stroke in a user of Thermadrene: A case study in alternative medicine. *Clin Pharmacol Ther* 2002;72:343.

5. Schulz V, Hansel R, Tyler VE. *Rational Phytotherapy: A Physician's Guide to Herbal Medicine*. New York, NY: Springer-Verlag; 1998:104.

GUGGAL

See SALAI GUGGAL.

GYMNEMA

■ SOURCE, DESCRIPTION, USES

Gymnema (*Gymnema sylvestre*, family Asclepiadaceae) is a woody, climbing vine native to India and elsewhere in southeast Asia, that has been used for centuries as an herb for the treatment of diabetes (*madhu meha*, or "honey urine") in traditional Ayurvedic medicine. Its common name there is *gurmar* ("sugar destroyer"), because chewing the leaves blocks the ability of the taste buds to discriminate sweetness (and bitterness) in foods.[1] Traditional uses include as a stomachic, diuretic, refrigerant, astringent, and tonic.[1] Western use has included as a diet aid.

■ PHARMACOLOGY

Gymnema contains a number of potentially active principles, including resins, gymnemic acids, saponins, stigmasterol, quercitol, and the amino acid derivatives betaine, choline, and trimethylamine.[1] There is evidence, both experimental and clinical, of gymnema's antidiabetic activity. Saponins have exhibited antisweet activity,[2] and the aqueous portion of an alcoholic extract of the leaves was shown to have a hypoglycemic effect in both normal and streptozotocin diabetic rats.[3] This extract also was shown to lower muscle glycogen content in rats and to be additive to insulin in this regard.[4] The mechanism of action may involve stimulation of insulin secretion from the β cells of the islets of Langerhans, as has been demonstrated in a number of cultured cell lines.[5] Most, but not all, animal studies support an antidiabetic action for gymnema, with a variety of mechanisms being proposed.[6]

Two clinical studies have been reported. One involved 27 type 1 (insulin-dependent) diabetic patients who received 400 mg/day of a standardized extract for up to 30 months in addition to their regular insulin therapy, and 37 others who continued on insulin alone. Gymnema extract decreased the insulin requirement by about 50% and the blood glucose from 232 mg/dL to 152 mg/dL. Glycosylated hemoglobin (HbA_{1c}) also decreased significantly compared with the control group, which did not have a decline in insulin requirement.[7]

In a second study by this group, 22 type 2 (non–insulin dependent) diabetic patients received this dose in addition to their regular oral medication for 18 to 20 months. They experienced significant reductions in blood glucose and HbA_{1c} levels and were able to reduce their dosage of prescription oral hypoglycemics. Five patients were able to discontinue this oral medication entirely.[8]

■ ADVERSE EFFECTS AND INTERACTIONS

No adverse reactions other than hypoglycemia were reported in the previously described studies. Obviously, anyone taking this herb must monitor blood glucose closely because dosage of insulin or oral hypoglycemic drugs likely will have to be adjusted. The safety of this herb in pregnancy has not been established.

In summary, gymnema shows promise as an aid in the treatment of diabetes, but the studies described here are small and relatively short term, given the lifelong need to treat this condition. More controlled studies are required before making a final judgment. See also Appendix X.

■ REFERENCES

1. Gymnema sylvestre monograph. *Altern Med Rev* 1999;4:46.
2. Ye W, Liu X, Zhang O, Che CT, Zhao S. Antisweet saponins from Gymnema sylvestre. *J Nat Prod* 2001;64:232.
3. Chattopadhyay RR. A comparative evaluation of some blood sugar lowering agents of plant origin. *J Ethnopharmacol* 1999;67:367.
4. Chattopadhyay RR. Possible mechanism of antihyperglycemic effect of Gymnema sylvestre leaf extract, Part I. *Gen Pharmacol* 1998;31:495.
5. Persaud SJ, Al-Majed H, Raman A, Jones PM. Gymnema sylvestre stimulates insulin release in vitro by increased membrane permeability. *J Endocrinol* 1999;163:207.
6. Grover JK, Yadav S, Vats V. Medicinal plants of India with anti-diabetic potential. *J Ethnopharmacol* 2002;81:81.
7. Shanmugasundaram ER, Rajeswari G, Baskaram K, Rajesh Kumar BR, Radha Shanmugasundaram K, Kizar Ahmath B. Use of Gymnema sylvestre leaf in the control of blood glucose in insulin-dependent diabetes mellitus. *J Ethnopharmacol* 1990;30:281.

8. Baskaran K, Ahamath BK, Radha Shanmugasundaram K, Shanmugasundaram ER. Antidiabetic effect of a leaf extract from Gymnema sylvestre in non-insulin-dependent patients. *J Ethnopharmacol* 1990;30:295.

HAWTHORN

■ SOURCE, DESCRIPTION, USES

The fruit, leaves, and flowers of the hawthorn (*Crataegus* spp.) have been used medicinally for centuries and were in use by North American Indians before the arrival of Europeans.[1] Hawthorn has a long history of use in traditional Chinese medicine.[2] Although *C. oxyacantha* and *C. monogyna*, species of European shrubs, are generally named as the source of hawthorn extracts, Petrides[3] points out that the number of hawthorn species native to North America has been variously estimated from 100 to 1000 with considerable hybridization, making identification difficult. It is likely that all species of these shrubs and low trees possess similar chemical constituents. Indeed, Chang and colleagues[2] list six species of hawthorn that are used medicinally around the world. Other names for hawthorn are haw, may bush, and whitethorn. Hawthorns are members of the Rosaceae family.

Historically, hawthorn has been used as a cardiotonic, diuretic, appetite stimulant, and astringent for sore throat; as well as for hypertension, atherosclerosis, congestive heart failure, and arrhythmias. Current interest centers on hawthorn's cardiac actions.

■ PHARMACOLOGY

The main ingredients isolated from hawthorn include flavonoids, procyanidins, catechins, triterpenoids, aromatic carboxylic acids, cardioactive amines, and amino and purine derivatives, among others compounds.[2,4] Flavonoids and oligomeric proanthocyanidins are believed to be responsible for the cardiovascular effects of hawthorn.[2] (See Chang and colleagues[2] for structural formulae.) Marked cardiotonic activity has been confirmed, with positive inotropic and negative chronotropic actions. Increased coronary blood flow, increased cardiac output, and reduced oxygen consumption are believed to be related to phosphodiesterase inhibitory effect.[2,4] Potassium channel activation also has been reported.[4] Inhibition of thromboxane synthesis has been reported,[5] and vasodilation has been attributed to blockade of angiotensin-converting enzyme.[6]

Other activities of hawthorn include antiarrhythmic effect, hypotensive action, hyperlipidemic activity, and antioxidative action.[2,5] Several clinical studies have confirmed that hawthorn is potentially useful in early congestive heart failure, hypertension, angina, and minor arrhythmia.[2,6,7] No effect on diastolic blood pressure was seen in some studies.[2] Antilipidemic effect also has been confirmed in clinical studies of patients with New York Hospital Association stage II congestive heart failure or hyperlipidemia. Not all of these were well controlled.

■ ADVERSE EFFECTS AND INTERACTIONS

Although hawthorn shows obvious potential for the treatment of milder forms of congestive heart failure, angina, and hyperlipidemia, and, indeed, it is thus used in Germany and other parts of Europe and Asia,[2,3] there is an equally obvious potential for interactions with conventional heart medications. Monitoring of digoxin medication could be complicated by hawthorn. Many cardiac glycosides exist in nature and could be present in other herbal medications, unbeknownst to the user or physician. Interference with anticholesterolemic medication could occur, and little is known about the results of concurrent administration of calcium channel blockers or beta-blockers.

Given the multiple pharmacological actions of hawthorn, it should be used cautiously, if at all, in the presence of conventional drugs for heart disease, hypertension, or hyperlipidemia until more information is available. Side effects of treatment with hawthorn alone appear to be minimal.[2,6] Tannin-containing herbs such as hawthorn may interfere with iron absorption.[8] This may not be a serious problem clinically but should be considered in anemic patients, and it is advisable to avoid taking iron and the herbal preparation together. See also Appendix VII.

■ REFERENCES

1. Rigelsky JM, Sweet BV. Hawthorn: pharmacology and therapeutic uses. *Am J Health Syst Pharm* 2002;59:417.
2. Chang Q, Zuo Z, Harrison F, Chow MS. Hawthorn. *J Clin Pharmacol* 2002;42:605.
3. Petrides GA. *Trees and Shrubs: Roger Tory Peterson Field Guides.* Norwalk, Conn: Easton Press; 1986:197.
4. Schulz V, Hansel R, Tyler VE. *Rational Phytotherapy: A Physician's Guide to Herbal Medicine.* New York, NY: Springer-Verlag; 1998:89.
5. Mashour NH, Lin GI, Frishman WH. Herbal medicine for the treatment of cardiovascular disease. *Arch Intern Med* 1998;158:2225.
6. Morelli V, Zoorob RJ. Alternative therapies: Part II. Congestive heart failure and hypercholesterolemia. *Am Fam Physician* 2000;62:1325.

7. Rigelsky JM, Sweet BV. Hawthorn: pharmacology and therapeutic uses. *Am J Health Syst Pharm* 2002;59:417.

8. Miller LG. Herbal medicinals: Selected clinical considerations focusing on known or potential herb-drug interactions. *Arch Intern Med* 1998;158:2200.

HENBANE

■ SOURCE, DESCRIPTION, USES

All parts of henbane (*Hyoscyamus niger*, family Solanaceae) are used in herbal preparations. The plant grows widely throughout Europe and western Asia and was naturalized in North America more than 300 years ago.[1] Synonyms include hog's-bean, Jupiter's-bean, symphonica, and others. This is an extremely toxic plant, the use of which as an herbal remedy is highly questionable. Nevertheless, it appears on many websites and is generally available in the wild state. A local garden club actually lists it as an herbal remedy in a book it has published as a fund-raiser. Traditional medical uses include as a sleep aid, to relieve pain, as a poultice to soothe local injuries, for nervous conditions, and as a diuretic, to name a few applications.[1,2] Given the anti–motion sickness properties of scopolamine, a major component of henbane, herbal use of the plant for this purpose may also occur. The plant is branching, grows up to 80 cm in height, and has hairy leaves that spring from the base. The yellow flowers have a nauseating odor.

■ PHARMACOLOGY

As with many members of the Solanaceae family, henbane contains the so-called belladonna alkaloids atropine (hyoscyamine) and scopolamine (hyoscine). These are anticholinergic, muscarinic blocking agents. Scopolamine predominates in henbane, whereas atropine is the major alkaloid in deadly nightshade (*Atropa belladonna*) and in jimsonweed or Jamestown weed (*Datura stramonium*).[3] Plants such as henbane and stramonium are often employed as recreational drugs, especially by teenagers, because the central effects of hyoscine include sedation and euphoria.

The pharmacology of muscarinic blocking agents is well known and can be found in any good pharmacology textbook.[3]

■ ADVERSE EFFECTS AND INTERACTIONS

Signs and symptoms of henbane (and stramonium) poisoning are summarized in the rhyme that describes the anticholinergic toxidrome: "red as a beet, blind as a bat, mad as a hatter, hotter than hell." This rhyme highlights the peripheral vasodilation, extreme pupillary dilation, lack of perspiration, incoherence and hallucinations, and elevated temperature caused by impaired temperature regulation. To this list can be added tachycardia, with heart rates exceeding 150, and possibly seizures. Poisonings in Australia have resulted from people chewing henbane flowers in the hope of producing euphoria.[4] In Denver, two patients demonstrated typical anticholinergic syndrome after ingesting a wild plant. It required chemical analysis of plants collected from the same location to identify the probable cause as henbane poisoning.[5] Poisonings with the seeds of jimsonweed (stramonium) are becoming fairly common throughout North America because the plant is easy to recognize, grows freely on waste ground, even in cities, and the word about possible euphoric effects has spread quickly among youths (see JIMSONWEED and MANDRAKE). One characteristic of poisonings with jimsonweed (stramonium) is hallucinations in which the intoxicated individual sees little people. This has been called the Lilliputian syndrome, and some consider it to be virtually diagnostic.[6]

Although no specific drug interactions seem to have been reported for henbane, it is evident that there is a potential to interact with any agent acting in the autonomic or central nervous systems. These would include tranquilizers, sedatives, narcotic analgesics, cholinesterase inhibitors, adrenergic drugs, and cholinergic drugs, among others (see also Appendix II). Treatment usually requires the use of cholinesterase inhibitors such as physostigmine to increase levels of acetylcholine, because the effect at muscarinic receptors is competitive.

■ REFERENCES

1. Henbane. In: Grieve M. *A Modern Herbal.* Botanical.com website. Available at: http://www.botanical.com/botanical/mgmh/h/henban23.html.
2. Henbane. Available at: www.purplesage.org.uk/profiles/henbane.htm.
3. Brown JH, Taylor P. Muscarinic receptor agonists and antagonists. In: Hardman JG, Limbird L, Gilman AG, eds. *Goodman and Gilman's The Pharmacological Basis of Therapeutics.* 10th ed. New York, NY: McGraw-Hill; 2001:162.
4. Sands JM, Sands R. Henbane chewing. *Med J Aust* 1976;10:55.
5. Spoerke DG, Hall AH, Dodson CD, Stermitz FR, Swanson CH Jr, Rumack BH. Mystery root ingestion. *J Emerg Med* 1987;5:385.
6. Grim P. Runaway heart. *Discover* 1999;Apr:40.

HOPS

■ SOURCE, DESCRIPTION, USES

Hops, the dried fruit of the plant *Humulus lupulus*, have been used as flavoring in beer for centuries, possibly millennia.[1] The use of hops as an
herbal remedy may be somewhat more recent, based on the observation
that hops pickers tired easily, possible from inhaling the volatile oil.[2] *H.
lupulus* is a relative of the stinging nettle and a member of the family
Urticaceae. It is native to the British Isles, where it grows wild, and is cultivated in many parts of the world.[1] Infusions and tinctures of the above-
ground plant are used as a sedative-hypnotic and tranquilizer in Europe and
as a tonic, aromatic bitter, and diuretic.[1,2]

■ PHARMACOLOGY

Although a component of hops, methyl butanol, has been shown to have
sedative properties in mice, it is too volatile to persist in stored glands
(fruit), flowers, or oil.[2] Clinical trials have not been suggestive of sedative-
hypnotic effect. There does not appear to be convincing evidence of sedative efficacy for hops.

Hops do, however, contain phytoestrogens, and some women have taken
hops for breast enhancement.[3] Milligan and colleagues[3] examined a series of
structurally related naringenin flavonoids from hops for ability to compete
with estrogen and estradiol at their receptors and for progestenic and
androgenic activity, High estrogenic activity was identified for 8-prenyl-
naringenin. Neither the rest of the flavonoids nor polyphenolic extracts displayed significant noteworthy hormonal activity.

■ ADVERSE EFFECTS AND INTERACTIONS

The high estrogenic activity of hops creates the possibility for interference
with estrogen replacement therapy, oral contraception, and breast cancer
therapy (see also PHYTOESTROGENS AND PHYTOPROGESTINS). In
view of evidence that other naringenin isomers are competitive inhibitors of
cytochrome P450 3A4[4] and can interfere with the metabolism of felodipine
and other drugs, caution is advisable when hops is taken in the presence of
prescription medication. There do not appear to be any reports of adverse

effects from the use of hops alone, although excessive use has the potential to disrupt the normal estrus cycle.

■ REFERENCES

1. Hops. In: Grieve M. *A Modern Herbal*. Botanical.com website. Available at: http://www.botanical.com/botanical/mgmh/h/hops—32.html.
2. Shulz V, Hansel R, Tyler VE. *Rational Phytotherapy: A Physician's Guide to Herbal Medicine*. New York, NY: Springer-Verlag; 1998:81.
3. Milligan SR, Kalita JC, Pocock V, et al. The endocrine activities of 8-prenylnaringenin and related hop (Humulus lupulus L.) flavonoids. *J Clin Endocrinol Metab* 2000;85:4912.

HORSE CHESTNUT

■ SOURCE, DESCRIPTION, USES

The horse chestnut, *Aesculus hippocastanum* (family Hippocastanaceae), is an imported species often found growing wild in northeastern North America. The buckeyes are related native species of the genus *Aesculus* that tend to grow further west.[1] Horse chestnuts have seven to nine wedge-shaped, toothed leaves and large, sticky end buds, whereas buckeyes have five leaves and smooth, nonsticky end buds.[1] Extracts of the seeds of the ornamental horse chestnut (horse chestnut seed extract, HCSE) have been used traditionally for arthritic and rheumatic complaints for decades in Europe. More recently, attention has centered on the use of the extract for treating chronic venous insufficiency (CVI) and hemorrhoids.[2]

■ PHARMACOLOGY

In pharmacological studies, HCSE has been shown to reduce venous capillary permeability.[3] The active ingredient is aescin (or escin), a triterpene glycoside, and controlled clinical trials support the beneficial effects (e.g., reduction of lower leg volume).[3] Symptoms such as leg pain, fatigue, and pruritus also were reduced. Some studies have indicated that HCSE is more effective in the early stages of CVI.[4] In one study,[5] HCSE (Venostasin) was compared with Pycnogenol (French maritime pine bark extract, PBE) for efficacy in CVI. Although PBE significantly reduced lower leg circumference and subjective symptoms and lowered blood cholesterol and low-density lipoprotein values, the effects of Venostasin were moderate and not statistically significant. In another study, HCSE was found to be as effective as compression stockings in reducing lower leg volume.[6] Pharmacological effects reported for HCSE include the ability to close venular endothelial gaps,[5] improved entry of ions into channels to raise venous tension, release of prostaglandins, antagonism of serotonin and histamine, and reduced catabolism of tissue mucopolysaccharides.[7]

■ ADVERSE EFFECTS AND INTERACTIONS

The usual therapeutic doses appear to be well tolerated. High doses or parenteral administration have been associated with renal and hepatic toxicity and hematologic abnormalities.[2,8] Mild gastrointestinal symptoms, headache, and pruritus have been reported rarely.[2] One product, Venocuran (now withdrawn), contains horse chestnut and has been associated with a pseudolupus syndrome.[8] See also Appendix VII.

Horse chestnut is thought to contain coumarin or coumarin derivatives; therefore, there is a potential to increase the effect of oral anticoagulants and, possibly, antiplatelet agents.[9]

■ REFERENCES

1. Petrides GA. *Trees and Shrubs: Roger Tory Peterson Field Guides.* Norwalk, Conn: Easton Press; 1986:53, 64.
2. Rodblatt MD. Cranberry, feverfew, horse chestnut and kava. *West J Med* 1999;171:195.
3. Pittler MH, Ernst E. Horse chestnut seed extract for chronic venous insufficiency. A criteria-based systematic review. *Arch Dermatol* 1998;134:1356.
4. Otillinger B, Greeske K. Rational therapy of chronic venous insufficiency—chances and limits of the therapeutic use of horse-chestnut seeds extract. *BMC Cardiovasc Disord* 2001;1:5.
5. Koch R. Comparative study of venostasin and pycnogenol in chronic venous insufficiency. *Phytother Res* 2002;16(suppl 1):S-1.
6. Diehm C. Comparison of leg compression stocking and oral horse-chestnut seed extract therapy in patients with chronic venous insufficiency. *Lancet* 1996;347:292.
7. Sirtori CR. Aescin: Pharmacology, pharmacokinetics and therapeutic profile. *Pharmacol Res* 2001;44:183.
8. Mashour NH, Lin GI, Frishman WH. Herbal medicine for the treatment of cardiovascular disease. *Arch Intern Med* 1998;158:2225.
9. Heck AM, Dewitt BA, Lukes AL. Potential interactions between alternative therapies and warfarin. *Am J Health Syst Pharm* 2000;57:1221.

IVY LEAF

■ SOURCE, DESCRIPTION, USES

The herb is prepared from the leaves (most often) and berries of common ivy (*Hedera helix*), a native of Europe and Central Asia.[1] This climbing plant has dark green, glossy leaves. Historically, ivy leaf has been used to treat dysentery, lung diseases (the spitting of blood), jaundice, and hangover.[1] Current use is primarily as an expectorant.[2]

■ PHARMACOLOGY

The expectorant action of ivy has been attributed to the presence of polar saponins. These substances are poorly absorbed from the gastrointestinal tract but apparently stimulate bronchial mucus secretion via parasympathetic reflexes.[2] In one recently published, German, open-label study,[3] 1350 patients, aged 4 years and older, who had chronic bronchitis (with or without airway obstruction) were treated with a commercial tablet containing a special extract of ivy (Prospan). The results were as follows: 92.2% reported that cough was reduced or eliminated; 94.2% reported expectoration; 83.1%, improved dyspnea; and 86.9%, improved respiratory pain. In each category, at least 38% reported complete elimination of the symptom. Conversely, a double-blind, placebo-controlled trial using dried ivy leaf extract was conducted in 24 children with bronchial asthma and reviewed recently.[4] Although there was no improvement in the 1-second forced expiratory volume, there was a significant decrease in airway resistance. The authors concluded that ivy extract might work in a secretolytic and bronchospasmolytic manner.

Recently, researchers isolated a natriuretic peptide from *H. helix* that is recognized by antibodies for atrial natriuretic peptide. They suggested that this peptide might be involved in ion transportation.[5]

■ ADVERSE EFFECTS AND INTERACTIONS

Large doses of saponins are known to cause gastrointestinal upset, and contact dermatitis also has been reported.[2] In the previously mentioned trial involving 1350 patients, only three reported adverse effects: two of these patients had eructation and one, nausea.[3] There are no reports of drug interactions. Given the detergent action of saponins, there is a theoretical possibility of interference with absorption of drugs from the gastrointestinal tract. Thus, patients should stagger doses of other medications to avoid taking simultaneously with ivy leaf.

■ REFERENCES

1. Ivy, common. In: Grieve M. *A Modern Herbal.* Botanical.com website. Available at: http://www.botanical.com/botanical/mgmh/i/ivycom15. html.
2. Schulz V, Hansel R, Tyler VE. *Rational Phytotherapy: A Physician's Guide to Herbal Medicine.* New York, NY: Springer-Verlag; 1998:155.
3. Hecker M, Runkel F, Voelp A. Treatment of chronic bronchitis with ivy leaf special extract—multicenter post-marketing surveillance study in 1,350 patients [in German]. *Forsch Komplementarmed Klass Naturheild* 2002;9:77.
4. Huntley A, Ernst E. Herbal medicines for asthma: A systematic review. *Thorax* 2000;55:925.
5. Billington T, Pharmawati M, Gehring CA. Isolation and immunoaffinity purification of a biologically active plant natriuretic peptide. *Biochem Biophys Res Commun* 1997;235:722.

JIMSONWEED

■ SOURCE, DESCRIPTION, USES

Jimsonweed is one of many names for *Datura stramonium* (family Solanaceae). Others include Jamestown weed, thorn-apple, devil's apple, angel's trumpet, and stink weed. An alien to North America (it is a native of Europe), jimsonweed now grows widely throughout the continent. It is a tall, erect plant, growing up to 1.5 m, with course-toothed leaves, white or violet flowers, and spiny seed pods.[1] The leaves have been used since colonial times in the treatment of a variety of conditions, including being smoked for asthma, and also were used as an antispasmodic. The seeds were used as a narcotic.[2] Current use is more likely to be for recreational purposes among teenagers, with poisoning as a frequent consequence.

■ PHARMACOLOGY

Atropine (hyosciamine) and scopolamine (hyoscine) are the active principles. The pharmacology and toxicology of jimsonweed are discussed under HENBANE, another member of the Solanaceae family that has the same active principles.

■ REFERENCES

1. Peterson RT, McKenny M. *Northeastern Wildflowers: Roger Tory Peterson Field Guides.* Norwalk, Conn: Easton Press; 1984:12.
2. Thornapple. In: Grieve M. *A Modern Herbal.* Botanical.com website. Available at: http://www.botanical.com/botanical/mgmh/t/thorna12.html.

JIN BU HUAN

■ SOURCE, DESCRIPTION, USES

Jin bu huan is a Chinese patent herbal medicine. The product, Jin bu huan Anodyne tablets, contains 36% levo-tetrahydropalmatine (L-THP) by weight. It is promoted as an analgesic, sedative, antispasmodic, and hypnotic and recommended for patients suffering from insomnia caused by pain.[1]

■ PHARMACOLOGY

Jin bu huan contains the single ingredient L-THP plus starch.[1] No information regarding the pharmacology of this ingredient was found. It is reputed to have opiate-like properties.[2]

■ ADVERSE EFFECTS AND INTERACTIONS

The herb of origin stated on the product package was *Polygala,* which does not contain L-THP. The active ingredient is present, however, in the genus *Stephania.*[1] Jin bu huan frequently has been associated with hepatitis. McCrae and colleagues[2] reviewed 11 such cases in adults associated with chronic use. A single acute ingestion in children has caused severe illness with neurologic and cardiovascular manifestations.[1,3] Fatalities have occurred in adults. The mechanism of hepatotoxicity is unclear; however, the structural formula of L-THP resembles that of pyrrolizidine alkaloids, which are known botanical hepatotoxins.[2]

In summary, jin bu huan should not be taken under any circumstances. It has been added to Poisindex, an international poison reference index.[1]

■ REFERENCES

1. Jin bu huan toxicity in children. *MMWR* 1993;42:633.
2. McRae CA, Agarwal K, Mutimer D, Bassendine MF. Hepatitis associated with Chinese herbs. *Eur J Gastroenterol Hepatol* 2002;14:559.
3. Horowitz RS, Feldhaus K, Dart DC, Stermitz FR, Beck JJ. The clinical spectrum of Jin Bu Huan toxicity. *Arch Intern Med* 1996;156:899.

KARELA

■ SOURCE, DESCRIPTION, USES

Karela is the Hindi name for what is called bitter gourd in English (*Mordica charantia*, family Cucurbitaceae).[1,2] Synonyms include karavella, kathilla, and cundeamor. Karela is native to India and southern Asia and also grows in South America. The fruit is about the size of a gherkin pickle, green in the middle and tapering to yellow ends. It is commonly used as a vegetable. In Indian Ayurvedic medicine, it has been used for centuries in the treatment of diabetes mellitus. Numerous other traditional uses include as an emetic, purgative, anthelmintic, and astringent, among others.[1]

■ PHARMACOLOGY

By the 1960s, pharmacologists in India had established that karela lowered blood glucose levels in both diabetic patients and experimental animals.[3] In 1981, Leatherdale and colleagues[4] reported on a small study involving nine patients with type 2 diabetes. One patient was treated with diet alone, three with diet plus chlorpropamide, three with tolbutamide, one with gliben-clamide, and one with glymidine. A standard glucose tolerance test was performed after withdrawing medication for 48 hours. Karela juice taken before the test reduced both plasma glucose levels and the area under the curve. Patients who ate fried karela daily for 8 to 11 weeks showed significant reduction in "glycosylated" (glycated) hemoglobin after this period. Because plasma insulin levels did not change, the authors concluded that increased insulin secretion was not the mechanism of action of karela. The juice was somewhat more effective than the fried karela. The authors also noted a hypoglycemic effect in rats.

More recently, both aqueous and alcohol extracts of karela were shown to reduce blood glucose levels in alloxan diabetic rats and streptozotocin (STZ) diabetic mice.[1] Although the effect was more pronounced when a significant number of β cells survived, it persisted when the majority had been destroyed, suggesting a direct insulinomimetic action. This is supported by findings that karela extract partially restored liver glycogen levels, indicating more effective glucose utilization. Karela also has been shown to attenuate renal damage in STZ diabetic mice.[5]

Other activities that have been shown for karela juice include the induction of some cytochrome P450–dependent monooxygenases in STZ diabetic rats[6] and antispermatogenic and androgenic effects in normal rats.[7]

■ ADVERSE REACTIONS AND INTERACTIONS

The question of whether karela should be considered as a food, a nutriceutical, or an herbal remedy is arbitrary because it is used as all three and drug interactions are possible in each case. There was an early report of a possible interaction with the oral hypoglycemic chlorpropamide.[8] An Indian woman taking this drug for diabetes mellitus experienced periodic glucosuria that did not occur when she ate a curry containing karela. Although no other reports of interactions with antidiabetic agents were found, this possibility cannot be overlooked and must be considered when managing diabetic patients, especially those of eastern or South American origin. Such an interaction could, theoretically, be exploited to lower the dose of oral hypoglycemic drugs and, potentially, the risk of an untoward effect. In one animal study,[2] no abnormalities were detected in any of several hematological parameters after 2 months of treatment.

The report of testicular and hormonal disturbances in rats[7] predicates caution when using concentrated preparations in men, especially in light of one report that testicular lesions (and hepatic damage) were observed in dogs given excessive amounts of cerasee, a component of wild karela.[9] More data are required regarding the potential use and hazards of this herb before an unqualified endorsement can be made, especially with respect to its use in conjunction with antidiabetic medications. See also Appendix X.

■ REFERENCES

1. Karela. Available at: http://www.himalayahealthcare.com/products/karela.htm.
2. Rathi SS, Grover JK, Vats V. The effect of Mormordica charantia and Muncuna pruriens in experimental diabetes and their effect on key metabolic enzymes involved in carbohydrate metabolism. *Phytother Res* 2002;16:236.
3. Pitchumoni CS. Karela and blood sugar. *Lancet* 1979;1:924.
4. Leatherdale BA, Panesar RK, Singh GH, Atkins TW, Bailey CJ, Bignell AH. Improvement in glucose tolerance due to Momordica charantia (karela). *B MJ* 1981;282:1823.

5. Grover JK, Vats V, Rathi SS, Dawar R. Traditional Indian anti-diabetic plants attenuate progression of renal damage in streptozotocin induced diabetic mice. *J Ethnopharmacol* 2001;76:233.

6. Raza H, Ahmed I, Lakhani MS, Sharma AK, Pallot D, Montague W. Effect of bitter melon (Momordica charantia) fruit juice on the hepatic cytochrome P450-dependent monooxygenases and glutathione S-transferases in streptozotocin-induced diabetic rats. *Biochem Pharmacol* 1996;52:1639.

7. Naseem MZ, Patil SR, Patil SR, Patil R, Patil SB. Antispermatogenic and androgenic activities of Momordica charantia (karela) in albino rats. *J Ethnopharmacol* 1998;61:9.

8. Aslam M, Stockley IH. Interaction between curry ingredient (karela) and drug (chlorpropamide). *Lancet* 1969;1:607.

9. Anderson RA. Chromium, glucose tolerance and diabetes. *Biol Trace Elem Res* 1992;32:19.

KAVA

■ SOURCE, DESCRIPTION, USES

From the plant *Piper methysticum* (literally intoxicating pepper), kava has been used throughout the South Pacific for centuries as a social and ceremonial drug with mildly intoxicating properties. It also was used to treat a variety of physical ailments. The effect has been compared with that of the benzodiazepines diazepam (Valium) and alprazolam (Xanax) in that it seems to potentiate the γ-aminobutyric acid (GABA)–mediated, inhibitory neurotransmitter system. Kava is one of the best selling herbals in the United States, with sales in 1998 growing at the rate of 437%.[1]

■ PHARMACOLOGY

The active agents are kavalactones (kavapyrones), which act on the same GABA receptors as benzodiazepines. Other pharmacologically active ingredients possessing local anesthetic and muscle-relaxing properties also may be present. In addition to its anxiolytic activity, kava appears to possess anticonvulsant properties.[2] In the 1980s, excessive use by Australian aboriginal people led to medical problems. Although the claim that it is nonaddictive is probably true, any agent that produces desirable central effects can be habit forming. Clinical studies have indicated that its short-term use is effective in reducing anxiety,[2,3] but there are risks associated with taking this potent agent.

■ ADVERSE EFFECTS AND INTERACTIONS

The U.S. Food and Drug Administration has issued warnings that the use of kava has been associated with 25 cases of serious hepatotoxicity in Germany and Switzerland, including cirrhosis, hepatitis, and liver failure,[3] and has advised the public not to take this herb. In the United States, a previously healthy young woman required a liver transplant after using kava.[3]

Numerous other adverse reactions have been reported. Extrapyramidal side effects and exacerbation of Parkinson's disease have occurred at doses of 100 to 450 mg/day.[4] Dry flaky skin, known as kava dermopathy, has occurred after long-term consumption of high doses of kava, and at least one case of photosensitivity has been reported.[5] Hair loss, hearing loss, and loss of appetite also have been reported with prolonged use of high doses.[2] Side effects at doses at or below 100 mg/day of standard extract are uncommon.[2]

The potential for drug interactions with this agent is high. It may be additive with any central nervous system depressant, including alcohol, leading to inebriation. One patient became disoriented and lethargic after taking kava with the prescription drugs alprazolam (Xanax), a benzodiazepine GABA agonist; cimetidine (Tagamet), a histamine H_2-receptor blocker; and terazosin (Hytrin), an antihypertensive.[6] Kava is contraindicated in patients taking benzodiazepines, barbiturates, or antipsychotic drugs, and in those who habitually consume alcohol. It also is contraindicated in patients with Parkinson's disease. Kava should be discontinued at least 24 hours before surgery because of its possible interaction with anesthetics.[7] The safety of kava in pregnant women and its effects on fertility have not been established. In August 2002, the Canadian government ordered the removal of all products containing kava from retail shelves because of the risks associated with its use.

Because kava is marketed under a plethora of names, as well as being an ingredient in herbal mixtures, patients may be unaware that they are taking it. Names include ava, ava pepper, ava long pepper, awa, goa, gi, intoxicating pepper, intoxicating long pepper, kao, kava-kava, kava root, kavain, kava pepper, kavapipar, kawa, kawa-kawa, kawa pepper, kawa pfeffer, kew, *Macropiper latifolium*, *Piper inebrians*, Maori kava, and numerous others.[3] See also Appendix II.

■ REFERENCES

1. Hirsch M. What are the uses and dangers of kava? *Harvard Mental Health Letter*. Nov 2000. Available at: http://www.health.harvard.edu/medline/Mental/M1100h.html.

2. Ernst E. The risk-benefit profile of commonly used herbal therapies: Ginkgo, St. John's wort, ginseng, echinacea, saw palmetto and kava. *Ann Intern Med* 2002;136:42.

3. Wooltorton E. Herbal kava: Reports of liver toxicity. *Can Med Assoc J* 2002;166:777.
4. Schelosky L, Raffauf C, Jendroska K, Poewe W. Kava and dopamine antagonism. *J Neurol Neurosurg Psychiat* 1995;58:639.
5. Jappe U, Franke I, Reinhold D, Gollnick HP. Sebotropic drug reaction resulting from kava-kava extract therapy: A new entity? *J Am Acad Dermatol* 1998;38:104.
6. Almedia JC, Grimsley EW. Coma from the health food store: Interaction between kava and alprazolam. *Ann Intern Med* 1996;125:940.
7. Ang-Lee MK, Moss J, Yuan C-S. Herbal medicines and perioperative care. *JAMA* 2001;286:208.

KELP

■ SOURCE, DESCRIPTION, USES

Kelp is the name applied to a variety of brown seaweeds that grow in the intertidal zone of the Atlantic and Pacific Oceans.[1] The two varieties that are most often referred to as herbal remedies are *Fucus vesiculosis* and various species of *Laminaria*, notably *L. japonica*. Given that the correct identification of these seaweeds requires some botanical expertise, it is likely that several species are actually used in the preparation of herbal remedies. According to one Internet supplier,[2] the whole plant is used for its so-called normalizing effects on most organs, especially the reproductive ones but also the heart and brain (purportedly because of its manganese content), to cleanse the colon, to relieve anemia, as a diuretic, and for its vitamin content. Current interest in kelp stems from the belief that it can assist in weight loss by stimulating the thyroid gland.[3] Kelp is dried and may be taken in the form of tablets or as flakes that can be added to salads and other foods.

■ PHARMACOLOGY

Kelp is rich in iodine as well as other minerals and vitamins. It is its iodine content, however, that imparts pharmacological, as opposed to purely nutritional, properties. The belief that kelp may assist in weight loss appears to stem from the knowledge that hyperthyroidism (thyrotoxicosis) is usually accompanied by weight loss and the knowledge that iodine can improve thyroid function in iodine-deficient goiter. By a leap of logic, it is assumed that if iodine can improve thyroid function in simple goiter, then it can do so to a normal or slightly deficient thyroid with accompanying weight loss. In moderate doses in the short term, kelp may actually correct hyperthyroidism by a mechanism not completely understood but which involves the inhibition of the synthesis of iodotyrosine and iodothyronine by iodide.[4] However, the effects of high doses over longer periods can be the opposite of what is expected.

Kelp may have other pharmacological properties. A crude extract has been shown to be hypotensive in rats and to relax potassium chloride–stimulated arterial strips. It also has been shown to have negative chronotropic effects on isolated right atria of rats.[5]

■ ADVERSE EFFECTS AND INTERACTIONS

Paradoxically, high doses of iodine over a protracted period can lead to myxedema in patients sensitive to iodide.[3,4] Regarding kelp, the problem first emerged in Japan, where kelp is consumed in large amounts in some locales. This problem has since been observed in the west in people taking kelp for weight loss.[3]

Interactions between kelp and thyroid medications, including levothyroxine and iodine salts, are a possibility. Caution also has been advised in patients taking central nervous system stimulants.[3]

Kelp may be a useful nutritional supplement, but the consumption of excessive amounts is not without risk.

■ REFERENCES

1. Gosner KL. *Atlantic Seashore: Roger Tory Peterson Field Guides.* Norwalk, Conn: Easton Press; 1984:29.
2. Kelp. Available at: http://www.formulamaster.com/kelp.htm.
3. Miller LG. Selected clinical considerations focusing on known or potential drug-herb interactions. *Arch Intern Med* 1998;158:220.
4. Farwell AP, Braverman LP. Thyroid and antithyroid drugs. In: Hardman JG, Limbird L, Gilman AG, eds. *Goodman and Gilman's The Pharmacological Basis of Therapeutics.* 10th ed. New York, NY: McGraw-Hill; 2001:1584.
5. Chiu KW, Fung AYL. Cardiovascular effects of green beans (Phaseolus aureus), common rue (Ruta graveolens) and kelp (Laminaria japonica) in rats. *Gen Pharmacol* 1997;29:859.

KOLA

Discussion of kola herbs can be confusing. Several herbal products incorporate the name kola, and they come from different botanical sources and have quite different pharmacological properties. The three major categories, African kola, *Garcinia kola,* and Gotu kola, are dealt with separately in the monographs that follow.

KOLA (NUT, AFRICAN)

■ SOURCE, DESCRIPTION, USES

African kola nut herb comes from the seed kernel of a large African tree (*Cola nitida* and *C. acuminata*). The dried, powdered nut contains 2% caffeine plus other methylxanthines[1] and tannins.[2] Kola nut is widely used in Africa and elsewhere as a stimulant beverage. Traditionally, it is used to increase the capacity for physical exertion as well as for migraine headache, "nervous debility," diarrhea, and depression. Synonyms include cola nut and kola nut. In North America, this herb may show up in some herbal weight-loss products.

■ PHARMACOLOGY

The pharmacology of kola is essentially that of the methylxanthines, notably caffeine. Effects include central nervous system stimulation, cardioacceleration, decreased peripheral resistance, bronchodilation, and mild diuresis.

■ ADVERSE EFFECTS AND INTERACTIONS

The effects of excessive use are those of caffeine overdose, including nervousness, restlessness, irritability, and insomnia. In more extreme cases, toxic effects may progress to mild delirium and emesis. Muscle tremors, tachycardia, extrasystole, and rapid respiration may occur. Toxic effects may occur with as little as 1 g of caffeine, and a dose of 10 g of caffeine has been fatal.[3]

A particular concern with herbs rich in tannins is the possibility that they may be carcinogenic. This already has been demonstrated for betel nut[2] and mat (see MATÉ) and is a concern for kola nut users. There is no information regarding safety during pregnancy. Use in pregnant women should be discouraged as should use in children.See also Appendix II.

■ REFERENCES

1. Schulz V, Hansel R, Tyler VE. *Rational Phytotherapy: A Physician's Guide to Herbal Medicine.* New York, NY: Springer-Verlag; 1998:104.
2. Morton JF. Widespread tannin intake via stimulants and masticatories, especially guarana, kola nut, betel vine, and accessories. *Basic Life Sci* 1992;59:739.
3. Rall TW. Drugs used in the treatment of asthma: The methylxanthines, cromolyn sodium, and other agents. In: Gilman AG, Rall TW, Nies AS, Taylor P, eds. *Goodman and Gilman's The Pharmacological Basis of Therapeutics.* 8th ed. New York, NY: Pergamon Press; 1990:618.

KOLA (BITTER)

See KOLA (GARCINIA).

KOLA (GARCINIA)

■ SOURCE, DESCRIPTION, USES

Garcinia kola, or bitter kola, comes from a large West African forest tree (*Garcinia kola*) a member of the Guttiferae family. It also is cultivated as a source of medicinals. Young branches are used as chew sticks for oral hygiene, the pulp and seed are eaten to promote health, and an extract of the seeds is used to treat bronchitis, colds, sore throats, headache, and dysentery.[1]

■ PHARMACOLOGY

Interest in the pharmacological properties of *Garcinia kola* began in the early 1980s. Iwu[2] demonstrated remarkable hepatoprotective activity of an extract, kolaviron, in mice given phalloidin intraperitoneally. Mice that received 100 mg/kg of kolaviron intraperitoneally had a survival rate of 100% compared with 5% for the untreated controls. A more recent study has confirmed this hepatoprotective effect in rats challenged with 2-acetylaminofluorene.[3] Lipid peroxidation induced by the challenge also was prevented. Kolaviron is a mixture of a bioflavonoid (GB2) and kolaflavone.[3]

In addition to the hepatoprotective effect, *Garcinia kola* extracts have been shown to possess antiviral and anti-inflammatory activity, to inhibit gastrointestinal motility, and to promote weight loss.[1]

Other *Garcinia* species, such as *G. mangostana* and *G. pedunculata,* are listed in various Internet sites as substitutes for *G. kola,* but there do not appear to be any useful data regarding their characteristics.

■ ADVERSE EFFECTS AND INTERACTIONS

Garcinia kola does not contain methylxanthines in significant amounts; therefore, the adverse effects of African kola are not relevant to this herb. There do not appear to be any adverse effects reported for *Garcinia kola* seed extract. However, one study in rabbits reported a complex biphasic effect on the pharmacokinetics and antibacterial action of ciprofloxacin.[1] The interaction was antagonistic at 1 and 2.5 hours but potentiative at other times. Until more is known of the pharmacokinetics and drug interactions of *Garcinia kola,* it would be prudent to avoid concomitant use with other medications. More data are required to make informed decisions regarding this potentially useful herb.

■ REFERENCES

1. Esimone CO, Nwafor SV, Okoli Co, et al. In vivo evaluation of interaction between aqueous seed extract of Garcinia kola Heckel and ciprofloxacin hydrochloride. *Am J Ther* 2002;9:275.
2. Iwu MM. Antihepatoxic constituents of Garcinia kola seeds. *Experientia* 1985;41:699.
3. Farombi EO, Tahnteng JG, Agboola AO, Nwankwo JO, Emerole GO. Chemoprevention of 2-acetylaminofluorene-induced hepatotoxicity and lipid peroxidation in rats by kolaviron—a Garcinia seed extract. *Food Chem Toxicol* 2000;38:535.

KOLA (GOTU)

■ SOURCE, DESCRIPTION, USES

Gotu kola is prepared from the aerial parts of *Centella asiatica* (family Umbelliferae), a plant native to India, where it has been used as a medicinal plant for centuries. It is mentioned in Ayurvedic medical texts based on ancient Hindu scriptures. The plant is low and creeping, with a round leaf about the size of an old English penny, giving rise to its common name, Indian pennywort. It favors low, swampy areas[1] and also is widely cultivated in India, Madagascar, Sri Lanka, China, and parts of Africa.[2] Traditional uses of gotu kola have included as a "stimulatory-nervine tonic," rejuvenant, and sedative-tranquilizer, to promote healthy skin, as a sleep aid or diuretic, for high blood pressure, and to improve cognitive function.[1,2]

▓ PHARMACOLOGY

Gotu kola contains no caffeine and should not be confused with kola nut.[3] Gotu kola has been shown to have sedative properties in animal studies, which have been attributed to saponin glycosides called brahmoside and brahminoside.[3] In studies using avoidance and maze techniques, aqueous extracts of gotu kola have been shown to enhance learning and memory in male rats, and the higher doses decreased brain malondialdehyde and increased glutathione levels.[4]

In a placebo-controlled, double-blind study of human volunteers, the acoustic startle response (ASR) was used to test the anxiolytic potential of gotu kola crude herb powder.[2] Powdered gotu (12 g) was mixed with 300 mL of grape juice. Compared with placebo, the gotu kola significantly reduced the ASR amplitude at 30 and 60 minutes posttreatment. It had no effect on blood pressure, heart rate, or self-rated mood. The ASR is augmented by fear and anxiety and by anxiogenic agents such as caffeine and yohimbine.[2]

Current theory holds that cholecystokinin (CCK) receptors in the brain play a role in the panic response, and that patients with panic disorder have enhanced sensitivity to agonists of this receptor. A number of centrally acting herbs act as antagonists of this receptor, and studies with gotu kola suggest that it may interact with CCK-A and CCK-B receptors. Further research in this field may yield useful treatments for panic disorder.

▓ ADVERSE EFFECTS AND INTERACTIONS

Gotu kola appears to be well tolerated, although there have been reports of photosensitivity and hypersensitivity, especially with topical applications for eczema and ulcers.[3] Given the central action of this herb, the possibility of interactions with other centrally acting agents, whether drugs or herbs, cannot be discounted. There do not appear to be any data regarding safety in pregnancy or for children.See also Appendix II.

▓ REFERENCES

1. Gotu kola. Herbal Information Center website. Available at: http://www.kcweb.com/herb/gotu.htm.

2. Bradwejn J, Zhou Y, Koszycki D, Shlik J. A double-blind, placebo-controlled study on the effects of Gotu Kola (Centella asiatica) on acoustic startle response in healthy subjects. *J Clin Psychopharmacol* 2000;20:680.
3. Cauffield JS, Forbes HJM. Dietary supplements used in the treatment of depression, anxiety, and sleep disorders. *Prim Care* 1999;3:290.
4. Veerendra Kumar MH, Gupta YK. Effect of different extracts of Centrella asiatica on cognition and markers of oxidative stress in rats. *J Ethnopharmacol* 2002;79:253.

KUDZU

■ SOURCE, DESCRIPTION, USES

Kudzu root, from *Pueraria lobata* and other *Pueraria* species (family Fabaceae), has been used in Chinese herbal medicine for more than 2000 years. It is a perennial leguminous vine, native to eastern Asia, and first introduced to America in 1876 from Japan.[1,2] Since then, it is has become widely dispersed throughout the southeastern states, where it is sometimes referred to as the "foot-a-night" vine in recognition of its rapid rate of growth. Traditional herbal uses included as an antipyretic, antidiarrhetic, diaphoretic, and antiemetic.[1] Modern interest has focused on its potential for treating alcoholism (dipsomania).

■ PHARMACOLOGY

Kudzu root is rich in a number of pharmacologically active substances. These include the isoflavones genistein, daidzein, and daidzin, all of which have estrogenic properties (see PHYTOESTROGENS AND PHYTOPROG-ESTINS), as well as quercetin, which has numerous activities,[3] and puerarin, also a phytoestrogen, which accounts for 80% of the phytoestrogen content of kudzu.[4]

The Syrian golden hamster is noted for preferring ethanol to water in a free choice situation; using this as a model for dipsomania, it has been shown that crude methanol extract of kudzu root as well as daidzein and daidzin given intraperitoneally suppressed ethanol consumption by 50% or more. Daidzin appeared to account for most of the activity of the extract.[1] The mechanism appears to involve inhibition of aldehyde dehydrogenase in liver mitochondria, which is also the site of action of disulfiram.[1] The daidzin treatment that suppressed alcohol consumption more than 50% in hamsters, however, had no effect on plasma acetaldehyde levels, suggesting that its mechanism differs from that of disulfiram.[1]

To determine if kudzu root extract would alter drinking habits of veterans in a substance abuse program, a randomized, placebo-controlled, double-blind study was conducted using 1.2 g of root extract or placebo twice daily. Sobriety and craving for alcohol were assessed using a questionnaire and a rating scale of 0–10. Twenty-one subjects who received kudzu and 17 who received placebo finished the 1-month trial. There were no statistically significant differences in sobriety or craving for alcohol between the two groups.[5]

■ ADVERSE EFFECTS AND INTERACTIONS

No adverse effects were reported for the previously described trial. The lack of adverse reaction to subsequent alcohol consumption seems to confirm the belief that the herb does not act in the same way as disulfiram. There does not appear to be any information regarding the potential for drug interactions with kudzu but, on a biochemical basis, it would seem likely that it could modify the effects of disulfiram and, possibly, other drugs that have a disulfiram-like action, such as the sulfonylurea oral hypoglycemic agents.

This line of research may lead to new antidipsotropic agents, but the present information regarding safety and efficacy is insufficient to make an informed judgment.

■ REFERENCES

1. Keung WM, Vallee BL. Kudzu root: An ancient Chinese source of modern antidipsotropic agents. *Phytochemistry* 1998;47:499.
2. Pappert RA, Hamrick LJ, Donovan LA. Genetic variation in Pueraria lobata (Fabaceae), an introduced, clonal, invasive plant of the southeastern United States. *Am J Bot* 2000;87:12450.
3. Dr. Duke's phytochemical and ethnobotanical databases. Available at: http://www.ars-grin.gov/duke/plants.html.
4. Benlhabib E, Baker JI, Keyler DE, Singh AK. Composition, red blood cell uptake, and serum protein binding of phytoestrogens extracted from commercial kudzu-root and soy preparations. *J Med Food* 2002;5:109.
5. Shebek J, Rindone JP. A pilot study exploring the effect of kudzu on the drinking habits of patients with chronic alcoholism. *J Altern Complement Med* 2000;6:45.

L-CARNITINE

■ SOURCE, DESCRIPTION, USES

L-carnitine is a nonessential amino acid that is obtained in the diet largely from animal products. Normal, healthy individuals are not likely to develop a carnitine deficiency unless they are on a vegan diet without nutritional supplementation.[1] In individuals with certain pathological conditions and in the newborn that is not being breast-fed, however, nutritional supplementation with carnitine is required. This is called a conditioned, or conditionally essential, nutritional requirement.[1,2] L-carnitine also is being taken in the belief that it will improve stamina and athletic performance or promote weight loss.[1] Pharmaceutical-grade carnitine is available for oral and parenteral administration.[1]

■ PHARMACOLOGY

L-carnitine can be synthesized in the body from other essential amino acids. It is required for certain steps in lipid metabolism and is essential for the transport of long-chain fatty acids from the cytoplasm to the mitochondria for β-oxidation.[2] It binds toxic acyl groups and releases free coenzyme A. The acylcarnitine diffuses out of the cell for elimination in the urine and the coenzyme A is available to participate in glycolysis and other metabolic processes.[2] There is considerable evidence that congestive heart failure depletes the myocardium of several nutrients, including L-carnitine, coenzyme Q, and taurine.[2,3] There is some clinical evidence that supplementation with these agents restores their myocardial levels and reduces left ventricular diastolic volume, which could be of benefit prior to surgical revascularization.[2,3]

L-carnitine has been included in infant formulas for some time. It was reported however, that the addition of 25 mg/kg per day to the diet of premature infants did not improve growth or protect from episodes of hypoglycemia. This was a double-blind, placebo-controlled trial with 86 infants born between 28 and 34 gestational weeks.[4]

There is some evidence to suggest that patients with chronic fatigue syndrome (CFS) might benefit from L-carnitine supplementation. Although serum carnitine levels do not appear to be a reliable indicator of carnitine metabolism, patients with CFS have shown reduced serum levels of acylcarnitine, suggesting that the process of cellular detoxification is not functioning properly.[5] Trials with carnitine supplementation, however, have yielded mixed findings, and it has been suggested that there may be responders and nonresponders.[5] More research is required to define the role of L-carnitine in CFS.

Patients with acquired immunodeficiency syndrome have been shown to have low levels of L-carnitine in their monocytes and to respond with improved metabolic and immunological function after receiving 6 g/day for 2 weeks.[5] This observation seems to warrant further investigation.

Because it is important in energy metabolism, L-carnitine has become popular as a supplement for athletes hoping to improve stamina and performance. At present, there does not appear to be conclusive evidence to justify this claim for normal, nondeficient adults.

■ ADVERSE REACTIONS AND INTERACTIONS

No reports of adverse reactions are available.

■ REFERENCES

1. Borum PR. Supplements: Questions to ask to reduce confusion. *Am J Clin Nutr* 2000;72(suppl):538S.
2. Sole MJ, Jeejeebhoy KN. Conditioned nutritional requirements: Therapeutic relevance to heart failure. *Herz* 2002;27:174.
3. Jeejeebhoy F, Keith M, Freeman M, et al. Nutritional supplementation with MyoVive repletes essential cardiac myocyte nutrients and reduces left ventricular size in patients with left ventricular dysfunction. *Am Heart J* 2002;143:1092.
4. Shortland GJ, Walter JH. Randomized controlled trial of L-carnitine as a nutritional supplement in preterm infants. *Arch Dis Child Fetal Neonatal Ed* 1998;78:F185.
5. Werbach MR. Nutritional strategies for treating chronic fatigue syndrome. *Altern Med Rev* 2000;5:93.

L-TRYPTOPHAN

■ SOURCE, DESCRIPTION, USES

L-tryptophan, an essential amino acid that is the biochemical precursor to 5-hydroxytryptamine (serotonin),[1] is a component of many plant and animal proteins. It is commonly taken as a sleep-aid supplement, for depression,[2] and to minimize jet lag.

■ PHARMACOLOGY

Low serum L-tryptophan levels have been associated with depression in some small studies.[2] Animal studies have shown that serotonin is an important neurotransmitter in the central nervous system and an important modulator of a number of emotional and behavioral elements, including mood, sleep, aggression, pain, anxiety, and numerous physiological functions.[3,4] Release of serotonin from neurons appears to be greater when the subject is agitated or aggressive,[4] suggesting that a feedback loop may be operating. There have been studies indicating that L-tryptophan levels are depressed in a majority of individuals with chronic fatigue syndrome and fibromyalgia, whose plasma levels were inversely related to the severity of pain.[5] L-tryptophan supplementation has been shown to produce a mild analgesic response.[5] Pain relief was experienced to some degree by 50 fibromyalgia patients who received 100 mg three times daily of 5-hydroxytryptophan, a metabolite of L-tryptophan, for 3 months.[5]

■ ADVERSE EFFECTS AND INTERACTIONS

Concern over the use of L-tryptophan supplementation centers mainly on a condition known as eosinophilia-myalgia syndrome (EMS) that has been associated with it. In 1989, more than 1500 cases of EMS were identified in residents of New Mexico who had consumed a tryptophan supplement obtained from a single supplier in Japan.[2] In one series of 21 patients, all but one was female and all but one was Caucasian.[6] They were frequently described as "health-conscious." Typically, the onset of EMS was gradual, starting with flu-like symptoms and progressing to more serious symptoms, including severe myalgia, weakness, arthralgia, fever, and respiratory problems.[6] Laboratory findings included eosinophilia, increased total white cell count, and elevated levels of serum aldolase and aspartate aminotransaminase.[6] Hepatomegaly frequently was present. Symptoms generally, but not always, cleared with time when the patient stopped taking the supplement; however, there were 28 deaths in the New Mexico outbreak.[2]. Although some contaminants of the supplement were identified, it has not been possible to conclusively demonstrate that they are the causative agent.[2] Interestingly, melatonin has been associated with a few cases of eosinophilia (although no major outbreaks), and similar contaminants have been identified in commercial melatonin products.[7] (See also MELATONIN.) The U.S. Food and Drug Administration recalled all products containing L-tryptophan, but it is still available from several Internet sites. Also available is 5-hydroxytryptophan.

A "serotonin syndrome" has been described in patients who took tryptophan supplements along with serotonin uptake inhibitors or monoamine oxidase inhibitors.[2] The syndrome involves cardiovascular disturbances and Parkinson-like symptoms.

Until much more is known about the cause of ESR, the use of L-tryptophan supplements is a highly questionable practice, and use in conjunction with drugs that affect neurotransmitter function is contraindicated. See also Appendix II.

■ REFERENCES

1. Lefkowitz RJ, Hoffman BB, Taylor P. Neurohumoral transmission: The autonomic and somatic motor nervous systems. In: Gilman AG, Rall TW, Nies AP, Taylor P, eds. *Goodman and Gilman's The Pharmacological Basis of Therapeutics.* 8th ed. New York, NY: Pergamon Press; 1990:84.
2. Cauffield JS, Forbes HJM. Dietary supplements used in the treatment of depression, anxiety, and sleep disorders. *Prim Care* 1999;3:290.
3. Sandyk R. L-tryptophan in neuropsychiatric disorders. *Int J Neurosci* 1992;67:127.
4. Young SN, Teff KL. Tryptophan availability, 5-HT synthesis and 5-HT function. *Prog Neuropsychopharmacol Biol Psychiat* 1989;13:373.
5. Werbach MR. Nutritional strategies for treating chronic fatigue syndrome. *Altern Med Rev* 2000;5:93.
6. Philen RM, Eidson M, Kilbourne EM, Sewell CM, Voorhees R. Eosinophilia-myalgia syndrome: A clinical series of 21 patients. *Arch Intern Med* 1991;151:533.
7. Williamson BL, Tomlinson AJ. Structural characterization of contaminants found in commercial preparations of melatonin: Similarities to case-related compounds from L-tryptophan associated with eosinophilia-myalgia syndrome. *Chem Res Toxicol* 1998;11:234.

LAVENDER

■ SOURCE, DESCRIPTION, USES

Several species of lavender have been used herbally, including *Lavandula angustifolia* (English lavender), *L. officinalis, L. spica, L. stoechas* (French lavender), *L. dentata, L. latifolia,* and *L. pubescens.* Lavenders are indigenous to the western shores of the Mediterranean basin but are widely cultivated throughout Europe. None is native to North America.[1] The plants are aromatic evergreen shrubs, and the essential oil and extracts of the flowers have been used for centuries in scents and as folk remedies.[1,2]

Traditional uses, apart from use as a scent, included as a carminative (mainly English lavender) and "nervine" (to relieve nervous disorders), taken as a tea for headache (mainly French lavender), and topically as a disinfectant for wounds. *L.latifolia* has been used as an abortifacient, and *L. angustifolia* as a diuretic.[3]

■ PHARMACOLOGY

The main constituents of lavender are linalool, linalyl acetate, 1,8-cineole, cis and trans β-ocimene+, terpinen-4-ol, and camphor.[3] The content of the essential oil may vary, depending on the type of lavender as well as the extraction process, growing conditions, and so forth. The following discussion summarizes the main effects of lavender for which some documented evidence exists.

CENTRAL NERVOUS SYSTEM

Essential oil of lavender is used primarily for aromatherapy and as a body massage. There is evidence that linalool and linalyl acetate are absorbed rapidly through the skin and reach peak plasma levels within 20 minutes.[3] Linalool can alter acetylcholine release and ion channel activity at the neuromuscular junction. Both linalool and linlyl acetate were shown to have central nervous system depressant activity, including sedation and narcotic action, and have been shown experimentally to affect central neurotransmitters.[3] In one double-blind, placebo-controlled study, 15 patients with severe dementia and agitated behavior were exposed to aromatherapy. A 2% lavender essential oil steam was given in the ward for a 2-hour period daily, alternating with water alone every second day for ten treatment sessions. Ten Pittsburgh Agitation Scale (PAS) scores were obtained for each patient. Nine patients (60%) showed improvement, five (30%) showed no difference, and one (7%) became worse with the therapy. The group mean PAS score was significantly better ($p = .016$) than the control mean score.[4] In another controlled study, 17 patients in a cancer hospice were exposed to lavender oil 3% aromatherapy, water humidification only (control), or no treatment. They were assessed for vital signs as well as levels of pain, anxiety, depression, and sense of well being before and after each 60-minute session. Pain and anxiety levels were decreased compared with controls, but there were no differences in the other parameters. Blood pressure and heart rate were slightly lowered in both groups.[5] Lavender oil added to bath water has been reported to lessen postpartum discomfort.[3] Other studies have reported that lavender oil as a massage or as aromatherapy assisted elderly people to sleep better.[2,3,6]

There are obvious difficulties in interpreting data that rely heavily on subjective measures, but, taken together, the results suggest a modest benefit with little associated risk.

GASTROINTESTINAL AND UROGENITAL SYSTEMS

Animal studies have shown antispasmodic effect of lavender on both intestinal, and uterine, smooth muscle.[3] This effect was thought to be related to an intracellular increase in cyclic adenosine monophosphate. The oral administration of an aqueous extract of lavender has been shown to have diuretic properties in rats.[7]

OTHER ACTIVITIES

Lavender has been shown to possess antimicrobial and mosquito-repellant activity.[3,8] Lavender species also have been shown to possess significant antioxidant activity that correlates with the phenolic content of the extract.[9]

■ ADVERSE REACTIONS AND INTERACTIONS

No reports of adverse reactions or interactions are available. The effect of lavender on drug-metabolizing enzymes is not known. The use of lavender oil for aromatherapy or massage would seem to involve little risk, given the short-term and intermittent nature. More research is needed to confirm their possible benefits, and there is currently little known regarding the risks or benefits of oral administration.

■ REFERENCES

1. Lavenders. In: Grieve M. *A Modern Herbal*. Botanical.com website. Available at: http://www.botanical.com/botanical/mgmh/l/lavend13.html.
2. Cauffield J, Forbes HJM. Dietary supplements used in the treatment of depression, anxiety, and sleep disorders. *Prim Care* 1999;3:290.
3. Cavanagh HMA, Wilkinson JM. Biological activities of lavender essential oil. *Phytother Res* 2002;16:301.
4. Holmes C, Hopkins V, Hensford C, MacLaughlin V, Wilkinson D, Rosenvinge H. Lavender oil as a treatment for agitated behaviour in severe dementia: A placebo controlled study. *Int J Geriat Psychiat* 2002;17:305.
5. Louis M, Kowalski SD. Use of aromatherapy with hospice patients to decrease pain, anxiety, and depression and to promote an increased sense of well-being. *Am J Hosp Palliat Care* 2002;19:381.
6. Gyllenhaal C, Merritt S, Peterson SD, Block KI, Gochenour T. Efficacy and safety of herbal stimulants and sedatives in sleep disorders. *Sleep Med Rev* 2000;4:229.
7. Elhajili M, Baddouri K, Elkabbaj S, Meiouat F, Settaf A. Diuretic activity of the infusion of flowers from Lavandula officinalis [in French]. *Reprod Nutr Dev* 2001;41:393.

8. Choi WS, Park BS, Ku SK, Lee SE. Repellant activities of essential oils and monoterpenes against Culex pipiens pallens. *Am Mosq Control Assoc* 2002;18:348.
9. Parejo I, Viladomat F, Bastida J, et al. Comparison between the radical scavenging activity and antioxidant activity of six distilled and nondistilled Mediterranean herbs and aromatic plants. *J Agric Food Chem* 2002;50:6882.

LEI GONG TENG

See TRIPTERYGIUM WILFORDII.

LICORICE

■ SOURCE, DESCRIPTION, USES

The licorice plant, *Glycyrrhiza glabra*, is a member of the legume family native to China and India, where is has been cultivated for centuries. The root has been, and is, used as an expectorant and to soothe sore throats. It also was used in a paste to treat peptic ulcers, and licorice extract is still used for this purpose in many parts of Europe. Other applications have included rheumatoid arthritis and Addison's disease.[1] American wild licorice (*G. lepidota*) grows extensively throughout the western United States and Canada[2] and has similar properties. Licorice candy may contain artificial flavoring or low levels of natural-source licorice extract as indicated on product labels.

■ PHARMACOLOGY

Early on in the use of licorice paste for peptic ulcers, it was observed that some patients developed edema, and further investigation revealed that these high doses could lead to a syndrome resembling hyperaldosteronism with hypertension.[1] Glycyrrhetinic acid, the main triterpenoid present in licorice as a glycoside, inhibits gastric secretion. It was used to develop a drug, carboxolone sodium succinate, that is widely used in Europe to treat peptic ulcers. It is believed to inhibit prostaglandin synthesis and lipoxygenase.[3] Licorice appears to potentiate the effects of adrenocorticotropic hormone and corticosteroids, accounting for its effects in rheumatoid arthritis.[1]

Licorice root also contains phytoestrogens (see PHYTOESTROGENS AND PHYTOPROGESTINS) and possibly also antiestrogens.[1]

■ ADVERSE EFFECTS AND INTERACTIONS

Because of its aldosterone-like activity, licorice root extract is contraindicated in the presence of hypertension, hypokalemia, renal failure, and pregnancy. It also is contraindicated in liver disorders.[3] Excessive use can lead to a hyperaldosteronism-like syndrome. Children with apparent mineralocorticoid excess are usually hypertensive, and this should be considered an absolute contraindication to licorice root preparations.[1] Patients receiving corticosteroids likely will have to have dosage adjustment if they are taking licorice root. It has been shown to decrease plasma clearance and increase plasma levels of glucocorticoids, and to cause hypertension, edema, and hypokalemia in women taking oral contraceptives.[4]

The following mixtures of Chinese herbal medicines contain glycyrrhizin: sho-saiko-to, saibuku-to, and sairei-to. Homma and colleagues[5] conducted studies of the effects of these medicines on the pharmacokinetics of prednisolone in volunteers. Surprisingly, the results varied considerably. Sho-saiko-to decreased the area under the curve of prednisolone, saiboku-to increased it, and sairei-to had no effect. The authors suggest that unknown active principles or their metabolites might be responsible for these discrepancies. Several other herbs are present in these mixtures. See also Appendix VII.

■ REFERENCES

1. Davis EA, Morris DJ. Medicinal uses of licorice through the millennia: The good and plenty of it. *Molec Cell Endocrinol* 1991;78:3.
2. Niehaus TF, Ripper CL, Savage V. *Southeastern and Texas Wildflowers: Roger Tory Peterson Field Guides.* Norwalk, Conn: Easton Press; 1984:94.
3. Schulz V, Hansel R, Tyler VE. *Rational Phytotherapy: A Physician's Guide to Herbal Medicine.* New York, NY: Springer-Verlag; 1998:184.
4. Fugh-Berman A. Herb-drug interactions. *Lancet* 2000;355:134.
5. Homma M, Oka K, Ikeshima K, et al. Different effects of traditional Chinese medicines containing similar herbal constituents on prednisolone pharmacokinetics. *J Pharm Pharmacol* 1995;47:687.

LIQOURICE

See LICORICE.

LOBELIA

■ SOURCE, DESCRIPTION, USES

Lobelia inflata (family Lobelioideae) is the most common of several species of lobelia that grow throughout most of northeastern North America. It is a tall, slim plant having alternating lobate, toothed leaves and flowers that nestle at the stem of the uppermost leaves.[1] All are considered a subfamily of the bluebell family.[1] Synonyms include Indian-tobacco, pukeweed, gagroot, and asthma weed.[2] Traditionally, lobelia has been used as an expectorant, a diaphoretic, an emetic, and an antiasthmatic. Topically, it has been used for sprains and bruises.[2] The dried, flowering herb and seeds are used as the herbal remedy.

Current use of lobelia is mainly as an aid to smoking cessation. Evidence for the efficacy of this practice is scanty.

■ PHARMACOLOGY

The active principle of lobelia is the alkaloid α-lobeline. It has the same pharmacological activity as nicotine but is less potent. It stimulates nicotinic, cholinergic receptors in the autonomic ganglia and at the neuromuscular junction.[3] In the bronchial tree, this has the same bronchodilatory effect as would an adrenergic agonist; hence its use as an herbal remedy for asthma. Some studies suggest that lobeline acts not as a classical nicotine agonist but rather by potently inhibiting dopamine uptake into synaptic vesicles.[4] Another ingredient of lobelia, β-amyrin palmitate, has antidepressant activity and stimulates norepinephrine release.[5,6]

A recent study found that Hispanic parents were more likely than parents of other cultural groups to use potentially toxic herbal products such as lobelia to treat childhood asthma.[7]

■ ADVERSE EFFECTS AND INTERACTIONS

Because lobeline stimulates the sympathetic and the parasympathetic system as well as the neuromuscular junction, the signs and symptoms of lobelia intoxication are numerous and dose dependent. They can include progressive vomiting, weakness, tremor, pinpoint pupils, stupor, and unconsciousness. Tachycardia and respiratory stimulation may occur. Smoking lobelia leaves has been reported to cause hallucinations.[8,9]

There is an obviously high likelihood for lobelia to interact with other centrally acting drugs and herbal remedies. See also Appendix II. This is a potentially dangerous herb.

■ REFERENCES

1. Peterson RT, McKenny M. *Northeastern Wildflowers: Roger Tory Peterson Field Guides.* Norwalk, Conn: Easton Press; 1984:130.
2. Lobelia. In: Grieve M. *A Modern Herbal.* Botanical.com website. Available at: http://www.botanical.com/botanical/mgmh/l/lobeli38.html.
3. Taylor P. Agents acting the neuromuscular junction and autonomic ganglia. In: Hardman JG, Limbird L, Gilman AG, eds. *Goodman and Gilman's The Pharmacological Basis of Therapeutics.* 10th ed. New York, NY: McGraw-Hill; 2001:208.
4. Teng LT, Crooks PA, Dwoskin LP. Lobeline displaces [^{3}H] dihydrotetrabenzine binding and releases [^{3}H] dopamine from rat striatal synaptic vesicles: Comparison with d-amphetamine. *J Neurochem* 1998;71:258.
5. Subarnas A, Tadano T, Oshima Y, Kisara K, Ohizumi Y. Pharmacological properties of beta-amyrin palmitate, a novel centrally acting compound, isolated from Lobelia inflata leaves. *J Pharm Pharmacol* 1993;45:545.
6. Subarnas A, Tadano T, Nakahata N, et al. A possible mechanism of antidepressant activity of beta-amyrin palmitate isolated from Lobelia inflata leaves in the forced swimming test. *Life Sci* 1993;52:289.
7. Mazur LJ, De Ybarrondo L, Miller J, Colasurdo G. Use of alternative and complementary therapies for pediatric asthma. *Tex Med* 2001;97:64.
8. Dreisbach RH. *Handbook of Poisoning.* Los Altos, Calif: Lange; 1983:553.
9. Fisher CR, Veronneau SJH. Herbal preparations: A primer for the aeromedical physician. *Aviat Space Environ Med* 2000;71:45.

MA HUANG

See EPHEDRA.

MANDRAKE

■ SOURCE, DESCRIPTION, USES

The European mandrake (*Atropa mandragora*, family Solinaceae) also is known as *Mandragora officinarum*, mandragora, or Satan's apple.[1] It is a native of southern Europe and the eastern Mediterranean.[1] The plant is described as having a deep root 1 m or more in length, very large leaves (25 by 12 cm) that lie flat to the ground, and flowers resembling a primrose on a single stalk 10 to 15 cm in height.[1] Traditionally, the leaves have been used topically as a cooling poultice, in ointments, or boiled in milk as a poultice for skin conditions and ulcers. The root and root bark have been used as an emetic and a purgative.[1] The ancients had many uses for mandrake, including as a sedative, for melancholy, and for convulsions.

■ PHARMACOLOGY

As with many members of the Solanaceae family, mandrake contains anticholinergic belladonna alkaloids (muscarinic blocking agents), mainly scopolamine (hyoscine) and some atropine (hyosciamine). Other Solanaceae that contain these alkaloids include deadly nightshade (*Atropa belladonna*) and, to a lesser extent, common nightshade (*Solanum nigrum*) and bittersweet or woody nightshade (*Solanum dulcamara*). Jimsonweed (*Datura stramonium*) is another Solanaceae that contains large amounts of scopolamine, as is henbane (*Hyosciamus niger*). It is the scopolamine that imparts the central effects to mandrake, notably sedation.

■ ADVERSE EFFECTS AND INTERACTIONS

Adverse effects are those of muscarinic blocking activity and are dose related. See HENBANE for discussion of these effects. The anticholinergic toxidrome "red as a beet, blind as a bat, mad as a hatter, hotter than hell" describes the major signs and symptoms of intoxication.

It is well known that children are especially sensitive to the effects of these agents, and there have been cases of toxic psychoses after transdermal absorption of scopolamine in children and the elderly.[2]

Another problem associated with European mandrake is the risk that people may mistake American mandrake for the European variety. American mandrake, *Podophyllum pelatum* of the (unrelated) family Berberidaceae, is very toxic, containing a microtubule-dissolving podophyllotoxin that acts as a powerful emetic and purgative and can cause degenerative changes in the liver, kidney, and brain.[3] Cases of mistaken identity, even by suppliers of health food supplements, have resulted in poisonings.[4]

There is an obvious potential for mandrake to interact with other drugs that work in the central nervous system or the autonomic nervous system. See also Appendix II.

■ REFERENCES

1. Mandrake In: Grieve M. *A Modern Herbal.* Botanical.com website. Available at: http://www.botanical.com/botanical/mgmh/m/mandra10.html.
2. Brown JH, Taylor P. Muscarinic receptor agonists and antagonists. In: Hardman JG, Limbird L, Gilman AG, eds. *Goodman and Gilman's The Pharmacological Basis of Therapeutics.* 10th ed. New York, NY: McGraw-Hill; 2001:167.
3. Driesbach RH. *Handbook of Poisoning.* Los Altos, Calif: Lange; 1983:474.
4. Frasca T, Brett AS, Yoo SD. Mandrake toxicity: A case of mistaken identity. *Arch Intern Med* 1997;157:2007.

MARIGOLD

See CALENDULA.

MARSH MALLOW

■ SOURCE, DESCRIPTION, USES

Marsh mallow (*Althaea officinalis*, family Malvaceae) is a native of Europe that has been introduced to North America and that now grows extensively throughout the northeast. It favors the edges of swamps and has coarse-toothed, velvety, gray-green leaves and pink, five-petaled flowers.[1] Traditional use included as a demulcent, an emollient, a treatment for urinary tract infections, and, especially, for gastrointestinal upsets including diarrhea. The stem, leaves, and root are employed in herbal remedies.[2] The plant also has been used as a food source, especially the roots.[2]

■ PHARMACOLOGY

The soothing properties of marsh mallow are attributed to its high mucilage content. A recent study showed that an extract of marsh mallow inhibited endothelin-1–induced activation of human melanocytes as well as the secretion of endothelin-1 by keratinocytes.[3] These authors suggested that marsh mallow extract might be useful as a whitening agent.

■ ADVERSE EFFECTS AND INTERACTIONS

Marsh mallow would appear to be an innocuous plant. There has been a suggestion that it might inhibit the absorption of some drugs.[4]

■ REFERENCES

1. Peterson RT, McKenny M. *Northeastern Wildflowers: Roger Tory Peterson Field Guides.* Norwalk, Conn: Easton Press; 1984:258.
2. Mallow, marsh. In: Grieve M. *A Modern Herbal.* Botanical.com website. Available at: http://www.botanical.com/botanical/mgmh/m/mallow07.html.
3. Kobayashi A, Hachiya A, Ohuchi A, Kitahara T, Takema Y. Inhibitory mechanism of an extract of Althaea officinalis L. on endothelin-induced melanocyte activation. *Biol Pharm Bull* 2002;25:229.
4. Fisher CR, Veronneau SJH. Herbal preparations: A primer for the aeromedical physician. *Aviat Space Environ Med* 2000;71:45.

MATÉ

■ SOURCE, DESCRIPTION, USES

Maté comes from a white-flowered shrub, *Ilex paraguayensis* (or *araguariensis*), native to South America, mainly Paraguay. A tea made from the dried, powdered leaves of the plant is widely used in South America as a caffeinated beverage. Synonyms include Yerba maté, Paraguay tea, and Jesuit's tea, among others.[1] In Brazil it is called *chimarrao*. It is used as a tonic, diaphoretic, and powerful stimulant, as well as a social beverage.

■ PHARMACOLOGY

The principle ingredient is caffeine. Tannins also are present.[1] The dried herb has been reported to contain 0.5% to 1.5% caffeine.[2] By comparison, tea may contain 2.5% to 5.5% caffeine.[2] The pharmacological actions of maté are those of caffeine: central nervous stimulation, cardioacceleration, and mild diuresis, to name but a few.[3] An herbal combination consisting of maté, guarana, and damiana has been tested as an aid to weight loss. This product, YGD, delayed gastric emptying and led to significant weight loss over 45 days compared with a placebo.[4]

■ ADVERSE EFFECTS AND INTERACTIONS

The effects of excessive use of are those of caffeine overdose. They include nervousness, restlessness, irritability, and insomnia; in more extreme cases, toxic effects may progress to mild delirium and emesis. Muscle tremors, tachycardia, extrasystole, and rapid respiration may occur. Toxic effects may occur with as little as 1 g of caffeine, and a dose of 10 g has been fatal.[3] Because of the relatively low caffeine content of maté, severe toxicity is unlikely, but the large amounts that are consumed can cause mild symptoms of intoxication.

The greatest concern regarding use of this herb relates to the likelihood that it contains carcinogens. Numerous studies have shown that heavy use of maté beverage is associated with a significant increase in the risk of several cancers, notably of the oropharyngeal cavity, larynx, and esophagus. In one Brazilian study, the relative risk factors for oral and laryngeal cancers were 1.9 and 2.2 for heavy users.[5] In a study in Uruguay, there was a dose-related increase of the risk of bladder cancer in maté drinkers.[6] When individuals who consumed less than 0.5 L daily were taken as an odds ratio (OR) of 1, those who consumed 0.5 to 0.99 L had an OR of 1.9, and those who consumed in excess of 1.5 L had an OR of 13.7. Renal cancer, too, has been shown to be higher in heavy users in Uruguay, who had a renal carcinoma relative risk of 3.0.[7]

There has been considerable debate over whether the cancers of the upper aerodigestive tract are due to thermal injury or to the presence of a carcinogen. The drink is consumed through a metal, filtered tube and is taken at a very high temperature. To date, no carcinogen or mutagen has been isolated from maté. These facts would seem to argue in favor of thermal injury, but the association of increased risk of kidney and bladder cancers are more suggestive of a carcinogen. In one study, there appeared to be a synergistic effect between the amount consumed and high temperature.[8] Although most other hot beverages also increased risk, black coffee did not. A diet rich in vegetables, fruits, and cereals had a protective effect. It seems unlikely that maté consumption would pose a serious risk for cancer in North America, except perhaps in some subpopulations of South American origin. There is no information regarding safety during pregnancy. Use in pregnant women should be discouraged, as should use in children.

Centrally acting agents, whether herbal remedies, prescription drugs, or over-the-counter (OTC) medications, carry a significant risk of adverse effects and interactions. OTC nasal decongestants, sedating antihistamines, and antinausea agents may interact with caffeine-rich beverages (see also Appendix II).

■ REFERENCES

1. Paraguay tea. In: Grieve M. *A Modern Herbal*. Botanical.com website. Available at: http://www.botanical.com/botanical/mgmh/p/partea05.html.
2. Schulz V, Hansel R, Tyler VE. *Rational Phytotherapy: A Physician's Guide to Herbal Medicine*. New York, NY: Springer-Verlag; 1998:104.
3. Undem BJ, Lichtenstein LM. Drugs used in the treatment of asthma. In: Hardman JG, Limbird L, Gilman AG, eds. *Goodman and Gilman's The Pharmacological Basis of Therapeutics*. 10th ed. New York, NY: McGraw-Hill; 2001:746.
4. Anderson T, Fogh J. Weight loss and delayed gastric emptying following a South American herbal preparation in overweight patients. *J Hum Nutr Diet* 2001;14:243.
5. Pintos J, Franco EL, Oliveira BV, Kowalski LP, Curado MP, Dewar R. Mate, coffee and tea consumption and risk of cancers of the upper aerodigestive tract in southern Brazil. *Epidemiology* 1994;5:583.
6. De Stefani E, Correa P, Fierro L, Fontham E, Chen V, Zavala D. Meat intake, Black tobacco, mate and bladder cancer. A case-control study from Uruguay. *Cancer* 1991;67:536.
7. De Stefani E, Fierro L, Correa P, et al. Meat intake, 'mate' drinking and renal cell cancer in Uruguay: A case-control study. *Br J Cancer* 1998;78:1239.
8. Castellsague X, Munoz N, De Stefani E, Victora CG, Castelletto R, Rolon PA. Influence of mate drinking hot beverages and the diet on esophageal cancer risk in South America. *Int J Cancer* 2000;88:658.

MEADOW SAFFRON

See COLCHICUM.

MEADOWSWEET

■ SOURCE, DESCRIPTION, USES

Meadowsweet (*Filipendula ulmaria*, formerly *Spiraea ulmaria*) is a member of the Rosaceae family and native to northern Europe. The herb consists of dried flowers and unopened buds.[1] It is used in teas, alone or with other herbs, as an antipyretic for colds and flu. Related North American species, native to the northeast, are *Spiraea latifolia* and *S. alba*.[2]

■ PHARMACOLOGY

Meadowsweet flowers contain several substances with pharmacological potential, including the flavonol glycoside quercetin-4-glycoside (spiraeoside), tannins, salicylaldehyde, and methyl salicylate.[1] Phenolic components have been identified as having potent antioxidant properties.[3] Some quercetin glycosides have been shown to be hypotensive.[4] Salicylate levels are not thought to be high enough to account for the diaphoretic activity of meadowsweet, according to some authors,[1] whereas others[5] list the salicylate content as high.

■ ADVERSE EFFECTS AND INTERACTIONS

Heck and colleagues[5] note a potential for potentiation of warfarin by meadowsweet and attribute this to inhibition of platelet function by the salicylates in the herb. Russian investigators, however, have found significant anticoagulant and fibrinolytic activity in both the flowers and the seeds of meadowsweet.[6] This activity was noted after oral administration in experimental animals, as well as in vitro, which is not suggestive of a coumarin type of agent. Meadowsweet should not be given to anyone taking oral anticoagulants and probably not to anyone taking platelet-inhibiting drugs. See also Appendices I, VII and VIII.

■ REFERENCES

1. Shulz V, Hansel R, Tyler VE. *Rational Phytotherapy: A Physician's Guide to Herbal Medicine.* New York, NY: Springer-Verlag; 1998:143.
2. Peterson RT, McKenny M. *Northeastern Wildflowers: Roger Tory Peterson Field Guides.* Norwalk, Conn: Easton Press; 1984:284.
3. Kahkonen MP, Hopia AI, Vuorela HJ, et al. Antioxidant activity of plant extracts containing phenolic compounds. *J Agric Food Chem* 1999;47:3954.
4. Wang HX, Ng TB. Natural products with hypoglycemic, hypotensive, hypocholesterolemic, antiatherosclerotic and antithrombotic activities. *Life Sci* 1999;65:2663.
5. Heck AM, deWitt BA, Lukes AL. Potential interactions between alternative therapies and warfarin. *Am J Health Syst Pharm* 2000;57:1221.
6. Liapina L, Koval'chuk GA. A comparative study of the action on the hemostatic system of extracts from the flowers and seeds of the meadowsweet (Filipendula ulmaria [L.] Maxim.) [in Russian]. *Izv Akad Nauk Ser Biol* 1993;4:625.

MELATONIN

■ SOURCE, DESCRIPTION, USES

Melatonin is a hormonal substance produced by the pineal gland that regulates the sleep cycle. Its synthesis is inhibited by light, and a burst of melatonin is secreted at night, peaking in the early hours of the morning.[1] Melatonin is widely consumed as a sleep aid.

■ PHARMACOLOGY

In all mammals, the circadian cycle is modulated by a so-called internal clock, a molecular oscillator centered in the suprachiasmatic nucleus (SCN) of the hypothalamus.[2] The autonomic nervous system links the SCN to the periphery. Melatonin is synthesized in the SCN according to the following pathway: dietary tryptophan → serotonin→ melatonin.[1] It activates α- and β-adrenoreceptors. Both alpha- and beta-blocking drugs can disrupt the process. Melatonin is the humoral link between the SCN and the peripheral organs, and it also acts on melatonin receptors in the SCN, relaying temporal, light-dark signals from the periphery. Clinical studies indicate that persons who are long sleepers have a longer so-called biological night, as indicated by nocturnal high plasma melatonin levels and also by high plasma cortisol levels and lowered body temperature.[3] Melatonin has other physiological properties that have been identified experimentally, such as free radical scavenging and reduction of bone loss associated with aging.[4]

Clinical evidence of the efficacy of melatonin as a sleep aid is equivocal. In a survey of over-the-counter sleep aids, Chung and colleagues[5] reviewed several clinical studies of melatonin and concluded that the evidence was not conclusive. Several studies found no relief of insomnia using subjective measures, nor did one study that used objective measures. Several other studies that used objective measures found significant improvement in quality and quantity of sleep. In a study of dementia patients who experienced agitation during night-time, Serfaty and colleagues[6] found no evidence that 2 weeks of low-dose melatonin treatment (6 mg slow-release tablets/day) produced any improvement in sleep patterns. Studies in neurologically impaired children found that 2.5 to 5.0 mg improved sleep patterns whereas lower doses had no effect.[1]

■ ADVERSE EFFECTS AND INTERACTIONS

Gastrointestinal disturbances have been reported with high doses of melatonin,[1] as has lethargy and a "hung over" feeling. Animal studies have shown that melatonin can cause coronary and cerebral arterial vaso-constriction,[7] a potential cause for concern in some patients. Exacerbation of symptoms in depressed patients is also a concern.[7] Other effects that have been noted include hypothermia, depressed libido, and retinal damage. Little is known about potential interactions with other drugs that act in the central nervous system, but this cannot be dismissed as a potential problem. A particular concern is the eosinophilia that has been observed in cancer patients receiving melatonin. Analysis of melatonin preparations found the same chemical contaminants that have been identified in L-tryptophan.[8] L-tryptophan has been the cause of outbreaks of sometimes-fatal eosinophilia-myalgia, the cause of which is poorly understood. To date, no similar outbreaks have been reported for melatonin, but more data and a better understanding of the phenomenon are required.

In summary, melatonin might be a useful aid to sleep when taken in a controlled and monitored environment, but the attendant risks would seem to argue against its indiscriminate use as a proprietary sleep aid.

■ REFERENCES

1. Cauffield JS, Forbes HJM. Dietary supplements used in the treatment of depression, anxiety, and sleep disorders. *Prim Care* 1999;3:290.

2. Mutoh T, Shibata S, Korf HW, Okamura H. Melatonin modulates the light-induced sympathoexcitation and vagal suppression with participation of the suprachiasmatic nucleus in mice. *J Physiol* 2003;547(pt 1):317.

3. Aeschbach D, Sher L, Postolache TT, Matthews JR, Jackson MA, Wehr TA. A longer biological night in long sleepers than in short sleepers. *J Clin Endocrinol Metab* 2003;88:26.

4. Cardinali DP, Ladizesky MG, Boggio V, Cutrera RA, Mautalen C. Melatonin effects on bone: Experimental facts and clinical perspectives. *J Pineal Res* 2003;34:81.

5. Chung KF, Lee CKY. Over-the-counter sleeping pills: A survey of use in Hong Kong and a review of their constituents. *Gen Hosp Psychiat* 2002;24:430.

6. Serfaty M, Kennell-Webb S, Warner J, Blizard R, Raven P. Double blind randomised placebo controlled trial of low dose melatonin for sleep disorders in dementia. *Int J Geriat Psychiat* 2002;17:1120.

7. Lamberg L. Melatonin potentially useful but safety, efficacy remain uncertain. *JAMA* 1996;276:1011.

8. Williamson BL, Tomlinson AJ, Mishra PK, Gleich GJ, Naylor S. Structural characterization of contaminants found in commercial preparations of melatonin: Similarities to case-related compounds from L-tryptophan associated with eosinophilia-myalgia. *Chem Res Toxicol* 1998;11:234.

MENISPERMUM SPECIES

■ SOURCE, DESCRIPTION, USES

A number of *Menispermum* species (family Menispermaceae) have been used as herbal medicines. One, *M. canadense*, is native to North America. It is a woody climbing vine with rounded, slightly lobular leaves. Small clusters of flowers develop into black, grape-like fruit,[1] which could be mistaken for wild grape. Synonyms include Canada moonseed, yellow parilla, Texas sarsaparilla, and vine maple.[2] Traditional use for the dried roots, in small doses, included as a tonic, diuretic, or laxative. Larger doses were claimed to stimulate appetite and increase bowel activity, and high doses acted as a purgative and induced vomiting.[2]

M. dauricum grows throughout much of China, and the root and rhizome are listed in the Chinese Pharmacopoeia as analgesics and antipyretics.[3] They have been used in traditional Chinese medicine for centuries.

■ PHARMACOLOGY

All species are rich in biologically active alkaloids. Among these, acutamine has been shown to inhibit the growth of cultured human T–cells.[3]. Dauricoside, an alkaloid glycoside, dauricine, and daurisoline inhibited platelet aggregation induced by adenosine diphosphate.[4] Daurisoline also has been shown to block P-type calcium channels in rat cerebellar slices.[5] A mixture of phenolic alkaloids offered some protection against ischemia-reperfusion injury in rabbits.[6] Oxoisoaporphine alkaloids have shown cytotoxic activity against a variety cancer cell lines, and showed experimental anticancer activity.[7]

■ ADVERSE EFFECTS AND INTERACTIONS

Given the number of active principles present in *Menispermum,* it is not surprising that there is a high risk of adverse reactions. The U.S. Food and Drug Administration lists *Menispermum* species among those containing aristolochic acids, the importation of which into the United States has been banned because of their toxicity.[8]

Several cases have been reported of end-stage renal failure and several of nephropathy associated with the use of Chinese herbal medicines for weight reduction. Unique histopathological changes in the kidneys (cortical interstitial fibrosis with relative preservation of the glomeruli) led to the coining of the term *Chinese herbal nephropathy* (CHN) for this condition. See ARISTOLOCHIA for more details.

This family of plants may yield useful pharmacological agents, but as herbal remedies they carry significant risks. See also Appendix III.

■ REFERENCES

1. Peterson RT, McKenny M. *Northeastern Wildflowers: Roger Tory Peterson Field Guides.* Norwalk, Conn: Easton Press; 1984:xix, 76.
2. Parilla, yellow. In: Grieve M. *A Modern Herbal.* Botanical.com website. Available at: http://www.botanical.com/botanical/mgmh/p/parill07.html.
3. Yu BW, Chen JY, Wang YP, Cheng KF, Li XY, Qin GW. Alkaloids from Menispermum dauricum. *Phytochemistry* 2002;61:439.
4. Hu SM, Xu SX, Yao XS, Cui CB, Tezuka Y, Kikuchi T. Dauricoside, a new glycosidal alkaloid having an inhibitory activity against blood-platelet aggregation. *Chem Pharm Bull (Tokyo)* 1993;41:1866.
5. Lu YM, Frostl W, Dreessen J, Knopfel T. P-type calcium channels are blocked by the alkaloid daurisoline. *Neuroreport* 1994;5:1489.
6. Wang F, Qu L, Lv Q, Guo LJ. Effect of phenolic alkaloids from Menispermum dauricum on myocardial-cerebral ischemia-reperfusion injury in rabbits. *Acta Pharmacol Sin* 2001;22:1130.
7. Yu BW, Meng LH, Chen JY, et al. Cytotoxic oxoisoaporphine alkaloids from Menispermum dauricum. *J Nat Prod* 2001;64:968.
8. U.S. Food and Drug Administration. Listing of botanical ingredients of concern. FDA/Center for Food Safety and Applied Nutrition. Available at: http://vm.cfsan.fda.gov/~dms/csds-bo2.html.

MILK THISTLE (SILYBUM)

■ SOURCE, DESCRIPTION, USES

The milk thistle (*Silybum marianus*) is native to Europe and North Africa and has been introduced elsewhere, including to North America.[1] It is an annual or biennial plant of the Asteraceae family, growing up to 2 m in height.[2] Used for centuries in European folk medicine for liver problems, it was called Marian thistle in early Christian tradition.[1] It also is known as sylibum. The herbal remedy is prepared from the fruit of the plant, the crude preparation consisting of the ripe fruit from which the pappus (downy appendage) has been removed.[2] The fruits contain about 15% to 30% fatty oil and 20% to 30% protein.[2] The active constituents comprise about 2% to 3% of the dried herb.

■ PHARMACOLOGY

The references cited here represent a small fraction of the extensive literature that has developed regarding milk thistle's active principles. The mixture of active principles, called silymarin, is comprised of four isomers. The main one is silybinin (50%), a polyphenolic flavonoid and the agent of main therapeutic interest. It is spelled in several ways. The others are isosylibinin, silydianin, and silychristin.[2,3] Silymarin is not water-soluble and cannot be taken as a tea. It usually is taken in gelatin capsules.[4]

One of the most widely confirmed uses for silymarin is in the treatment of poisoning with the mushroom *Amanita phalloides* and other *Amanita* species. This protective action has been repeatedly demonstrated and may be effective up to 3 days after the ingestion of the mushrooms.[4] Hepatoprotective activity has been demonstrated, by reductions in serum enzyme levels and long-term survival rates, in chronic hepatitis, acute alcohol poisoning, chronic alcoholic liver disease, and alcoholic cirrhosis.[2,4]

The hepatoprotective action of silymarin has not been confirmed in all clinical studies of alcoholic liver disease, and use of silymarin in that condition remains somewhat controversial. Luper[4] cites a French study that failed to demonstrate that 420 mg/day of silymarin for 3 months altered the course of proven alcoholic hepatitis. Langmead and Rampton[5] reviewed several, controlled clinical trials and concluded that together, they made it unlikely that silymarin would be of significant use in treating alcoholic liver disease. Angulo and colleagues[5] described a study of 27 patients with primary biliary cirrhosis who had been on ursodeoxycholic acid for prolonged periods and showed persistent elevations of alkaline phosphatase activity more than 2 times upper-normal values. Silymarin, 140 mg three times daily, was added to the regimen for 1 year but failed to alter serum enzyme, bilirubin, or albumin values or Mayo risk scores.

Studies in experimental animals confirm a wide variety of pharmacological activities. These include inhibition by silybinin of growth of human prostate carcinoma cells in athymic nude mice,[3] prevention of ultraviolet-induced immune suppression and oxidative damage in mouse skin (strain C3H/HeN) by silymarin,[7] increase in the expression of transforming growth factors by silymarin,[8] protection by silymarin against skin tumors induced by prompters in mice,[9] and protection against azoxymethane-induced colon cancer in F344 rats.[10]

Recently, it was shown that silymarin inhibited inducible nitric oxide synthase (iNOS), and hence nitric oxide (NO) synthesis, in mouse macrophages after being given orally to the mice.[11] iNOS is highly expressed in macrophages, and NO synthesis plays an important role in inflammatory processes. Inhibition of iNOS could thus account for part of the anti-inflammatory activity of silymarin.

It is conceivable that, in the future, this herbal agent may lead to the development of useful therapeutic agents.

■ ADVERSE EFFECTS AND INTERACTIONS

Oral silymarin appears to be well tolerated. There have been some reports of mild gastrointestinal distress associated with its use.[2,4] There is one report of a woman who experienced severe abdominal pain, diarrhea, vomiting, weakness, and collapse every time she took a preparation containing milk thistle.[12] The possibility that some other ingredient in the capsules was the offending agent could not be ruled out.

By far the greatest potential problem with milk thistle and silymarin is their ability to inhibit several of the cytochrome P450 (CYP450) drug metabolizing enzymes. The major flavonolignans of silymarin have been shown to inhibit CYP2D6, CYP3A4, CYP2E1, and CYP2C9 in a dose-dependent manner at micromolar concentrations.[13,14] Inhibition of these drug-metabolizing enzymes could lead to unexpected increases in plasma levels of many drugs. Despite this possibility, one study failed to demonstrate clinically significant decreases in blood levels of indinavir in healthy volunteers given 153 mg of silymarin three times daily for 13 weeks,[15] although modest reductions in the area under the curve were noted. Nevertheless, extreme caution should be exercised in using silymarin with prescription drugs until more information is available regarding interactions. The lessons of St. John's wort, that inhibition of drug metabolizing enzymes can have serious consequences, should be heeded. See also Appendix VI.

The usual caveats regarding the use of this herb in children and pregnant mothers pertain.

■ REFERENCES

1. Milk thistle. Herbal Information Center website. Available at: http://www.kcweb.com/herb/milkt.htm.
2. Schulz V, Hansel R, Tyler VE. *Rational Phytotherapy: A Physician's Guide to Herbal Medicine.* New York, NY: Springer-Verlag; 1998:214.
3. Singh RP, Dhanalakashmi S, Tyagi AK, Chan DC, Agarwal C, Agarwal R. Dietary feeding of silibinin inhibits advance human prostate carcinoma growth in athymic nude mice and increases plasma insulin-like growth factor-binding protein-3 levels. *Cancer Res* 2002;62:3063.
4. Luper S. A review of plants used in the treatment of liver disease: Part 1. *Altern Med Rev* 1998;3:410.
5. Langmead L, Rampton, DS. Review article: Herbal treatment in gastrointestinal and liver disease—benefits and dangers. *Aliment Pharmacol Ther* 2001;15:1239.
6. Angulo P, Patel T, Jorgensen RA, Therneau TM, Lindor KD. Silymarin in the treatment of primary biliary cirrhosis with a suboptimal response to ursodeoxycholic acid. *Planta Med* 2000;32:897.

7. Katiyar SK. Treatment of silymarin, a plant flavonoid, prevents ultraviolet light-induced immune suppression and oxidative stress in mouse skin. *Int J Oncol* 2002;21:1213.

8. He Q, Osuchowski MF, Johnson VJ, Sharma RP. Physiological responses to a natural antioxidant flavonoid mixture, silymarin, in BALB/c mice: I induction of transforming growth factor beta 1 and c-myc in liver with marginal effects on other genes. *Planta Med* 2002;68:676.

9. Ahmad N, Gali H, Javed S, Agarwal R. Skin cancer chemopreventive effects of a flavonoid antioxidant silymarin are mediated via impairment of receptor tyrosine kinase signaling and perturbation in cell cycle progression. *Biochem Biophys Res Comm* 1998;248:294.

10. Kohno H, Tanaka T, Kawabata K, et al. Silymarin, a naturally occurring polyphenolic antioxidant flavonoid, inhibits azoxymethane-induced colon carcinogenesis in male F344 rats. *Int J Cancer* 2002;101:461.

11. Kang JS, Jeon YJ, Kim HM, Han SH, Yang KH. Inhibition of inducible nitric-oxide synthase expression by silymarin in lipopolysaccharide-stimulated macrophages. *J Pharmacol Exp Ther* 2002;302:138.

12. Adverse Drug Reactions Committee. An adverse reaction to the herbal medication milk thistle (Silybum marianum). *Med J Aust* 1999;170:218.

13. Zuber R, Modriansky M, Dvorak Z. Effect of silybin and its congeners on human liver microsomal cytochrome P450 activities. *Phytother Res* 2002;16:632.

14. Beckmann-Knopp S, Rietbrock S, Weyhenmeyer R, et al. Inhibitory effects of silibinin on cytochrome P-450 enzymes in human liver microsomes. *Pharmacol Toxicol* 2000;86:250.

15. Piscitelli SC, Formentini E, Burstein AH, Alfaro R, Jagannatha S, Falloon J. Effects of milk thistle on the pharmacokinetics of indinavir in healthy volunteers. *Pharmacotherapy* 2002;22:551.

MISTLETOE (EUROPEAN)

■ SOURCE, DESCRIPTION, USES

European mistletoe (*Viscum album*) is a semiparasitic shrub of the family Loranthaceae that is native to much of Europe. It has shiny green leaves, small yellow flowers, and sticky white berries. Ancient beliefs attributed aphrodisiacal powers and the ability to protect against poisons to mistletoe. It was believed to possess mystical powers and played an important role in many ancient cultures, including the Celts, Germans, and Greeks. The name is a corruption of two Anglo-Saxon words, *mistel,* meaning dung, and *tan,* meaning twig. The name derived from the observation that the plant often grew on branches where bird droppings had been deposited. The droppings contained seeds from berries eaten by the birds.[1] American mistletoe (*Phoradendron flavescens*) is very similar in appearance to the European variety,[2] but its medicinal characteristics have not been elucidated. Current herbal usage of European mistletoe (EM) is focused on its potential as an immunostimulant and anticancer agent.

■ PHARMACOLOGY

The most important active principles in EM appear to be lectins.[3] Stimulation of T lymphocytes and phagocytosis have been demonstrated in animal studies.[3] Iscador, a total extract or EM, was first used to treat cancer in 1922.[4] Since that time, numerous clinical trials have been conducted with mixed results, but it remains the most widely used complementary cancer treatment in Germany.[4] In one large, nonrandomized, matched pair study (396 pairs), survival time was prolonged in the Iscador-treated group compared with the control group for patients diagnosed with several cancers. These were carcinoma of the stomach, colon, rectum, breast (without metastases, with axillary metastases, and with distal metastases), and small-cell and non—small-cell bronchogenic carcinoma. The differences were statistically significant ($p < .05$ to $p < .01$) for six of these eight diagnoses. Two small, randomized studies supported these findings but were not well controlled. There also was evidence that a minimum period of treatment was necessary to yield the effect. In a randomized, controlled study of EM lectin given subcutaneously (the usual route of administration) to patients undergoing transurethral resection for bladder cancer, there was no difference between treated and control groups after 18 months with regard to number of recurrences, time to first recurrence, or recurrence-free outcomes.[5] EM extract also was studied as adjunctive therapy in a randomized, controlled trial involving 477 patients with head and neck squamous cell carcinoma who received surgery with or without radiotherapy. Those receiving the EM extract showed no difference to 5-year survival rate and no detectable differences in cellular immune responses or quality of life.[6] A review of clinical studies with EM lectins concluded that there was not yet convincing evidence of inhibition of tumor progression or prolongation of survival time, but there was perhaps some improvement of quality of life.[7]

There is much laboratory evidence that EM lectins possess pharmacological properties suggestive of antineoplastic activity. Such activities include cytotoxicity through stimulation of natural killer cells, immunostimulation, and tumor-suppressing activity in animals.[8,9] Nevertheless, convincing clinical evidence for antineoplastic activity remains elusive. Other species of mistletoe currently are being investigated and have shown a variety of activities in the laboratory.[10–12]

■ ADVERSE EFFECTS AND INTERACTIONS

Although side effects do not seem to be common, EM extract and its lectins are cytotoxic and, therefore, potentially hazardous. Chills, fever, headache, chest pain, and orthostatic hypotension have been reported.[3] Allergic reactions occur, including anaphylaxis,[13] and hypereosinophilia has been reported.[14]

The use of EM extract for the treatment or amelioration of cancer should be considered to be in the experimental stage. If EM is used, it should be under the supervision of an oncologist. There is a danger that individuals who self-medicate with the herb could interfere with their prescribed therapy and possibly put themselves at risk from adverse effects or therapeutic failure. It must be kept in mind that patients may take the herb for other conditions such as arthritis and not be aware of its cytotoxic properties.

■ REFERENCES

1. Available at: Mistletoe at: http://www.ag.usask,ca/cofa/departments/hort/hortinfo/misc/mistleto.html.
2. Petrides G. *Trees and Shrubs: Roger Tory Peterson Field Guides.* Boston, Mass: Houghton Mifflin; 1984:69.
3. Schulz V, Hansel R, Tyler VE. *Rational Phytotherapy: A Physician's Guide to Herbal Medicine.* New York, NY: Springer-Verlag; 1998:278.
4. Grossarth-Maticek R, Kiene H, Baumgartner SM, Ziegler R. Use of Iscador, an extract of European mistletoe (Viscum album), in cancer treatment: Prospective nonrandomized and randomized matched-pair studies nested within a cohort study. *Altern Therap* 2001;7:57.
5. Goebell PJ, Otto T, Suhr J, Rubben H. Evaluation of an unconventional treatment modality with mistletoe lectin to prevent recurrence of superficial bladder cancer: a randomized phase II trial. *J Urol* 2002;168:72.
6. Steuer-Vogt MK, Bonkowsky V, Ambrosch P, et al. The effect of adjuvant mistletoe treatment programme in resected head and neck cancer patients: A randomized controlled clinical trial. *Eur J Cancer* 2001;37:23.
7. Stauder H, Kreuser ED. Mistletoe extracts standardized in terms of mistletoe lectins (ML I) in oncology: Current state of clinical research. *Onkologie* 2002;25:374.
8. Mengs U, Gothel D, Leng-Peschlow E. Mistletoe extracts standardized to mistletoe lectins in oncology: Review on current status of preclinical research. *Anticancer Res* 2002;22:1399.
9. Tabiasco J, Pont F, Fournie JJ, Vercellone A. Mistletoe viscotoxins increase natural killer cell-mediated cytotoxicity. *Eur J Biochem* 2002;269:2591.

10. Deeni YY, Sadiq NM. Antimicrobial properties and phytochemical con-
    stituents of the leaves of African mistletoe (Tapinanthus dodoneifolius
    (DC) Danser) (Loranrhaceae): An ethnomedical plant of Hausaland,
    northern Nigeria. *J Ethnopharmacol* 2002;83:235.
11. Lin J-H, Chiou Y-N, Lin Y-L. Phenolic glycosides from Viscum angula-
    tum. *J Nat Prod* 2002;65:638.
12. Li SS, Gullbo J, Lindholm P, et al. Ligatoxin B, a new cytotoxic protein
    with a novel helix-turn-helix DNA-binding domain from the mistletoe
    Phoradendron liga. *Biochem J* 2002;366:405.
13. Hutt N, Kopferschmitt-Kubler M, Cabalion J, Purohit A, Alt M, Pauli G.
    Anaphylactic reactions after therapeutic injection of mistletoe (Viscum
    album L.). *Allergol Immunopathol* 2001;29:201.
14. Huber R, Barth H, Schmitt-Graff A, Klein R. Hypereosinophilia induced
    by a high-dose intratumoral and peritumoral mistletoe application to a
    patient with pancreatic carcinoma. *J Altern Complement Med* 2000;6:305.

MOSS (ICELAND)

■ SOURCE, DESCRIPTION, USES

Iceland moss (*Cetraria islandica*) is not a true moss but is, rather, a lichen.
It is common throughout arctic and subarctic areas and further south in
mountainous regions. It has a high starch content and also contains some
sugar, fumaric acid, oxalic acid, and other chemicals.[1] It is used traditionally
as a demulcent, tonic, and nutritive.[1] It has been used for treating ulcers, as
well as for tuberculosis, tumors, chronic pulmonary troubles, and catarrh.

■ PHARMACOLOGY

Numerous biologically active agents have been isolated from Iceland moss.
An alkali-soluble polysaccharide has been shown to possess immunostimu-
latory properties.[2] Anticancer and antibacterial activities also have been
demonstrated, including against *Helicobacter pylori*, the causative agent of
peptic ulcer. The active component was identified as protolichesterinic acid.[3]

■ ADVERSE EFFECTS AND INTERACTIONS

No reports of adverse effects are available, but theoretically, Iceland moss
could affect the absorption of drugs from the gastrointestinal tract.

REFERENCES

1. Moss, Iceland. In: Grieve M. *A Modern Herbal.* Botanical.com website. Available at: http://www.botanical.com/botanical/mgmh/m/mosice52.html.
2. Ingolfsdottir K, Jurcic K, Fischer B, Wagner H. Immunologically active polysaccharide from Cetraria islandica. *Planta Med* 1994;60:527.
3. Ingolfsdottir L, Hjalmarsdottir MA, Sigurdsson A, Gudjonsdottir GA, Bryanjolfsdottir A, Steingrimsson O. In vitro susceptibility of Helicobacter pylori to protolichesterinic acid from the lichen Cetraria islandica. *Antimicrob Agents Chemother* 1997;41:215.

MOTHERWORT

SOURCE, DESCRIPTION, USES

Motherwort, sometimes called motherworth (*Leonurus cardiaca*), is a member of the mint (Labiatae) family. It is a native of Europe but a common alien species throughout northeastern North America.[1,2] Growing to 1 m on a single, erect stem, it has wedge-shaped, opposed leaves that often are held horizontally with three major points and minor notches. Flowers are pink-lilac and form rosettes at the axils (where leaf joins stem).[1] The genus name, *Leonurus,* comes from the Greek for lion's tail and refers to the similarity of the plant in some observer's eyes.

The aboveground plant is cut and dried to prepare the herb. Traditional uses include as a diaphoretic, an antispasmodic, a tonic, a "nervine," an emmenagogue, and for female "weakness and disorders" (hence the common name, motherwort).[2] It was taken most often as a conserve but also was used as an infusion; however, the latter was very unpleasant in taste.[2] It also has been used for cardiac disorders (hence the species name, *cardiaca*).[3] The herb is available as a tincture, an extract, and in bulk in North America.[4]

PHARMACOLOGY

Several chemicals with potential biological activity have been identified in motherwort, including alkaloids, leonurine, diterpenes, prehispanolone, flavonoids, and cafeic acid.[4] Milkowska-Leyck and colleagues[3] conducted an extensive investigation of a dried extract (chloroform/methanol) of the herb. They isolated a complex molecule identified as lavandulifolioside and examined its cardiovascular pharmacology and toxicity. This molecule reduced the heart rate and coronary blood flow in the isolated rat heart and induced electrocardiographic changes (widening of the QRS and prolongation of Q-T interval). A single dose ($1/20$ LD_{50}) had no effect on blood pressure or heart rate of anesthetized rats, but a higher dose ($1/13$ LD_{50}) reduced both diastolic and systolic pressure. Oral (intragastric) administration to mice caused some decrease in spontaneous locomotor activity. The acute oral toxicity in mice was $LD_{50} > 2000$ mg/kg. The authors concluded that the action of lavandulifolioside is more akin to that of quinidine than to the cardiac glycosides that also are known to be present in motherwort.

Other activities that have been ascribed to motherwort include anti-inflammatory, antianxiety, and anticoagulant effects.[4] Zou and colleagues[5] studied 105 subjects with hyperviscosity after they were given the herb intravenously daily for 15 days (10 mL of 5 g/mL) and found significant reductions in circulating levels of fibrinogen and a reduction in blood viscosity. Although this was clinically beneficial for these patients, it would have a negative impact on hemostasis for normal subjects, especially because reduced platelet aggregation also was observed. These effects were attributed to a chemical component of the extract called prehispanolone.

■ ADVERSE REACTIONS AND INTERACTIONS

Given the pharmacological actions of this herb, there is a strong potential to interact with many prescription and over-the-counter drugs. Concomitant administration with oral anticoagulants, cardiac drugs, nonsteroidal anti-inflammatory drugs, and possibly antidepressants is ill advised. Despite the common name of this herb, the possibility of adverse effects in pregnant women must be considered. Nursing mothers should probably avoid this herb as well. See also Appendices I, II, VII, and VIII.

■ REFERENCES

1. Peterson RT, McKenny M. *Northeastern Wildflowers: Roger Tory Peterson Field Guides*. Norwalk, Easton Press;1984:280.
2. Motherwort. In: Grieve M. *A Modern Herbal*. Botanical.com website. Available at: http://www.botanical.com/botanical/mgmh/m/mother55.html.
3. Milkowska-Leyck K, Filipik B, Strzelecka H. Pharmacological effects of lavandulifolioside from Leonurus cardiaca. *J Ethnopharmacol* 2002;80:85.
4. Abebe W. Herbal medication: Potential for adverse interactions with analgesic drugs. *J Clin Pharm Ther* 2002;27:391.
5. Zou QZ, Bi RG, Li JM, et al. Effect of motherwort on blood hyperviscosity. *Am J Chin Med* 1989;17:65.

MYRRH

■ SOURCE, DESCRIPTION, USES

Genuine myrrh comes from the bush *Commiphora myrrha* (family Burseraceae), also known as *C. myrrha var. molmol* or *C. molmol*. It is described as a stout bush growing to nearly 2 m in height and native to "Arabia and Somaliland."[1] An oleo-gum resin from the stem is used to prepare an essential oil. In addition to being used as a fragrance in incense and perfumes, its traditional herbal use includes as an astringent, a healing agent, a tonic, a stimulant, an emmenagogue, an expectorant, and a carminative, as well as for dyspepsia.[1] It also has been used for peptic ulcer because of the mucilage present in the gum[2] and is a traditional treatment for diabetes in the Middle East. Synonyms include gugulipid and guggal gum.

■ PHARMACOLOGY

C. myrrha is one of about 150 related species.[3] Many of these are used as substitutes or adulterants for true myrrh. The plethora of chemical constituents and the fact that they may differ from species to species has made the identification of active principles difficult. Dekebo and colleagues[3] analyzed the constituents from several *Commiphora* species. Over two dozen were found in *C. myrrha* alone.

There has been a resurgence of interest in myrrh. One Egyptian trial studied its use for the treatment of schistosomiasis, a parasitic infection that has become increasingly resistant to schistosomicidal drugs such as praziquantel. In this trial, 204 infected patients were given 10 mg/kg per day for 3 days. A cure rate of 91.7% was reported, and subjects who did not respond were retreated, raising the cure rate to 98%. Six months after treatment, biopsies were performed on 20 cases and none showed ova.[4]

Some promising results also have been obtained in the treatment of *Fasciola hepatica* liver fluke infestation. Seven infected patients were given a preparation consisting of 8 parts resin and 3.5 parts volatile oils of myrrh (12 mg/kg per day for 6 days). There was a marked improvement in signs and symptoms and all feces were egg-free within 3 weeks.[5] The oil extract also has been shown to be molluscicidal against some species of snails, the intermediate hosts for liver flukes.[6]

There has been some experimental evidence from studies in rats that myrrh (gugalipid) possesses lipid-lowering properties by stimulating low-density lipoprotein receptor activity in hepatocytes.[7]

■ ADVERSE EFFECTS AND INTERACTIONS

The small clinical trials described earlier did not report any but mild and transient side effects, mostly gastrointestinal, and stated that the treatment was well tolerated. Allergic contact dermatitis has been reported following exposure to myrrh.[8] No information appears regarding interactions with other drugs.

■ REFERENCES

1. Myrrh. In: Grieve M. *A Modern Herbal.* Botanical.com website. Available at: http://www.botanical.com/botanical/mgmh/m/myrrh-66.html.
2. Borrelli F, Izzo AA. The plant kingdom as a source of anti-ulcer remedies. *Phytother Res* 2000;14:581.
3. Dekebo A, Dagne E, Sterner O. Furanosesquiterpenes from Commiphora sphaerocarpa and related adulterants of true myrrh. *Fitoterapia* 2002;73:48.
4. Sheir Z, Nasr AA, Massoud A, et al. A safe, effective herbal antischistosomal therapy derived from myrrh. *Am J Trop Med Hyg* 2001;65:700.
5. Massoud A, el Sisi S, Salama O, Massoud A. Preliminary study of therapeutic efficacy of a new fasciolicidal drug derived from Commiphora molmol (myrrh). *Am J Trop Med Hyg* 2001;65:96.
6. Allam AF, el Sayad MH, Khalil SS. Laboratory assessment of the molluscicidal activity of Commiphora molmol (myrrh) on Biomphalaria alexandrina, Bulinus truncatus and Lymnaea cailliaudi. *J Egypt Soc Parasitol* 2001;31:683.
7. Singh V, Kaul S, Chander R, Kapoor NK. Stimulation of low density lipoprotein receptor activity in liver membrane of guggal-sterone-treated rats. *Pharmacol Res* 1990;22:37.
8. Gallo R, Rivera G, Catterini G, Cozzani E, Guarrera M. Allergic contact dermatitis from myrrh. *Contact Dermatitis* 1999;41:230.

NETTLE (STINGING)

■ SOURCE, DESCRIPTION, USES

Originally a native of Europe, the stinging nettle (*Urtica dioica*, family Uticaceae) grows throughout the world, including most of North America. It is usually about 0.5 to 2 m in height, unbranched, with toothed, heart-shaped leaves and tiny, greenish flowers. The leaves and stem are covered with, short, stinging hairs.[1,2] Traditional herbal use has employed all parts of the plant. The leaves and stem lose their stinging properties upon cooking, and a tea made from them was used as a poultice to stop bleeding during the American Civil War.[1] Peterson[3] describes how the leaves and stems can be eaten, after simmering, in soups and teas. Medieval herbals state that the dried root is useful as a diuretic and for arthritic conditions.[4] Numerous other claims have been made for this herb. Current interest centers on its potential for use in the treatment of benign, prostatic, hyperplasia (BPH).

■ PHARMACOLOGY

The stinging property of nettle results from the presence of formic acid, histamine, serotonin, and choline in the short surface hairs.[1] In the treatment of BPH, ethanol and methanol extracts are generally used, and these have been shown to contain phytosterols, triperpene acids, lignans, polysaccharides, and simple phenols.[4] Pharmacological properties that have been demonstrated and that could contribute to nettle root's anti-BPH activity include inhibition of prostatic aromatase, competitive binding to sex hormone–binding globulin (SHBG), and anti-inflammatory properties.[4] Several of the lignans present in nettle root have been shown to bind with high affinity to SHBG.[5]

Other activities that have been demonstrated experimentally include the inhibition of prostatic Na^+-K^+-ATPase,[6] inhibition of proliferation of cultured human epithelial and lymph node carcinoma cells, and inhibition of stromal cells by methanol extract and its polysaccharide components.[7,8] Experimentally induced prostate hyperplasia in mice was reduced by one third by a 20% methanol extract of nettle root.[9] A few controlled clinical studies have been conducted and seem to indicate that treatment with nettle root extract improves urine flow but not necessarily subjective symptoms.[4]

One recent, randomized, double-blind, clinical trial compared finesteride with a combined preparation of nettle root and sabal extracts. Subjects (n = 431) were patients with prostate volumes greater than 40 mL. Both treatments resulted in a significant increase in urine flow after 24 weeks, and there was no statistically significant difference between them.[10] The International Prostate Symptom Score also improved in both groups. The finesteride group reported more side effects. It thus appears that there may be a place for herbal therapy in treating BPH, but this area is still evolving.

■ ADVERSE EFFECTS AND INTERACTIONS

Nettle root extract appears to be well tolerated. In one German study involving 4087 patients taking 600 to 1200 mg daily for 6 months, only 35 reported adverse effects, mostly gastrointestinal disturbances.[4] Some allergic reactions also were reported. There does not yet appear to be any information regarding drug interactions, but combining treatment with prescription drugs for BPH should be approached cautiously until more data are available. Tannin-containing herbs such as stinging nettle may interfere with iron absorption.[11] This may not be a serious problem clinically but should be considered in anemic patients, and it is advisable to avoid taking iron and the herbal preparation together. See also Appendix VIII.

■ REFERENCES

1. Nettles. Available at: http://www.rain-tree.com/nettles.htm.
2. Peterson RT, McKenny M. *Northeastern Wildflowers: Roger Tory Peterson Field Guides.* Norwalk, Conn: Easton Press;1984:382.
3. Peterson LA. *Edible Wild Plants: Roger Tory Peterson Field Guides.* Norwalk, Conn; 1984:150.
4. Schulz V, Hansel R, Tyler VE. *Rational Phytotherapy: A Physician's Guide to Herbal Medicine.* New York, NY: Springer-Verlag; 1998:228.
5. Schottner M, Gansser D, Spiteller G. Lignans from the roots of Urticaria dioica and their metabolites bind to human sex hormone binding globulin (SHBG). *Planta Med* 1997;63:529.
6. Hirano T, Homma M, Oka K. Effects of stinging nettle extracts and their steroidal components on the Na^+-K^+-ATPase of the benign prostatic hyperplasia. *Planta Med* 1994;60:30.
7. Lichius JJ, Lenz C, Lindermann P, Muller HH, Aumuller G, Konrad L. Antiproliferative effect of a polysaccharide fraction of a 20% methanolic extract of stinging nettle roots upon epithelial cells of the human prostate (LNCaP). *Pharmazie* 1999;54:768.
8. Konrad L, Muller HH, Lenz C, Laubinger H, Aumuller G, Lichius JJ. Antiproliferative effect on the human prostate cancer cells by a stinging nettle root (Urticaria dioica) extract. *Planta Med* 2000;66:44.
9. Lichius JJ, Renneberg H, Blaschek W, Aumuller G, Muth C. The inhibiting effects of components of stinging nettle roots on experimentally induced prostatic hyperplasia in mice. *Planta Med* 1999;65:666.
10. Sokeland J. Combined sabal and Urtica extract compared with finesteride in men with benign prostate hyperplasia: Analysis of prostate volume and therapeutic outcome. *BJU Int* 2000;86:439.
11. Miller LG. Herbal medicinals: Selected clinical considerations focusing on known or potential drug-herb interactions. *Arch Intern Med* 1998;158:2200.

NONI

■ SOURCE, DESCRIPTION, USES

Noni, also called Tahitian noni juice (TNJ), is the concentrated fruit juice of a small evergreen plant, *Morinda citrifolia,* or nonu, native to Polynesia. The plant favors the volcanic soil of Hawaii, where it was introduced by ancient Polynesians. The fruit is described as being lumpy, growing to about 12 cm in length and having a very unpleasant smell. It has been used throughout the islands for 2000 years for a variety of conditions that include diabetes, heart trouble, cancer, nervousness, and arthritis, as well as to promote weight loss.[1,2] The leaves also are used in teas.

■ PHARMACOLOGY

Wang and Su studied the effects of TNJ on the formation of DNA adducts induced by 12-dimethylbenz(a)anthracine (DMBA) in female Sprague-Dawley rats and found that 10% in drinking water prevented DMBA-DNA adducts in several organs, including lungs and livers. They attributed this anticancer effect to inhibition of superoxide radical formation. Both a polysaccharide-rich substance[3] and two novel glycosides[4] have been proposed as the antitumor agents. The former has been shown to be immunomodulatory. Thus, there is some laboratory evidence in support of claims of anticancer properties for TNJ. No doubt more data will be forthcoming in the future.

Noni juice extract has been shown to inhibit the oxidation of low-density lipoproteins (LDLs) and to upregulate hepatic LDL receptors, both activities that would be useful in controlling hyperlipidemia.[5]

■ ADVERSE EFFECTS AND INTERACTIONS

There is one case report of a man suffering from chronic renal insufficiency who presented at a hospital with hyperkalemia despite apparently adhering to a low-potassium diet. It subsequently emerged that he had been self-medicating with TNJ, which, on analysis, was found to contain 56.3 mEq/L of potassium, a level similar to that of orange juice and tomato juice.[6] Individuals requiring dietary restrictions for potassium should be cautioned against using noni juice. There is presently no available information regarding drug interactions or effects in pregnancy. Caution should be used until more is known about this potentially useful herbal remedy.

■ REFERENCES

1. Noni. Available at: http://www.hmt.com/noni/canoe.html.
2. Wang My, Su C. Cancer preventive effects of Morinda citrifolia (noni). *Ann N Y Acad Sci* 2001;952:161.
3. Hirazumi A, Furusawa E. An immunomodulatory polysaccharide-rich substance from the fruit Morinda citrifolia (noni) with antitumour activity. *Phytother Res* 1999;13:380.
4. Liu G, Bode A, Ma WY, Sang S, Ho CT, Dong Z. Two novel glycosides from the fruits of Morinda citrifolia (noni) inhibit AP-1 transactivation and cell transformation in the mouse epidermal JB6 cell line. *Cancer Res* 2001;61:5749.
5. Salleh MN, Runnie I, Roach PD, Mohamed S, Abeywardena MY. Inhibition of low-density lipoprotein oxidation and up-regulation of low-density liporeceptor in HepG2 cells by tropical plant extracts. *J Agric Food Chem* 2002;50:3693.
6. Mueller BA, Scott MK, Sowinski KM, Prag KA. Noni juice (Morinda citrifolia): Hidden potential for hyperkalemia? *Am J Kidney Dis* 2000;35:330.

OMEGA-3 FATTY ACIDS

■ SOURCE, DESCRIPTION, USES

Omega-3 fatty acids (OFAs) are essential fatty acids that achieved prominence two decades ago with the discovery that they were metabolized largely to the antithrombotic prostaglandin I_2 (PGI_2, prostacyclin) and that a diet rich in OFAs reduced the risk of a thrombotic event. Since that time, dietary supplementation has become popular for other applications as well, based in part on the antioxidant properties of OFAs. Ocean scale fish, especially from colder northern waters, and flaxseed oil are dietary sources rich in OFAs. They also are present in leafy green vegetables and olives. OFA supplements in the form of capsules containing concentrated oils also are available.[1]

■ PHARMACOLOGY

Mammals cannot synthesize OFAs, which are polyunsaturated fatty acids (PUFAs) with a double bond three carbons from the methyl terminal.[1] They are synthesized to 3-series prostaglandins (PGI_3) and leukotrienes and to thromboxane A_3 (TXA_3). The advantage of this is that PGI_3 has the same platelet-inhibiting properties as the PGI_2 (prostacyclin) made by endothelial cells but TXA_3 lacks the platelet-aggregating properties of TXA_2 made by platelets.[2] This shifts the balance in favor of antithrombotic activity. Fish and fish oil are normally rich in the OFAs eicosapentaenoic acid (EPA) and docosahexaenoic acid (DHA), which the fish acquire from the planktonic base of the marine food web.[2] (Farmed fish fed an artificial diet may lack similar levels of OFAs.) α-Linolenic acid, a precursor of EPA and its metabolite DHA, is found in flaxseed oil and green leafy vegetables.[3]

In addition to their beneficial effects in reducing the risk of cardiovascular disease, OFAs have been shown to be beneficial in patients with rheumatoid arthritis in a number of clinical studies.[3] This effect appears to be related to reduced synthesis of the inflammatory mediators interleukin-1β, thromboxane B_2 (TXB_2), and prostaglandin E_2 (PGE_2).[3] In the case of the latter two, this may be the result of selective inhibition of cyclooxygenase-2.

There is some evidence that people with chronic fatigue syndrome (CFS) have low levels of PUFAs and that supplementation with OFAs results in a diminution of their symptoms. This evidence is not conclusive, however, and more research is needed before a definitive conclusion can be reached regarding the usefulness of such supplementation in CFS.[4]

Other conditions that appear to benefit from dietary supplementation with OFAs (mostly as fish oil) are chronic inflammatory diseases such as nephropathies, Raynaud's disease, osteoarthritis,[1] and possibly systemic lupus erythematosus.[5]

It has been suggested that the ratio of 6 series to 3-series PUFAs in the western diet approaches 10 and that a ratio nearer 5 would be healthier.[6] Manipulating dietary PUFAs could be used to modify a number of factors, including fertility and reproduction in domestic livestock.[6]

ADVERSE EFFECTS AND INTERACTIONS

Inuit from western Greenland who pursue a traditional lifestyle have a diet high in OFAs and a low incidence of cardiovascular disease.[2] They also have an increased incidence of minor bleeding disorders and of platelet dysfunction. There is, thus, the possibility that a high intake of fish oil could lead to an increased risk of bruising and bleeding and that there could be an even greater risk in individuals who are taking nonsteroidal anti-inflammatory drugs or platelet-inhibiting drugs such as clopidogrel (Plavix), a platelet adhesion protein receptor blocker. One study of normal, healthy young men found that a diet containing numerous foods rich in OFAs could induce significant increases in the levels of EPA and decreases in TXB_2 and PGE_2 without resorting to fish oil supplement.[3] Such an approach could minimize the risk of an untoward reaction or interaction. See also Appendices I and VIII.

■ REFERENCES

1. Massey PB. Dietary supplements. *Med Clin North Am* 2002;86:127.
2. Philp RB. Possible drug strategies in combating atheroembolic disorders. In: Warren BA, ed. *Atheroembolism.* Boca Raton, Fla: CRC Press; 1986:103.
3. Mantzioris E, Cleland LG, Gibson RA, Neumann MA, Demasi M, James MJ. Biochemical effects of a diet containing foods enriched with n-3 fatty acids. *Am J Clin Nutr* 2000;72:42.
4. Werbach MR. Nutritional strategies for treating chronic fatigue syndrome. *Altern Med Rev* 2000;5:93.
5. Patavino T, Brady DM. Natural medicine and nutritional therapy as an alternative treatment in systemic lupus erythematosus. *Altern Med Rev* 2001;6:460.
6. Abayasekara DRE, Wathes DC. Effects of altering dietary fatty acid composition on prostaglandin synthesis and fertility. *Prostaglandins Leukot Essent Fatty Acids* 1999;61:275.

PAPAYA

■ SOURCE, DESCRIPTION, USES

Papaya (*Carica papaya*) is a popular tropical fruit that has received considerable scientific attention in recent years because it contains numerous substances of pharmacological interest. In Africa, the fruit traditionally has been made into a paste for the treatment of burns, skin infections, ulcers, and other skin conditions.[1] Throughout Africa, Asia, and South America, the seeds are crushed and used as an anthelmintic for both humans and farm animals.[2] The fruit also is used to treat liver disorders.[3]

■ PHARMACOLOGY

The pulp of the papaya fruit is effective as a dressing for debriding wounds and preventing infection. It helps provide a granulating surface for skin grafts.[1] Antibacterial activity has been demonstrated against some opportunistic organisms, and proteolytic enzymes are believed to play a role in this activity.[1] Extracts of the crushed seeds have been shown to be effective against *Caenorhabditis elegans* and other helminths.[2] The active ingredients are thought to be benzyl isothiocyanate (BITC) and carpain, principally the former. An enzyme myrosinase (thioglucosidase) acts on glucosinolate to yield BITC. The enzyme and its substrate normally are compartmentalized in the seed but are brought into contact by crushing.

Ethanol and aqueous extracts of the dried fruit were evaporated and administered to rats in gum acacia for 7 days before liver damage was induced by carbon tetrachloride (CCl_4). Serum enzymes were monitored and liver histopathology conducted 36 hours after the CCl_4 administration. The extracts provided significant protection against hepatotoxicity as manifested by a reduction in serum enzymes and lack of liver damage compared with untreated controls.[3]

Shoots of the papaya, extracted by methanol, inhibited oxidation of low-density lipoproteins, which would reduce oxidative damage,[4] theoretically a useful activity in hyperlipidemia. Antioxidant activity also has been demonstrated for a cocktail derived from fermentation of several botanical ingredients, including papaya.[5] Other ingredients were unpolished rice, seaweed, and several fermentation microorganisms. The extract protected rats against renal damage induced by oxidation of fatty acids.

■ ADVERSE EFFECTS AND INTERACTIONS

Both seed extract and BITC irreversibly inhibited phenylephrine- or potassium chloride–induced contraction of canine carotid artery strips and relaxed precontracted strips. The effect was not dependent on the presence of endothelial cells, and the authors of this study speculated that the effect resulted from increased calcium uptake, an action known to be associated with some anthelmintics. They concluded that papaya seed extract was not totally selective for helminths and that some mammalian cytotoxicity could result.[2]

One of the concerns regarding papaya has been its possible abortifacient action. Its use in pregnancy is commonly avoided in Asia because of this concern. Indeed, studies in rats showed that high doses of aqueous extract resulted in 30% resorption of fetuses.[6] Other studies have shown that crude papaya latex induced contractions of uterine smooth muscle similar to those induced by oxytocin and prostaglandin $F_{2\alpha}$. Unripe and semiripe papaya are rich in latex whereas ripe ones are not, and these authors felt that eating ripe papaya during pregnancy did not constitute a risk whereas unripe ones should be avoided.[7] Until the question of papaya's safety in pregnancy is clearly established, it would be best to err on the side of caution.

There is one report suggesting that papaya can increase the risk of bleeding in patients who take warfarin.[8]

In summary, papaya (fruit pulp) appears to be very useful for treating and preventing wound infections of the skin, possibly useful for its hepatoprotective effect, an effective anthelmintic (crushed seeds) but possibly with some toxicity, and best avoided during pregnancy and in patients taking oral anticoagulants. Moderate intake of the fruit or juice probably poses few risks otherwise.

■ REFERENCES

1. Edwards-Jones V, Greenwood JE. What's new in burn microbiology? James Laing memorial prize essay 2000. *Burns* 2003;29:15.
2. Wilson RK, Kwan TK, Kwan CY, Sorger GJ. Effects of papaya seed extract and benzyl isothiocyanate on vascular contraction. *Life Sci* 2002;71:497.
3. Rajkapoor B, Jayakar B, Kavimani S, Murugesh N. Effect of dried fruits of Carica papaya Linn on hepatotoxicity. *Biol Pharm Bull* 2002;25:1645.
4. Salleh MN, Runnie I, Roach PD, Mohamed S, Abeywardena MY. Inhibition of low-density lipoprotein oxidation and up-regulation of low-density lipoprotein receptor in HepG2 cells by tropical plant extracts. *J Agric Food Chem* 2002;50:3693.
5. Aruoma OI, Deiana M, Rosa A, et al. Assessment of the ability of the antioxidant cocktail-derived from fermentation of plants with effective microorganisms (EM-X) to modulate oxidative damage in the kidney and liver of rats in vivo: Studies upon the profile of poly- and mono-unsaturated fatty acids. *Toxicol Lett* 2002;135:209.
6. Oderinde O, Noronha C, Oremosu A, Kosumiju T, Okanlawon OA. Abortifacient properties of aqueous extract of Carica papaya (Linn) seeds on female Sprague-Dawley rats. *Niger Postgrad Med J* 2002;9:95.
7. Adebiyi A, Adaikan PG, Prasad RN. Papaya (Carica papaya) consumption is unsafe in pregnancy: Fact or fable? Scientific evaluation of a common belief in some parts of Asia using a rat model. *Br J Nutr* 2002;88:199.
8. Fugh-Berman A. Herb-drug interactions. *Lancet* 2000;355:134.

PASSIONFLOWER

■ SOURCE, DESCRIPTION, USES

Passionflower (*Passiflora incarnata*, family Passifloraceae), also known as maytop, is one of many related species that share in common a flat, many-petaled flower growing from a vine or shoot along with a three-lobed leaf.[1] The name comes from the plant's similarity to a crown of thorns.[2] Passionflower is native to the southeastern United States, as far west as eastern Texas. Traditional use was as a sedative and narcotic, to control diarrhea, for dysmenorrhea, and for insomnia.[2] The dried plant, collected after the berries have appeared, was used as the herb.[2] It is claimed that passionflower is the most popular ingredient in herbal sedative preparations in Great Britain today.[3]

■ PHARMACOLOGY

The herb contains 2.5% flavonoids, including vitexin, kaempferol, apigenin, and chrysin. The latter two have been shown to bind to benzodiazepine receptors.[3,4] Alcohol and aqueous extracts have been shown to have sedative and hypnotic effects in mice.[3,5] A clinical trial compared passionflower extract (45 drops/day) to oxazepam for controlling anxiety in two groups of outpatients diagnosed with generalized anxiety disorder. In this double-blind, randomized pilot study, passionflower extract and oxazepam were equally efficacious in controlling anxiety but more adverse reactions were associated with oxazepam.[6] These reactions were related principally to impairment of performance on the job. In another double-blind study, the same researchers showed that extract of passionflower was helpful in controlling the mental symptoms associated with opiate withdrawal in addicts.[7] Animal studies have shown that a benzoflavone from passionflower restored normal sexual activity to rats given delta-9-tetrahydrocannabinol chronically for 30 days, causing loss of libido.[8]

■ ADVERSE EFFECTS AND INTERACTIONS

Passionflower extract can contain coumarin; therefore, a potential exists for interaction with oral anticoagulants.[9] See also Appendix I. There is one case on record of a 34-year-old woman who experienced severe nausea, vomiting, drowsiness, and episodes of ventricular tachycardia after self-administration of a passionflower herbal remedy at recommended doses. She required hospitalization for cardiac monitoring and fluid therapy.[10]

Interactions with centrally acting drugs, such as sedatives and tranquilizers, are a theoretical possibility. See also Appendix II. Safety in children and pregnant women has not been established.

In summary, passionflower extract may well have anxiolytic properties but additional well-designed clinical studies are required to clearly define its efficacy and toxicity.

■ REFERENCES

1. Niehaus TF, Ripper CL, Savage V. *Southwestern and Texas Wildflowers: Roger Tory Peterson Field Guides.* Norwalk, Conn: Easton Press; 1984:344.
2. Passion flower. In: Grieve M. *A Modern Herbal.* Botanical.com website. Available at: http://www.botanical.com/botanical/mgmh/p/pasflo14.html.
3. Gyllenhaal C, Merritt S, Peterson SD, Block KI, Gochenour T. Efficacy and safety of herbal stimulants and sedatives in sleep disorders. *Sleep Med Rev* 2000;4:229.

4. Speroni E, Minghetti A. Neuropharmacological activity of extracts from Passiflora incarnata. *Planta Med* 1988;54:488.
5. Cauffield JS, Forbes HJM. Dietary supplements used in the treatment of depression, anxiety, and sleep disorders. *Prim Care* 1999;3:290.
6. Akhondzadeh S, Naghavi HR, Vazirian M, Shayeganpour A, Rashidi H, Khani M. Passionflower in the treatment of generalized anxiety: A pilot double-blind randomized controlled trial with oxazepam. *J Clin Pharm Ther* 2001;26:363.
7. Akhondzadeh S, Kashani L, Mobaseri M, Hosseini SH, Nikzad S, Khani M. Passionflower in the treatment of opiates withdrawal: A double-blind randomized controlled trial. *J Clin Pharm Ther* 2001;26:369.
8. Dhawan K, Sharma A. Restoration of Δ-9-THC-induced decline in sexuality in male rats by a novel benzoflavone moiety from Passiflora incarnata Linn. *Br J Pharmacol* 2003;138:117.
9. Heck AM, DeWitt BA, Lukes AL. Potential interactions between alternative therapies and warfarin. *Am J Health Syst Pharm* 2000;57:1221.
10. Fisher AA, Purcell P, Le Couteur DG. Toxicity of Passiflora incarnata L. *J Toxicol Clin Toxicol* 2000;38:63.

PATCHOULI

■ SOURCE, DESCRIPTION USES

The fragrant herb *Pogostemon cablin* (*P. patchouli*) is a member of the mint (Labiatae) family and is native to both the East and West Indies and parts of South America.[1] It has opposed, ovate leaves, a square stem, and white flowers and can grow to 0.6 m. The entire herb is distilled to yield an essential oil. Traditional uses include a decoction or juice from the leaves, taken orally for cough and asthma; a lotion from the roots, applied topically for rheumatism; and a poultice of leaves, for boils and headache.

Patchouli oil has been used for centuries in Asia and India as a fragrant ingredient in perfumes and soaps. It is currently employed in aromatherapy.

■ PHARMACOLOGY

The active principle is generally considered to be a tricyclic sesquiterpene alcohol, patchoulol, which is the characteristic component of patchouli essential oil and is synthesized from the precursor farnesyl pyrophosphate.[2] Much of the interest in the chemistry of patchouli oil relates to the perfume industry, but some biological activities have been identified, including antibacterial [3] and antiemetic action of a number of extracted components.[4]

■ ADVERSE EFFECTS AND INTERACTIONS

No current information is available. The early herbal literature states that patchouli sometimes causes loss of appetite, loss of sleep, and nervous attacks.[1]

■ REFERENCES

1. Patchouli. In: Grieve M. *A Modern Herbal.* Botanical.com website. Available at: http://www.botanical.com/botanical/mgmh/p/patcho15.html.
2. Croteau R, Munck SL, Akoh CC, Fisk HJ, Satterwhite DM. Biosynthesis of the sesquiterpene patchoulol from farnesyl pyrophosphate in leaf extracts of Pogostemon cablin (patchouli) mechanistic considerations. *Arch Biochem Biophys* 1987;256:56.
3. Pattnaik S, Subramanyam VR, Kole C. Antibacterial and antifungal activity of ten essential oils in vitro. *Microbios* 1996;86:237.
4. Yang Y, Kinoshita K, Koyama K, et al. Anti-emetic principles of Pogostemon cablin (blanco) Benth. *Phytomedicine* 1999;6:89.

PAU D'ARCO

■ SOURCE, DESCRIPTION, USES

Pau d'arco is a giant tree (*Tabebuia avellanedae*, family Bignoniaceae) native to the Caribbean and to Central and South America. Indigenous peoples have long claimed that it possessed remarkable medicinal properties. A tea made from the inner bark is said to have anti-inflammatory, analgesic, anti-neoplastic, diuretic, and anti-infective properties. It was taken internally and also used as a poultice for wounds and skin conditions.[1] Synonyms include taheebo, ipe roxo, ipes, lapacho, lapacho morado, and tabebuia.[1,2]

■ PHARMACOLOGY

The pharmacological properties of pau d'arco are thought to derive from the numerous active principles present, such as saponins, flavonoids, coumarins, and especially lapachol,[3] a naphthoquinone long recognized as having anti-neoplastic properties.[2] In one study using animal models of pain and inflammation,[3] an aqueous extract of the inner bark was shown to inhibit carrageenan-induced rat paw edema and mouse writhing after intraperitoneal acetic acid injection. In an older study by Rau and colleagues,[4] lapachol was shown to be active against Walker carcinoma 256 in mice but not against carcinoma 755, leukemia L-1210, P-1534, or sarcoma 180 at subtoxic doses. A more recent study has shown activity of lapachol and another principle against erythroleukemia (clone 3-1) cells.[5] The activity of lapachol was antagonized by vitamin K_1. Another active substance was present but not chemically identified.

■ ADVERSE EFFECTS AND INTERACTIONS

Studies have not shown that pau d'arco has an effect on human cancer. In early studies of oral lapachol as an investigational new drug (IND), it was found that it was poorly absorbed and that when significant plasma levels were attained, side effects nearly always followed. Nausea and vomiting occurred even at low doses, and higher doses could cause bruising and bleeding because of the antagonism of vitamin K. Interest in lapachol as an IND waned.[2] The American Cancer Society, in reviewing herbal anticancer treatments, strongly urged cancer patients not to use so-called nutritional treatments as the sole or primary means of cancer therapy.[2]

This herb should not be used for patients taking oral anticoagulants or nonsteroidal anti-inflammatory drugs such as acetylsalicylic acid (see also Appendix I). Use in children and pregnant women should be discouraged.

There is one report of fatal hepatic failure in a patient taking a combination of skullcap and pau d'arco[6] but there is no information concerning hepatotoxicity of pau d'arco alone (see also Appendix III).

■ REFERENCES

1. Pau d'arco. Available at: http://www.pau-d-arco.com/doctorsaid.html
2. American Cancer Society. Questionable methods of cancer management: 'Nutritional' therapies. *CA Cancer J Clin* 1993;43:309.
3. Miranda FG, Vilar JC, Alves IA, Cavalcanti SC, Antoniotti AR. Antinociceptive and antiedematogenic properties and acute toxicity of Tabebuia avellanedae Lor. Ex Griseb. Inner bark aqueous extract. *BMC Pharmacol* 2001;1:6.
4. Rau KV, McBride TJ, Oleson JJ. Recognition and evaluation of lapachol as an antitumor agent. *Cancer Res* 1968;28:1952.
5. Dinnen RD, Ebisuzaki K. The search for novel anticancer agents: A differentiation-based assay and analysis of a folklore product. *Anticancer Res* 1997;17:1027.
6. Hullar TE, Sapers BL, Ridker PM, Jenkins RL, Huth TS, Farraye FA. Herbal toxicity and fatal hepatic failure. *Am J Med* 1999;106:267.

PENNYROYAL

■ SOURCE, DESCRIPTION, USES

Pennyroyal is the common name for a small species of mint, *Mentha pulegium* (formerly *Pulegium regium*), native to Europe and the British Isles.[1] A related species, *Hedeoma pulegoides* (American pennyroyal), is native to northeastern North America.[2] Both are used as herbal remedies. Infusions, fluid extracts, and oils have been prepared for use from the leaves of the plant. Traditional uses have included as a carminative, a diaphoretic, a stimulant, an emmenagogue (to induce menses), and for spasms, hysteria, and flatulence. It also has been used as a flavoring agent, but it is too strong for most tastes. Synonyms for pennyroyal include Pulegium, run-by-the-ground, lurk-in-the-ditch, and pudding grass.[1] American pennyroyal is sometimes called squawmint.[3] Current interest in pennyroyal is as an abortifacient and for juvenile asthma. It must be emphasized that there is no scientific or clinical evidence to support either application. Other uses are as an insecticide and as a treatment for fleas in dogs.

■ PHARMACOLOGY

Pennyroyal contains several monoterpenes common to all mints, but in higher concentrations. This accounts for its much stronger aroma and flavor. One of these monoterpenes, the monoterpene ketone, (R)-(+)-pulegone, is the major constituent of pennyroyal oil and its main toxic component.[4] Menthofuran is a metabolite formed by cytochrome P450 (CYP450) oxidative enzymes. Earlier studies[5] showed that inhibition of CYP450 eliminated or reduced hepatotoxicity of pennyroyal in mice. Both pulegone and menthofuran are hepatotoxic, the former by depletion of glutathione and the latter by a different mechanism.[3] A recent study in rats identified 14 metabolites of pugelone.[4]

■ ADVERSE EFFECTS AND INTERACTIONS

Fulminant hepatic necrosis has been reported repeatedly following the use of pennyroyal, often to induce abortion, and several fatalities have resulted from such use.[3] Anderson and colleagues reviewed 24 typical cases.[6] One involved a 24-year-old woman who ingested very large amounts of pennyroyal oil and (phytoestrogen-containing) black cohosh to induce abortion. She went into cardiopulmonary arrest 7.5 hours later and was resuscitated successfully. The patient remained comatose, however, and died 46 hours after the pennyroyal ingestion. At autopsy, the liver showed centrolobular necrosis and degeneration. Degenerative changes in the proximal renal tubules also were noted, as were coagulopathic changes. Menthofuran metabolites adducted to microsomal proteins were found.

Toxic effects manifested shortly (1.5 to 3 hours) after ingestion of large amounts of pennyroyal include vomiting, dizziness, seizures, mydriasis, confusion, agitation, hallucinations, and, eventually, coma.[6]

People of Hispanic extraction traditionally have used herbal mint teas, called yerba buena, to treat colic and minor digestive ailments in infants.[7] These are generally not toxic, but the accidental inclusion of pulegone-containing mints such as pennyroyal or American pennyroyal can have serious consequences. Bakerink and colleagues reported on two infant fatalities resulting from such accidental misuse.[7]

It is difficult to see any legitimate application for using pennyroyal oil, and the consequences of such use can be catastrophic. Although no herb-drug interactions appear to have been reported, impaired liver function obviously could affect the biotransformation of many drugs.

■ REFERENCES

1. Pennyroyal. In: Grieve M. *A Modern Herbal.* Botanical.com website. Available at: http://www.botanical.com/botanical/mgmh/p/pennyr23.html.

2. Peterson RT, McKenny M. *Northeastern Wildflowers: Roger Tory Peterson Field Guides.* Norwalk, Conn: Easton Press; 1984:348.

3. Stickel F, Egerer G, Seitz HK. Hepatotoxicity of botanicals. *Public Health Nutr* 2000;3:113.

4. Chen LJ, Lebetkin EH, Burka LT. Metabolism of (R)-(+)-pulegone in F344 rats. *Drug Metab Dispos* 2001;29:1567.

5. Mizutani T, Nomura H, Nakanishi K, Fujita S. Effects of drug metabolism modifiers on pulegone-induced hepatotoxicity in mice. *Res Commun Chem Pathol Pharmacol* 1987;58:75.

6. Anderson IB, Mullen WH, Meeker JE, et al. Pennyroyal toxicity: measurement of toxic metabolite levels in two cases and review of the literature. *Ann Intern Med* 1996;124:726.

7. Bakerink JA, Gospe SM Jr, Dimand RJ, Eldridge MW. Multiple organ failure after ingestion of pennyroyal oil from herbal tea in two infants. *Pediatrics* 1996;98:944.

PEPPERMINT

■ SOURCE, DESCRIPTION, USES

Peppermint (*Mentha piperita*) grows throughout much of the world and is native to all of North America, favoring wet meadows and streambanks.[1] It also is grown commercially as a flavoring agent. It has been used, worldwide, for digestive problems as a tea or steam-extracted oil.[2]

■ PHARMACOLOGY

The active ingredients are volatile oils such as menthol, menthone, and menthyl acetate. Its current use is mainly for colic and irritable bowel syndrome. Enteric, coated capsules of a standardized oil have been shown to be effective against irritable bowel syndrome in placebo-controlled trials,[2,3] relieving or improving all symptoms of the disorder.[2] The topical use of peppermint oil for postherpetic neuralgia was found to be beneficial in one report.[4]

■ ADVERSE EFFECTS AND INTERACTIONS

Peppermint may relax the lower esophageal sphincter and, therefore, is contraindicated for patients with reflux disease. Peppermint should probably not be used in patients with biliary tract obstruction, cholecystitis, or severe liver damage.[2] Children may choke on the menthol fumes. Hypersensitivity reactions are rare but have been reported.[5] Peppermint oil has been shown to be a moderately potent inhibitor of cytochrome P450 3A4, raising the possibility that it, like grapefruit juice, also may inhibit the metabolism of felodipine.[6] Interactions with conventional drugs do not otherwise seem to be a problem.

■ REFERENCES

1. Peterson LA. *Edible Wild Plants: Roger Tory Peterson Field Guides.* Norwalk, Conn: Easton Press; 1985:118.
2. Hadley SK, Petry JJ. Medicinal herbs: A primer for primary care. *Hosp Pract* 1999;34:105.
3. Thompson Coon J, Ernst A. Herbal medicinal products for non-ulcer dyspepsia. *Aliment Pharmacol Ther* 2002;16:1698.
4 Davies SJ, Harding LM, Baranowski AP. A novel treatment of postherpetic neuralgia using peppermint oil. *Clin J Pain* 2002;18:200.

5. Nair B. Final report on the safety assessment of Mentha piperita (peppermint) oil, Mentha piperita (peppermint) leaf extract, and Mentha piperita (peppermint) leaf water. *Int J Toxicol* 2001;20(suppl):61.

6. Dresser GK, Wacher V, Wong S, Wong HT, Bailey DG. Evaluation of peppermint oil and ascorbyl palmitate as inhibitors of cytochrome C450 3Λ4 activity in vitro and in vivo. *Clin Pharmacol Ther* 2002;72:247.

PHYTOESTROGENS AND PHYTOPROGESTINS

■ SOURCE, DESCRIPTION, USES

Phytoestrogens are substances with estrogenic properties found in plants. Since their initial identification in 1926, several hundred plants have been shown to contain phytoestrogens.[1] They may be present in foodstuffs (e.g., cereal grains, soy milk and protein, vegetables or fruit) or taken in herbal supplements to relieve hot flashes and other menopausal signs. Herbal remedies containing phytoestrogens include alfalfa, black cohosh, chaparral, dong quai (dang guai), fenugreek (a spice), licorice, Panax ginseng, red clover, and wild yam. Panoxosides (ginsenosides) in ginseng have been reported to have estrogen-like activity by a different mechanism, possibly involving promoting the synthesis of endogenous estrogens. The natural functions of phytoestrogens are thought to involve fungicidal action, regulation of plant hormones, and protection against ultraviolet radiation, and they also may serve as a deterrent to herbivores.[2]

■ PHARMACOLOGY

The two major classes of phytoestrogens are lignans and isoflavones. Lignans are present in whole grains, flaxseed, and a variety of fruit and vegetables, and are converted to the active forms enterolactone and enterdione by intestinal flora.[2] Legumes are rich in isoflavones. These include formononitin (which may be metabolized to daidzein), daidzein, genistein, and biochanin A (which may be metabolized to genistein).[2] A third class, the coumestans, includes possibly the most potent of the phytoestrogens, coumestrol. In a test comparing the potency of coumestrol, daidzein, and genistein with 17β-estradiol (E2) in an E2-sensitive, breast cancer cell culture (MCF-7 cells), the relative potencies were coumestrol, 0.03 to 0.2; genistein and daidzein, 0.001 to 0.01. The mycoestrogen zearalenone, responsible for reproductive problems in swine, had a relative potency of 0.001 to 0.1.[1] Thus, although none of the phytoestrogens is especially potent, there is a real possibility that their cumulative effects could exert physiologically significant estrogenic activity. Additive effects with environmental zenoestrogens, such as DDT, cannot yet be discounted. Predictions of both beneficial and adverse effects of phytoestrogens are further complicated by the fact that some, such as coumestrol, may have activity as both estrogenic agonists and antagonists.[3]

The plant content of phytoestrogens can vary significantly with season, climate, part of the plant consumed, and method of preparation. Thus, soy sprouts are rich in coumestrol, whereas the bean has high levels of isoflavones.[1] Capsules containing dried, powdered plants may be more potent than teas prepared from the same plants. Phytoestrogens and their metabolites have been identified in human urine, even in those not taking herbal supplements.[2]

There is convincing, if somewhat circumstantial, evidence that a diet rich in phytoestrogens has significant health benefits. Epidemiological studies comparing the incidence of a number of diseases in Asian populations with that in North America suggest that a high intake of soy protein is associated with a much lower incidence of breast cancer, prostate cancer, cardiovascular disease, and osteoporosis and a lower incidence of postmenopausal symptoms. There was a sixfold increase in the incidence of breast cancer in Asian women who migrated to the west.[2-4] Several reviews of the subject[4-6] discuss clinical trials of phytoestrogens in postmenopausal women. A similar decrease in hot flashes occurred in treated (soy flour) and control (wheat flour) groups, suggesting a placebo effect, whereas vaginal cell maturation was increased in women receiving a soy-enriched diet but not in those maintained on their regular diet. These findings were confirmed in a more recent Australian trial[7] in which there were no statistically significant differences between the placebo group and the treated group, either with respect to frequency of hot flashes or incidence of adverse effects.

There is considerable experimental evidence that coumestrol and genistein inhibit bone resorption, genistein and daidzein possess antioxidant properties, and genistein inhibits protein tyrosine kinases and DNA topoisomerases, which would promote cell differentiation and, hence, inhibit cancer cell proliferation. Studies suggest that phytoestrogens offer some protection against breast cancer development in rats.

In May 2002, the results of the Women's Health Initiative randomized controlled trial of hormone replacement therapy (HRT) were released after 5.2 years instead of completing the planned 8.5 years. Of the 16,608 postmenopausal women with an intact uterus, aged 50 to 79 years, who participated in the trial, 8505 received conjugated equine estrogens, 0.625 mg/day, plus medroxyprogesterone acetate, 2.5 mg/day, and 8102 received a matching placebo. The trial was stopped because of unacceptable increases over the global index for a number of adverse effects. The relative risks or estimated hazard ratios were 1.29 for coronary heart disease, 1.26 for breast cancer, 1.41 for stroke, and 2.13 for pulmonary embolism. Although there were reductions in the hazard ratios for other diseases, such as colorectal and endometrial cancers, the overall health risks of HRT exceeded the benefits.[8]

Doubtless the results of this trial will have a negative impact on women's attitude toward HRT, and many likely will turn to phytoestrogen supplements as a perceived-safer alternative. Thus, it will be increasingly important in coming years to know much more about the efficacy and long-term effects of these agents.

■ ADVERSE EFFECTS AND INTERACTIONS

There are numerous examples of phytoestrogens interfering with normal reproduction in domestic livestock. Sterility in Australian sheep was attributed to large amounts of formononetin, a precursor of the phytoestrogen equol, in subterranean clover; reproductive problems in swine have been traced to zearalenone; and both an estrogenic mycotoxin from *Fusarium* mold and phytoestrogens have been responsible for reproductive problems in California quail.[1,4] Laboratory studies have confirmed the ability of phytoestrogens to upset normal sexual development in mice.[4] Studies of human hepatoma cells transfected with the estrogen receptor and an estrogen-responsive luciferase reporter gene showed that genistein and estradiol were additive.[9] One group of researchers[10] studied the ability of phytoestrogens in common plants used as foods, herbs, and spices to compete with estrogen and progesterone at their respective receptors (ER and PR). The six plants with the highest ER-binding characteristics were soy, licorice, red clover, thyme, tumeric, hops, and verbena, and the six highest PR-binding plants were oregano, verbena, tumeric, thyme, red clover, and damiana. In terms of bioactivity, ER-binding plants tended to be agonists whereas PR-binding ones were neutral or antagonistic. These observations raise the possibility of adverse effects and of interactions with estradiol in humans.

The side effects of excessive phytoestrogen use would be expected to be similar to those of estrogen excess, such as nausea, bloating, hypotension, breast fullness and tenderness, headache, and edema. The paucity of reports of such side effects may in part be the result of lack of efficacy of many preparations. Although these effects remain largely theoretical, disturbances in the menstrual cycle have been associated with excessive phytoestrogen consumption.[11]

One area of concern has been the possibility that soymilk and soy-based formulas (SBFs) for infants might result in impaired sexual development later in life, given the experimental data discussed earlier. SBFs now comprise more than 25% of all infant formulas sold in the United States. Mendez and associates[12] reviewed the existing literature and found that infants fed modern SBFs had normal growth and development. There was some evidence that both SBF and (cow's) milk-based formulas were associated with a higher incidence of asthma in young adults who were fed the formulas as infants. These and other authors[13] suggest that longer-term studies are required to conclusively demonstrate the safety of SBFs.

Confirmed reports of interactions between phytoestrogen therapy and drugs are scarce. There are, however, good theoretical grounds to avoid their use in women taking estrogen-progestin replacement therapy, oral contraceptives, or those who are receiving antiestrogen therapy (tamoxifen, raloxifene) for breast cancer.

One area that may assist in determining the risks and benefits associated with the use of herbal estrogen supplement is the emerging knowledge of estrogen receptor (ER) subtypes. The classical nuclear ER binds 17β-estradiol, estriol, and estrone with high affinity and regulates specific target genes by binding to a response element in their promoter regions. The ER is part of a superfamily of receptors that includes receptors for other steroids, thyroid hormone, retinoic acid, and vitamin D_3.[14] In addition, a large number of receptors has been identified for which there is no known ligand. These so-called orphan receptors comprise about two thirds of the 70-odd members of the receptor superfamily. When knockout mice deficient in the classical ER were studied, specific binding sites for estrogens were still present. This gene knockout caused major defects in reproductive organs but had little effect on other tissues in which estrogens play an important role, such as the cardiovascular system and bone. These findings led to the concept of two receptor subtypes, ERα and ERβ. Both tissue and species differences in distribution of the subtypes occur, and different affinities for both natural and synthetic ligands have been observed.[14] This situation raises the possibility that phytoestrogens may differ in their affinity for the different subtypes, which could have implications for estrogen replacement therapy and treatment of breast cancer. A further subtype of the ER has been identified in fish and tentatively named ERγ. Several isoforms of ERβ protein also have been identified. Their function is as yet unclear.

ERβ is highly expressed in both reproductive and other human tissues. It has a fairly high affinity for some plant-derived estrogens and is distributed throughout the gastrointestinal tract. It has been speculated that this ER might be involved in the protective effect of phytoestrogens against colon cancer.[14] Other physiological functions have been assigned to this receptor.

The picture is further complicated by the finding that a receptor, common in many human breast cancers, may interact with estrogenic ligands. This peroxisome proliferator-activated receptor γ (PPARγ) responds to a variety of natural and synthetic ligands and can mediate the expression of estrogen target genes. It also has been shown that ERα and ERβ can reduce PPARγ reporter activity.[15] Obviously, much more knowledge of these genes and receptors is needed to determine their importance for estrogen physiology.

In conclusion, it is evident that much more data are required to make definitive statements about the long-term hazards of phytoestrogen use.

■ REFERENCES

1. Philp RB. Environmental hormone disrupters. In: Philp RB, ed. *Ecosystems and Human Health.* Boca Raton, Fla: CRC/Lewis Press; 2001:261.

2. Barrett J. Phytoestrogens: Friends or foes? *Environ Health Perspect* 2002;104:478.

3. Rudel R. Predicting health effects of exposure to compounds with estrogenic activity: Methodological issues. *Environ Health Perspect* 1997;105(suppl):655.

4. Golden RJ, Noller KL, Titus-Ernstoff L, et al. Environmental endocrine modulators and human health: An assessment of the biological evidence. *Crit Rev Toxicol* 1998;28:109.

5. Kurzer MS, Xu X. Dietary phytoestrogens. *Annu Rev Nutr* 1997;17:353.

6. Murkies AL, Wilcox G, Davis SN. Phytoestrogens. *J Clin Endocrinol Metab* 1998;83:297.

7. Davis SR, Briganti EM, Chen RQ, Dalais FS, Bailey M, Burger HG. The effects of Chinese medicinal herbs on postmenopausal vasomotor symptoms of Australian women. *Med J Aust* 2001;174:68.

8. Writing Group for the Women's Health Initiative Investigators. Risks and benefits of estrogen plus progestin in healthy postmenopausal women: Principal results from the Women's Health Initiative randomized controlled trial. *JAMA* 2002;288:321.

9. Casanova M, You L, Gaido KW, Archibeque-Engle S, Janszen DB, Heck HA. Developmental effects of dietary phytoestrogens in Sprague-Dawley rats and interactions of genistein and daidzein with rat estrogen receptors in vivo and in vitro. *Toxicol Sci* 1999;51:236.

10. Zava DT, Dolbaum CM, Blen M. Estrogen and progestin bioactivity of foods, herbs, and spices. *Proc Soc Exp Biol Med* 1998;217:369.

11. Smolinske SC. Dietary supplement-drug interactions. *J Am Med Womens Assoc* 1999;54:191.

12. Mendez MA, Anthony MS, Arab L. Soy-based formulae and infant growth and development: A review. *J Nutr* 2002;132:2127.

13. Sheehan D. Herbal medicines, phytoestrogens and toxicity: Risk-benefit considerations. *Proc Soc Exp Biol Med* 1998;217:379.

14. Enmark E, Gustafsson J-A. Characterization of human estrogen receptor β. In Gronemeyer H, Fuhrmann U, Parczyk K, eds. *Molecular Basis of Sex Hormone Receptor Function: New Targets for Intervention.* New York, NY: Springer; 1998:161.

15. Wang X, Kilgore M. Signal cross-talk between estrogen receptor alpha and beta and the peroxisome proliferator-activated receptor gamma in MDA-MB-231 and MCF-7 breast cancer cells. *Mol Cell Endocrinol* 2002;194:123.

PLANTAIN

■ SOURCE, DESCRIPTION, USES

Common or greater plantain (*Plantago major*, family Plantaginaceae) is a familiar if unwanted inhabitant of many suburban lawns. It is a low plant with broad, basal leaves and a long, tight flower head on a slender stalk.[1] It grows extensively throughout North America and Europe. In the Scottish highlands, it is known as *slan-lus*, Gaelic for "the plant of healing," elsewhere in Great Britain as Englishman's foot, and by many other names. In the United States, it has been called snake-weed, in the belief that it will cure snakebite.[2] The dried roots, leaves, and flower spikes are used as the herb.

Traditional uses include as a refrigerant, a diuretic, and an astringent; for inflammation of mucus membranes or intermittent fever; and, topically, for ulcers and sores.[2] Currently, it is used for bronchial congestion (phlegm) and for inflammation of the oropharangeal mucosa.[3] *P. lanceolata* (English plantain) is used in the same manner.

There is currently considerable interest in developing English plantain as a pasture plant for grazing livestock as part of an effort to reduce the use of antibiotics as growth promoters, and replace them with medicinal herbs or their active principles.[4]

■ PHARMACOLOGY

Plantain contains approximately 6% mucilage, which gives it the soothing property useful for inflamed mucus membranes. A number of individual glycosides have been isolated, including catalpol, an active diuretic principle found also in *Catalpa ovata* (Chinese catalpa) fruit, and aucubin, which promotes the removal of uric acid from tissues to blood and its renal excretion. Acteoside, another glycoside, has antioxidant properties.[4] Whether plantain herb has sufficient levels of these bioactive components to exert their therapeutic effect is questionable, but plantain may serve as a source of these components for research and further development.

■ ADVERSE EFFECTS AND INTERACTIONS

No reports of adverse effects are available..

■ REFERENCES

1. Peterson RT, McKenny M. *Northeastern Wildflowers: Roger Tory Peterson Field Guides*. Norwalk, Conn: Easton Press; 1984:62.
2. Plantain, common. In: Grieve M. *A Modern Herbal*. Botanical.com website. Available at: http://www.botanical.com/botanical/mgmh/p/placom43.html.
3. Schulz V, Hansel R, Tyler VE. *Rational Phytotherapy: A Physician's Guide to Herbal Medicine*. New York, NY: Springer-Verlag; 1998:27, 151.
4. Tamura Y, Nishibe S. Changes in the concentrations of bioactive compounds in plantain leaves. *J Agric Food Chem* 2002;50:2514.

POPLAR (TREMBLING)

■ SOURCE, DESCRIPTION, USES

The bark of *Populus tremuloides* (family Salicaceae), a species of poplar native to North America, is used in the same manner as its European relative, *Populus tremula*. Both contain the salicylic acid–yielding alkaloids salicin and populin and are similar in usage to willow bark. Other species of *Populus* also may be used.[1]

■ PHARMACOLOGY

See WILLOW BARK.

■ ADVERSE REACTIONS AND INTERACTIONS

The same concerns regarding interaction with oral anticoagulants pertain as with willow bark.[2] See WILLOW BARK; see also Appendices I and VIII.

■ REFERENCES

1. Poplar, trembling. In: Grieve M. *A Modern Herbal*. Botanical.com website. Available at: http://www.botanical.com/botanical/mgmh/p/poplar61.html.
2. Pribitkin E deA, Boger B. Herbal therapy: What every facial plastic surgeon must know. *Arch Facial Plast Surg* 2001;3:127.

PYCNOGENOL

See FRENCH MARITIME PINE BARK EXTRACT.

RAGWORTS

See GROUNDSEL SPECIES.

RED CLOVER

■ SOURCE, DESCRIPTION, USES

A forage plant, the leaves and blossoms of red clover (*Trifolium pratense*) are used as a tea.

■ PHARMACOLOGY

See PHYTOESTROGENS AND PHYTOPROGESTINS.

■ ADVERSE EFFECTS AND INTERACTIONS

These are the same as for phytoestrogens.

RED YEAST RICE

See CHOLESTIN.

ROSEMARY

■ SOURCE, DESCRIPTION, USES

Rosemary (*Rosemarinus officinalis*) is a blue-flowered plant that grows wild around the Mediterranean coast. There is no closely related North American wildflower. An infusion of the leaves has been used for centuries for a variety of conditions, as a tonic, an astringent, a diaphoretic, a stimulant, a carminative, and a rubefacient; for headache and stomach problems; in wine for a "weak" heart; and as a rinse to darken the hair.[1] Modern uses are for upset stomach,[2] to improve memory,[3] and in aromatherapy.[4]

■ PHARMACOLOGY

Although little is known about the pharmacological basis for rosemary's purported applications, there is considerable interest in its antioxidant and antineoplastic properties. A component of rosemary, carnosic acid quinone, or carnosol, has been shown to have antioxidant and anti-inflammatory properties.[5–7] An ethanol extract of rosemary has been shown to reduce DNA strand breaks in hydrogen peroxide– or visible light–stimulated, methylene blue–treated, cultivated colon cancer cells.[8] It also has been shown to inhibit nitrous oxide (NO) production by inhibiting synthesis of inducible NO synthase, possibly contributing to its anti-inflammatory and chemoprotective actions.[9] Further evidence of antioxidant activity comes from a recent study showing that rosemary ethanol extract was an effective scavenger of peroxynitrite ($ONNO^-$).[10]

■ ADVERSE EFFECTS AND INTERACTIONS

There do not appear to be any adverse effects or drug-herb interactions associated with rosemary as it is currently used. Future use as an anti-inflammatory or anticancer drug may require higher doses or purified ingredients, and more research is required regarding these applications. There is one intriguing report concerning another herb, nettle leaf extract, which also has anti-inflammatory properties. When used in conjunction with the nonsteroidal anti-inflammatory drug (NSAID) diclofenac in patients with acute arthritis, the same improvement in range of motion and subjective symptoms was noted in the treatment group as in the control group receiving twice the dose of diclofenac alone.[11] This raises the possibility that anti-inflammatory herbal remedies used in conjunction with NSAIDs may allow a reduction in dosage of the latter and a reduced incidence of side effects. It also, however, raises the possibility that, without a reduction in NSAID dosage, an increased risk of adverse reactions might occur. See also Appendix VIII.

■ REFERENCES

1. Rosemary. In: Grieve M. *A Modern Herbal.* Botanical.com website. Available at: http://www.botanical.com/botanical/mgmh/r/rosema17.html.
2. Shulz V, Hansel R, Tyler VE. *Rational Phytotherapy: A Physician's Guide to Herbal Medicine.* New York, NY: Springer-Verlag; 1998:27.
3. Perry EK, Pickering AT, Want WW, Houghton PJ, Perry NS. Medicinal plants and Alzheimer's disease: From ethnobotany to phytotherapy. *J Pharm Pharmacol* 1999;51:527.
4. Shulz V, Hansel R, Tyler VE. *Rational Phytotherapy: A Physician's Guide to Herbal Medicine.* New York, NY: Springer-Verlag; 1998:105.
5. Masuda T, Inaba Y, Maekawa T, Takeda Y, Tamura H, Yamaguchi H. Recovery mechanism of the antioxidant activity from carnosic acid quinone, an oxidized sage and rosemary antioxidant. *J Agric Food Chem* 2002;50:5863.
6. Wargovitch MJ, Woods C, Hollis DM, Zander ME. Cancer prevention and health. *J Nutr* 2001;131(suppl):3034S.
7. Huang MT, Ho CT, Wang ZT, et al. Inhibition of skin tumorigenesis by rosemary and its constituents carnosol and ursolic acid. *Cancer Res* 1994;54:701.
8. Slamenova D, Kuboskova K, Horvathova E, Robichova S. Rosemary-stimulated reduction of DNA strand breaks and FPG-sensitive sites in mammalian cells treated with H_2O_2 or visible light-excited methylene blue. *Cancer Lett* 2002;177:145.
9. Lo AH, Liang YC, Lin-Shiau SY, Ho CT, Lin JK. Carnosol, an antioxidant in rosemary, suppresses inducible nitric oxide synthase through down-regulating nuclear factor-kappaB in mouse macrophages. *Carcinogenesis* 2002;23:983.
10. Choi HR, Choi JS, Han YN, Bae SJ, Chung HY. Peroxynitrite scavenging activity of herb extracts. *Phytother Res* 2002;16:364.
11. Chrubasik S, Enderlein W, Bauer R. Evidence for antirheumatic effectiveness of stewed Herna urticae diocae in acute arthritis: A pilot study. *Phytomedicine* 1997;4:105.

RUE

■ SOURCE, DESCRIPTION, USES

From a perennial evergreen shrub, *Ruta graveolens* (family Rutaceae), rue also is known as herb of grace, herbygrass, and country man's treacle.[1] The shrub is frequently grown as an ornamental shrub, and in parts of South America it is believed to ward off evil.[1,2] It usually is taken as an infusion and has been recommended for insomnia, headaches, nervousness, abdominal cramps, and renal problems. The oil is a strong local irritant, and dermatitis has been observed in persons who handle the plant. In the past, it was used as an abortifacient and can induce uterine bleeding and contractions. Poisonings and fatalities have resulted from the high doses used in this application. A common herbal dose is 1 teaspoon of leaves in 250 mL (1 cup) of boiling water, not more than twice daily.[1]

■ PHARMACOLOGY

This plant is a veritable pharmacopoeia of biologically active chemicals. An extensive literature has evolved since the 1970s on the isolation, purification, and pharmacological investigation of these components. All parts of the plant contain toxic ingredients, but the leaves are most commonly used in herbal remedies.[1] The active principles include rutine (a glycoside), furocoumarins (psoralens), quinolone alkaloids, tannin, essential oils, and many others. The furocoumarins are responsible for most of the toxic effects of this herb, including photosensitivity and dermatitis, hepatotoxicity, and nephrotoxicity.[1,2] They also have been shown to be mutagenic in bacterial cell cultures and human lymphocytes.[3,4] An essential oil, methyl-nonyl-ketone, is the component that affects the uterus.[1]

■ ADVERSE EFFECTS AND INTERACTIONS

Acute accidental overdose can cause epigastric pain, vomiting, excessive salivation, central nervous system (CNS) excitation, and possible seizures. Hypotension, bradycardia, and shock may develop. Hepatic and renal insufficiency may occur after several days. Chronic exposure to lower but excessive doses can cause the same spectrum of signs and symptoms with delayed onset.[1] Poisonings are fairly common in South America, where medical abortion is not legal. This herb is absolutely contraindicated in pregnant women.[5]

As noted, phytophotodermatitis can occur after dermal contact.[6] Similar to other Rutaceae, rue may contain psoralens that cause the phytophotodermatitis. This is a photochemical reaction and not a true antibody-based allergic reaction. See AMMI for more details on phytophotodermatitis; also see Appendix XIII.

Drug interactions have not been reported, but it should be obvious that, given the wide spectrum of pharmacological and toxicological effects of this herb, coadministration of virtually any class of drugs should be avoided. This is likely especially true of antihypertensive agents, CNS depressants or stimulants, other photosensitizing agents, and stimulant laxatives.

■ REFERENCES

1. Pronczuk J. Ruta graveolens L. Chemical Safety Information for Intergovernmental Organizations. World Health Organization, United Nations Environment Programme, International Labour Organization. Available at: http://www.inchem.org.
2. Wessner D, Hoffmann H, Ring J. Phytodermatitis due to Ruta graveolens applied as a protection against evil spells. *Contact Dermatitis* 1999;41:232.
3. Abel G, Schimmer O. Mutagenicity and toxicity of furocoumarins: Comparative investigation in two test systems. *Mutat Res* 1981;90:451.
4. Paulini H, Eilert U, Schimmer O. Mutagenic compounds in an extract from ruta herb (Ruta graveolens L.). Mutagenicity is partially caused by furoquinoline alkaloids. *Mutagenesis* 1987;2:271.
5. Kong YC, Lau CP, Wat KH, et al. Antifertility principal of Ruta graveolens. *Planta Med* 1989;55:176.
6. Brener S, Friedman J. Phytodermatitis induced by Ruta graveolens. *Contact Dermatitis* 1985;12:230.

SACCHAROMYCES

■ SOURCE, DESCRIPTION, USES

Saccharomyces is the name for a genus of yeasts and also refers to a product consisting of dried, live yeast cells. Because yeasts are nucleated members of the plant kingdom, *Saccharomyces* can be regarded as an herbal remedy. *Saccharomyces cerevisiae* is brewer's yeast; the species name is from the Latin word for beer (*cerveza* in Spanish). *S. boulardii* is the medicinal strain. For years there was debate as to whether these two were identical, but recent work, based on protein fingerprinting, indicates that *S. boulardii* is a strain of *S. cerevisiae*.[1]

In the 1920s, it was discovered that dried yeast had antidiarrheal activity against acute diarrhea from a number of causes.[2] Since that time, it has become both an alternative remedy and a medication used in the hospital setting for treating diarrhea, especially that associated with antibiotic therapy. It is part of a new approach to the treatment of infectious diseases, called probiotics, in which a benign living organism is used to counteract a pathogenic one..

PHARMACOLOGY

Microorganisms are in a constant state of chemical warfare as they compete for ecological resources. Antibiotics are produced as a defensive mechanism by soil bacteria to ward off competitors, which often develop countermeasures. This competition is essential in the gastrointestinal tract, and nonpathogenic organisms normally have the upper hand. When pathogens take over, diarrhea is often the result. The administration orally of *S. boulardii* (Sb) attempts to restore the balance. The mechanisms involved include adhesion and entrapment of pathogens by sugar structures on the yeast cell, and stimulation of intestinal immune responses.[2] One study showed that Sb promoted an 18-fold increase in immunoglobulin A in mice challenged with *Clostridium difficile* by gavage and a 4.4-fold increase in specific antibody to the bacteria's toxin.[3]

A number of clinical trials have been conducted on the use of Sb for treatment or prevention of diarrhea associated with the use of antibiotics. A recent meta-analysis was carried out on four randomized, double-blind, placebo-controlled studies.[4] The odds ratio favoring the active treatment over placebo was 0.39 ($p < .001$). The authors concluded that Sb could be used to prevent antibiotic-associated diarrhea. A more recent randomized, double-blind, placebo-controlled study looked at the use of Sb to control diarrhea in asymptomatic patients treated with clarithromycin to eliminate *Helicobacter pylori*.[5] There was a significantly lower incidence of diarrhea in the treated group and better tolerance of treatment.

It should be noted that both the meta-analysis and the *Helicobacter* study also looked at *Lactobacillus*, a bacterial probiotic, and found essentially the same level of efficacy as for Sb.[4,5]

Not all trials have yielded positive findings. In one study, 69 elderly patients (> 65 years of age) receiving antibiotic therapy in medical wards were given 113 g of Sb or placebo twice daily and assessed for bowel habits and presence of *C. difficile*. No significant differences were detected between treated (34) and placebo (35) groups.[6]

ADVERSE EFFECTS AND INTERACTIONS

There have been reports of bloating and gastric distress associated with Sb. Allergic reactions to yeast also occur.[2] The most serious complication, however, is the development of a systemic mycotic infection (fungemia), mostly in debilitated or immunocompromised patients. In one report, an 8-month old infant with acute myeloid leukemia was given Sb to control diarrhea associated with chemotherapy. Despite antibiotic therapy, the child developed a fever and fungemia was confirmed. The child recovered with amphotericin B therapy.[7] Lherm and colleagues[8] described seven cases that occurred over the course of 28 months in a 12-bed intensive care unit. All of the patients were seriously ill, on mechanical ventilation, and being treated with broad-spectrum antibiotics. All but one were pretreated with Sb. Contamination of a central venous catheter could not be ruled out as a factor. The authors note the increased frequency of fungemia with *Saccharomyces* strains over the past decade and advise against using Sb in critically ill patients.

It would also seem wise to avoid giving Sb to patients who are seriously immunocompromised, such as those with acquired immunodeficiency syndrome. This is particularly so in light of the evidence that Sb works, in part, by stimulating the immune system in the gastrointestinal tract. The absence of an appropriate immune response could negate any benefit from the Sb as well as increase the likelihood of systemic mycosis. The therapeutic failure in elderly patients, described earlier,[6] also could be related to reduced immune responses.

In summary, Sb prophylaxis for antibiotic-related diarrhea appears to be useful in patients who are not critically ill and who have normal immune responses.

■ REFERENCES

1. Mitterdorfer G, Mayer HK, Kneifel W, Viernstein H. Protein fingerprinting of Saccharomyces isolates with therapeutic relevance using one- and two-dimensional electrophoresis. *Proteonics* 2002;2:1532.
2. Schulz V, Hansel R, Tyler VE. *Rational Phytotherapy: A Physician's Guide to Herbal Medicine.* New York, NY: Springer-Verlag; 1998:195.
3. Qamar A, Aboulola S, Warny M, et al. Saccharomyces boulardii stimulates intestinal immunoglobulin A immune response to Clostridium difficile toxin A in mice. *Infect Immun* 2001;69:2762.
4. D'Souza A, Rajkumar C, Cooke J, Bulpitt CJ. Probiotics in prevention of antibiotic associated diarrhoea: Meta-analysis. *BMJ* 2002;324:1361.
5. Cremonini F, Di Caro S, Covino M, et al. Effect of different probiotic preparations on anti-Helicobacter pylori therapy-related side effects: A parallel group, triple blind, placebo-controlled study. *Am J Gastroenterol* 2002;97:2744.
6. Lewis SJ, Potts LF, Barry RE, et al. The lack of therapeutic effect of Saccharomyces boulardii in the prevention of antibiotic-related diarrhoea in elderly patients. *J Infect* 1998;36:171.
7. Cesaro S, Chinello P, Rossi L, Zanesco L. Saccharomyces cervisiae fungemia in a patient treated with Saccharomyces boulardii. *Support Care Cancer* 2000;8:504.

8. Lherm T, Monet C, Nougierre B, et al. Seven cases of fungemia with Saccharomyces boulardii in critically ill patients. *Intensive Care Med* 2002;28:797.

S-ADENOSSYL-L-METHIONINE (SAMe)

■ SOURCE, DESCRIPTION, USES

This chemically synthesized nutriceutical has been in use in Europe for decades in the treatment of osteoarthritis, as an antidepressant, and for liver disease, especially alcoholic cirrhosis. It has become available more recently in North America as a very expensive nutritional supplement.[1,2] It also has gained interest as a so-called anti-aging product.[2] Synonyms include S-adenosylmethionine and ademetionine.

■ PHARMACOLOGY

SAMe is normally synthesized in the body from adenosine and methionine and is an intermediate product in many biochemical processes, such as the production of hormones, neurotransmitters, and cartilage.[2] It is important in transmethylation reactions in the central nervous system.[3] Both animal studies and clinical trials suggest that SAMe has modest benefits in osteoarthritis and may have chondroprotective activity. Normal individuals synthesize sufficient amounts of SAMe, but those deficient in folate, vitamin B_{12}, and methionine (e.g., patients with chronic liver disease) may be more likely to benefit from SAMe.[1]

In clinical studies in Europe, SAMe has been compared favorably with tricyclic antidepressants, having fewer side effects. These studies have been criticized for design flaws, however, and SAMe has not been compared with the newer antidepressants.[2] Some more recent clinical trials have been more convincing. In one double-blind, placebo-controlled, crossover study, SAMe was administered to ten elderly, normal, healthy volunteers to determine its effects on brain function and behavior.[3] Both acute and subacute administration resulted in measurable but different electroencephalographic changes compared with placebo. The changes were typical of those associated with antidepressants such as imipramine. The authors also reviewed several clinical studies that support antidepressant effects of SAMe. A recent multicenter study examined the efficacy and safety of SAMe in treating patients with major depression.[4] SAMe was compared with imipramine in a double-blind manner, with drugs given intramuscularly. Efficacy measures were not significantly different for the two treatments.

Adverse reactions were significantly less for the SAMe group (146 patients) than for the imipramine group (147 patients).

Fetrow and Avila[5] conducted an extensive review of clinical studies with SAMe. There appears to be convincing evidence of its efficacy as an antidepressant, although not all studies were placebo controlled, and some were quite small. Trials in patients with fibromyalgia were less convincing, less extensive, and not placebo controlled. With regard to osteoarthritis, early studies and laboratory results appeared to indicate reasonable efficacy, but more recent clinical trials have been less convincing.

There appears to be persuasive evidence, both clinical and from laboratory studies, of the usefulness of SAMe in hepatic disorders, including intrahepatic cholestasis. Experimental evidence indicated that it is as effective as *N*-acetylcysteine for treating paracetamol (acetaminophen) hepatotoxicity in mice,[6] and a recent report documented the successful treatment of accidental acetaminophen poisoning in a dog by a clinic at Cornell University's Veterinary College.[7]

Some of the discrepancies regarding clinical results with SAMe may relate to its pharmacokinetics. Absorption from the oral route is unreliable unless enteric-coated tablets are used, and first-pass metabolism is significant. Most hospital-based trials have used parenteral preparations to circumvent this problem.

ADVERSE EFFECTS AND INTERACTIONS

SAMe could, in theory, trigger a manic episode in a person with bipolar disorder.[2] There is a potential for interactions with other antidepressants and possibly other drugs that act in the central nervous system. At least one case of anaphylaxis has been reported in association with SAMe.[7] The most common adverse effects relate to the gastrointestinal tract. Cramps and diarrhea, sometimes serious, have occurred. These effects seem to have been reported with greater frequency in fibromyalgia studies. Psychoactivation also has been reported following parenteral administration.

In summary, the pharmacological profile of SAMe seems more akin to that of a prescription drug than a nutriceutical. It may be useful in mild depression and have fewer side effects than some of the other antidepressants, it could be helpful in certain liver disorders, and its usefulness in other conditions such as osteoarthritis is still open to question. Side effects can be a concern. Additional well-designed clinical trials are required. This does not appear to be a supplement that should be taken with other centrally acting drugs, and a physician's supervision would be advisable.

REFERENCES

1. Massey PB. Dietary supplements. *Med Clin North Am* 2002;86:127.

2. Anti-aging products, part 1: Can supplements rewind our body clocks? *Harvard Women's Health Watch* 2001;9:2.

3. Saletu B, Anderer P, Linzmayer L, et al. Pharmacodynamic studies on the central mode of action of S-adenosyl-L-methionine (SAMe) infusions in elderly subjects, utilizing EEG mapping and psychometry. *J Neural Transm* 2002;109:1505.

4. Pancheri P, Scapicchio P, Chiaie RD. A double-blind, randomized parallel-group, efficacy and safety study of intramuscular S-adenosyl-L-methionine1,4-butanedisulphonate (SAMe) versus imipramine in patients with major depressive disorder. *Int J Neuropsychopharmacol* 2002;5:287.

5. Fetrow CW, Avila JR. Efficacy of the dietary supplement S-adenosyl-L-methionine. *Ann Pharmacother* 2002;35:1414.

6. Carrasco R, Perez-Mateo M, Gutierrez, A, et al. Effect of different doses of S-adenosyl-methionine on paracetamol hepatotoxicity in a mouse model. *Methods Find Exp Clin Pharmacol* 2000;22:737.

7. Wallace KP, Center SA, Hickford FH, Warner KL, Smith S. S-adenosyl-methionine for the treatment of acetaminophen toxicity in a dog. *J Am Anim Hosp Assoc* 2002;38:246.

SAGE

■ SOURCE, DESCRIPTION, USES

There are many species of sage, but Spanish sage (*Salvia lavanduaefolia, S. officinalis*) is the one most used medicinally. It grows primarily along the Mediterranean coast of Spain. It has been used for many purposes, including as an expectorant and for digestive problems, appetite loss, and inflammation of the oropharyngeal mucosa.[1] It has been claimed to enhance memory.[2]

■ PHARMACOLOGY

Because of the memory-enhancing claim, Spanish sage has been investigated for possible usefulness in treating Alzheimer's disease. Spanish sage contains many monoterpenoids, several of which have been examined for pharmacological activity. Perry and associates[3] found that camphor and 1,8-cineole were noncompetitive inhibitors of erythrocyte acetylcholinesterase but were not particularly potent. In a subsequent paper, this group reported[4] that an ethanol extract and the monoterpenoids 1-8 cineole and α- and β-pinene had antioxidant activity in bovine brain peroxisomes. The extract, as well as α-pinene and geraniol, inhibited ecosanoid formation in rat leukocytes (possible anti-inflammatory activity). All of these pharmacological activities could be useful in treating patients with Alzheimer's disease. Possible estrogenic activity was suggested by inhibition of yeast cell galactosidase by the ethanol extract and geraniol. Because in most cases the extract generally was more potent than the individual monoterpenoids, the authors suggested that there might be an additive effect of the latter.

■ ADVERSE EFFECTS AND INTERACTIONS

Burkhard and colleagues[5] reported two cases of epileptic seizures associated with exposure to sage essential oil. In one, a 54-year-old woman had taken a spoonful daily for several years, always associated with epigastric distress, faintness, perfuse sweating, dizziness, and tachypnea. After consuming a higher than usual dose, these signs and symptoms were more pronounced and there were involuntary movements of the tongue. In the other, a 53-year-old man was given several drops by a coworker as a stimulant and experienced clonic-tonic seizures. Sage essential oil contains thujone, camphor, and cineole, which have been shown to possess convulsant activity.[5]

There is a theoretical possibility of an additive interaction with estrogens and phytoestrogens if sage has significant estrogenic activity.

■ REFERENCES

1. Schulz V, Hansel R, Tyler VE. Rational Phytotherapy: A Physician's Guide to Herbal Medicine. New York, NY: Springer-Verlag; 1995:27, 149.
2. Perry EK, Pickering AT, Wang WW, Houghton PJ, Perry NS. Medicinal plants and Alzheimer's disease: From ethnobotany to phytotherapy. *J Pharm Pharmacol* 1999;51:527.
3. Perry NS, Houghton PJ, Theobald A, Jenner P, Perry EK. In-vitro inhibition of human erythrocyte acetylcholinesterase by *Salvia lavandulaefolia* essential oil and constituent terpenes. *J Pharm Pharmacol* 2000;52:895.
4. Perry NS, Houghton PJ, Sampson J, et al. In-vitro activity of *S. lavandulaefolia* relevant to the treatment of Alzheimer's disease. *J Pharm Pharmacol* 2001;53:1347.
5. Burkhard PR, Burkhardt K, Haenggeli CA, Landis T. Plant-induced seizures: Reappearance of an old problem. *J Neurol* 1999;246:667.

ST. JOHN'S WORT

■ SOURCE, DESCRIPTION, USES

A yellow flowering plant, *Hypericum perforatum*, native to the eastern hemisphere and naturalized to North America, the herb consists of the dried, powdered, above-ground portion of the plant taken as a tea, tincture, tablet, or capsule. St. John's wort (SJW) is purported to have sedative, anxiolytic, and astringent properties, and it is taken internally for anxiety and depression and applied topically for wounds, minor burns, inflammation, and local pain.[1,2] In the past, it also has been used for bronchitis, cancer, enuresis, gastritis, hemorrhoids, hypothyroidism, insect bites, insomnia, kidney disease, and scabies.[3]

■ PHARMACOLOGY

Today, SJW is used almost exclusively for anxiety and depression, most often the latter. In 1998, sales were estimated at $400 million in the United States and $6 billion in Europe.[1] The plant contains a variety of bioactive chemicals, including hypericin (a naphthodianthrone) and hyperforin (a prenylated phloroglucinol)—these are believed to be the major constituents of pharmacological interest—as well as tannin and flavonoids. Weak inhibition of monoamine oxidases A and B has been shown for hypericin, but not by all investigators,[1,2] and binding affinity for a variety of neurotransmitter receptors has been demonstrated. These include receptors for serotonin (5-HT_1), γ-aminobutyric acid types A and B, adenosine, benzodiazepine, inositol triphosphate, and acetylcholine (muscarinic receptors).[1,2] It also has been shown to inhibit synaptosomal uptake of 5-HT, dopamine, and norepinephrine.[2] Other, neurotransmitter-related, effects have been shown for components of SJW, and it is clear that its pharmacology is complex. Antiviral and antibacterial activity has been demonstrated experimentally.[2] Commercial preparations often are standardized to 0.3% hypericin,[4] although hyperforin may be the more important active principle.

A number of double-blind clinical studies have shown that SJW is more effective than placebo in relieving the symptoms of depression and generally as effective as tricyclic antidepressants. This has been confirmed by meta-analysis of data from 1757 outpatients with mild to moderate depression.[1] These studies have been criticized for lack of diagnostic rigor and for relying on subjective assessment of outcome. Other problems with these studies also have been cited, including the use of subtherapeutic doses of the conventional drugs.[1] Although SJW may be useful in treating mild depression and is prescribed extensively in Europe for that purpose, it has not been shown to be effective in severe depression.[5] Moreover, it is now clear that it may interact with numerous prescription drugs, with potentially serious consequences.

ADVERSE EFFECTS AND INTERACTIONS

Clinical studies have shown that moderate doses of SJW, equivalent to 1 mg of hypericin daily, over a period of a few weeks produced an incidence of side effects similar to that of placebo (7.4 % versus 6.2 %).[2] Side effects generally are mild and include gastrointestinal disturbances, headache, fatigue, and skin rashes. Photosensitivity has been reported occasionally. Other studies have shown similar incidences of side effects of SJW with conventional therapies such as fluoxetine.[2] By far the greatest concern is the potential for interactions with many drugs. Interactions with other centrally acting agents are to be expected, but demonstration that SJW is capable of inducing many isozymes of the mixed function oxidases cytochrome P450 (CYP)[2] raised awareness that SJW could accelerate the biotransformation of many drugs, with resulting declines in therapeutic response. Of particular interest is the isozyme CYP3A4[6] in the wall of the intestine and in the liver. CYP3A4 is involved in the biotransformation of the immunosuppressive drug cyclosporine. One report[7] involves two kidney transplantation recipients who began to self-medicate with SJW, resulting in declines in plasma cyclosporine levels to subtherapeutic concentrations. One patient developed acute rejection. When SJW was discontinued, cyclosporine levels returned to the therapeutic range. Several similar cases were reviewed by Ernst.[8] P-glycoprotein, a transport protein involved in reducing intracellular drug concentrations, including cyclosporine, also has been shown to be induced by SJW.[6]

Many drugs are metabolized by the same pathway, including antiviral protease inhibitors, nonsedating antihistamines, calcium channel blockers, lipid-lowering inhibitors of 3-hydroxy-3-methylglutaryl coenzyme A (HMG-CoA) reductase, barbiturates, benzodiazepines, estrogen, macrolide antibiotics, carbamazepine, ketoconazole, cortisone, and warfarin.[1,2] In one study,[9] 300 mg of SJW three times daily in capsule form for 14 days lowered plasma levels of the HMG-CoA reductase inhibitor simvastatin and its metabolite but not the level of pravastatin, another HMG-CoA reductase inhibitor. Both drugs were given as a single dose to test and placebo groups. The effect on simvastatin was attributed to increased first-pass metabolism. Similar effects have been shown for amitryptyline[10] and digoxin[6] and no doubt occur with many other drugs. Both mania and hypomania have been reported as side effects of SJW. Pies reviewed several cases.[11]

The concomitant use of SJW with other antidepressants should be discouraged, and the coadministration of other centrally acting drugs is unwise given the potential for both pharmacological and biochemical interactions. The safety of SJW in pregnancy has not been established. It should be evident that if SJW is to be used, it should be in the absence of almost any other medications. Tannin-containing herbs such as SJW may interfere with iron absorption.[12] This may not be a serious problem clinically but should be considered in anemic patients, and it is advisable to avoid taking iron and the herbal preparation together.

■ REFERENCES

1. Greeson JM, Sanford B, Monti DA. St. John's wort (*Hypericum perforatum*): A review of the current pharmacological, toxicological, and clinical literature. *Psychopharmacology* 2001;153:402.

2. Barnes J, Anderson LA, Phillipson JD. St. John's wort (*Hypericum perforatum*): A review of its chemistry, pharmacology and clinical properties. *J Pharm Pharmacol* 2001;53:583.

3. Ernst E. The risk-benefit profile of commonly used herbal therapies: Ginkgo, St. John's wort, ginseng, echinacea, saw palmetto and kava. *Ann Intern Med* 2002;136:42.

4. Ang-Lee MK, Moss J, Yuan C-S. Herbal medicines and perioperative care. *JAMA* 2001;286:208.

5. Shelton RC, Keller MB, Gelenberg A, et al. Effectiveness of St. John's wort in major depression: A randomized controlled trial. *JAMA* 2001;285:1978.

6. Durr D, Stieger B, Kullak-Ublick GA, et al. St. John's wort induces intestinal P-glycoprotein/MDRI and intestinal and hepatic CYP3A4. *Clin Pharmacol Ther* 2000;68:598.

7. Turton-Weeks SM, Barone GW, Gurley BJ, Ketel BL, Lightfoot ML, Abul-Ezz SR. St. John's wort: A hidden risk for transplant patients. *Prog Transplant* 2001;11:116.

8. Ernst E. St. John's wort supplements endanger the success of organ transplantation. *Arch Surg* 2002;137:316.

9. Sugimoto K, Ohmori M, Tsuruoka S, et al. Different effects of St. John's wort on the pharmacokinetics of simvastatin and pravastatin. *Clin Pharmacol Ther* 2001;70:518.

10. Johne A, Schmider J, Brockmoller J, et al. Decreased plasma levels of amitriptyline and its metabolites on comedication with an extract of St. John's wort (Hypericum perforatum). *J Clin Psychopharmacol* 2002;22:46.

11. Pies R. Adverse neuropsychiatric reactions to herbal and over-the-counter "antidepressants". *J Clin Psychiatry* 2000;61:815.

12. Miller LG. Herbal medicinals; selected clinical considerations focusing on known or potential drug-herb interactions. *Arch Intern Med* 1998;158:2200.

SALAI GUGGAL

■ SOURCE, DESCRIPTION, USES

Salai guggal (SG) is an ancient Ayurvedic medicine from India. It is the gum resin from *Boswellia serrata,* a large, branching tree found in India, North Africa, and the Middle East.[1,2] In ancient Ayurvedic medical texts, SG was recommended for arthritis, rheumatism, diarrhea, dysentery, pulmonary disease, and ringworm.[2] Synonyms include Indian frankincense and boswellin.[2]

■ PHARMACOLOGY

SG contains up to 16% essential oil (mostly α-thujene and p-cymene), along with terpenoids and gum.[1] Four pentacyclic triterpene acids have been identified, the major one being β-boswellic acid, which is believed to be the main active principle. An ethanol extract of the gum resin is commonly used as the active substance. Animal studies have shown that it possesses anti-inflammatory activity in a variety of animal models, among them carrageenan-induced edema in rat paws (this effect also occurred in adrenalectomized rats, indicating that stimulation of the adrenal cortex is not part of its mechanism), and formaldehyde/adjuvant-induced arthritis in rats.[3] SG also prevents polymorphonuclear (PMN) leukocyte migration and infiltration, and inhibits antibody synthesis and the complement pathway.[4] The ethanol extract has been shown to block the synthesis of 5-lipoxygenase products. Rat PMN leukocytes were stimulated with calcium and calcium ionophore to produce leukotrienes (LTs) and 5-hydroxyecosatetraenoic acid (5-HETE) from arachidonic acid. SG extract caused a concentration-dependent inhibition of the synthesis of proinflammatory LTB4 and 5-HETE.[5] Disruption of sulfated glycosaminoglycans by nonsteroidal anti-inflammatory drugs can accelerate articular damage in arthritic diseases. A comparison was made between SG (SG and boswellic acids) and ketoprofen in this regard.[6] Although ketoprofen inhibited both the synthesis and the catabolism of glycosaminoglycans, SG inhibited only their catabolism, with the result that content was unchanged in the SG groups but reduced in the ketoprofen group. This finding suggests that SG might have a sparing effect on articular degeneration.

Leukotrienes are known to play a role in bronchial asthma, being powerful bronchoconstrictors.[7] One placebo-controlled, double-blind study was undertaken in 80 patients with bronchial asthma. Patients received 300 mg of a preparation of the gum resin three times daily for 6 weeks or matching placebo. Over the course of the trial, 70% of the 40 SG-treated patients showed improvement of symptoms and a decrease of the eosinophil count and erythrocyte sedimentation rate whereas only 27% of the 40 control subjects showed improvement.[8]

A triterpenoid, β-boswellic acid, has been shown to posses antineoplastic activity in a mouse cancer model, and addition of a number of pure agents from boswellin-inhibited DNA synthesis in human leukemia HL-60 cell cultures. Antihyperlipidemic activity also was demonstrated.[9]

■ ADVERSE EFFECTS AND INTERACTIONS

Adverse effects do not appear to be a serious problem with SG. One Internet site[2] lists diarrhea, skin rash, and nausea as rare side effects. Toxicology studies found no pathological changes in hematological, biochemical, or histological parameters in primates and rats at doses up to 1000 mg/kg.[1] Other than the trial noted earlier, no clinical studies appear to be extant at this time. There is no information regarding long-term effects or potential drug-herb interactions. Given the mechanism of SG's action, there is a theoretical possibility of interactions with both steroidal and nonsteroidal anti-inflammatory agents. It is conceivable that such an interaction might even be beneficial, given that SG appears to work in a manner unlike that of either category of drug. Because of the lack of hard data, however, the possibility of an adverse interaction cannot be ruled out at this time. Conjoint administration of SG with prescription drugs should be undertaken cautiously and monitored closely. No information regarding the effects on reproduction or fetal development could be obtained. See also Appendix VIII.

■ REFERENCES

1. Boswellia serrata, common name: Frankincense. *Altern Med Rev* 1998;3:306.
2. Boswellia. Holistic-online.com website. Available at: http://www.holistic-online.com/Herbal-Med/_Herbs/h34.htm.
3. Singh GB, Atal CK. Pharmacology of an extract of salai guggal ex-Boswellia serrata, a new non-steroidal anti-inflammatory agent. *Agents Actions* 1986;18:407.
4. Sharma ML, Khajuria A, Kaul A, Singh S, Singh GB, Atal CK. Effects of salai guggal extract of Boswellia serrata on cellular and humoral immune responses and leukocyte migration. *Agents Actions* 1988;24:161.
5. Ammon HP, Mack T, Singh GB, Safayhi H. Inhibition of leukotriene B4 formation in rat peritoneal neutrophils by an ethanolic extract of the gum resin exudate of Boswellia serrata. *Planta Med* 1991;57:203.
6. Reddy GK, Chandrakasan G, Dhar SC. Studies on the metabolism of glycosaminoglycans under the influence of new herbal anti-inflammatory agents. *Biochem Pharmacol* 1989;38:3527.

7. Piper PJ. Formation and actions of leukotrienes. *Physiol Rev* 1984;64:744.
8. Gupta I, Gupta V, Parihar A, et al. Effects of Boswellia serrata gum resin in patients with bronchial asthma: Results of a double-blind, placebo-controlled, 6-week clinical study. *Eur J Med Res* 1998;3:511.
9. Huang MT, Badmaev V, Ding Y, Liu Y, Xie JG, Ho CT. Anti-tumor and anti-carcinogenic activities of triterpenoid beta-boswellic acid. *Biofactors* 2000;13:225.

SANGRE DE GRADO

■ SOURCE, DESCRIPTION, USES

Similar to cat's claw, sangre de grado (there is no equivalent English name in common use) is native to the Amazonian rain forest of Peru. It is the dark red sap, or latex, of a large tree *Croton lechleri*. The Spanish name refers to the color of the sap. In traditional Amazonian medicine, the sap is used fresh or dried and powdered. It is used as a gargle for sore throats, a post-partum vaginal antiseptic, and a topical hemostatic, and is taken internally to promote wound healing, to protect the gastrointestinal mucosa, and for diarrhea.[1]

■ PHARMACOLOGY

It has been noted[1] that the ethnobotanical approach (i.e., investigating medicinal plants used by indigenous cultures) to the study of possible plant pharmaceuticals has yielded positive findings with a frequency that is orders of magnitude greater than the classical approach (i.e., studying plants because of their taxonomic relationship to known plant sources of active pharmacological principles). Sangre de grado is an example of this type of payoff. The plant contains phenols, diterpenes, phytosterols, proanthocyanidins, a dihydrobenzofuran, the alkaloid taspine, and doubtless many other active agents. Antibacterial activity has been confirmed, as has usefulness in wound healing (taspine) and antineoplastic activity (taspine).[1]

A novel proanthocyanidin, designated SP-303, has been shown in clinical trials to be useful in controlling diarrhea in patients with acquired immunodeficiency syndrome (AIDS). In a phase II, randomized, double-blind, placebo-controlled study of 51 patients with AIDS-associated diarrhea, the treated group had a significant reduction in daily stool weight after 4 days of treatment.[2]

Antiviral activity of an extract of sangre de grado has been demonstrated against influenza, parainfluenza, herpes simplex types 1 and 2, and hepatitis A and B viruses.[1] In one controlled, double-blind study, a topical application of a preparation containing SP-303 was administered to AIDS patients with genital herpes; 50% of the treated group were culture-negative after 21 days compared with 19% of the control group.[3] It was hypothesized that a combination of antibacterial, anti-inflammatory, and antioxidant activities might confer nonspecific immunomodulatory effect.

Topical anti-inflammatory/analgesic activity has been confirmed in a clinical trial. Pest control workers preferred sangre de grado balm over placebo for pain, itching, and inflammation of insect stings and bites (e.g., wasps, ants), reporting that relief was obtained within minutes.[4] Benefits also were reported for treating cuts and abrasions.

Animal studies have confirmed many of the proposed therapeutic effects of this botanical remedy. Facilitated healing of fundic ulcers in rats has been observed and attributed in part to the inhibition of ulcer-induced upregulation of tumor necrosis factor-α, inducible nitrous oxide synthase, and interleukin-6. The bacterial counts in the fundic ulcers also were decreased.[5] The benefits of topical application have been supported by studies with rat models of inflammation.[4] Other *Croton* species (e.g., *C. palanostigma*) can be a source of sangre de grado,[6] which has been shown to induce apoptosis in human gastrointestinal cells in a dose-dependent manner. This finding could have implications for an anticancer effect. Taspine hydrochloride has been shown to induce fibroblast migration, a possible explanation for its effect to promote wound healing.[7]

■ ADVERSE EFFECTS AND INTERACTIONS

Nausea and vomiting have occurred as a result of the bitter taste of the herb. Because of possible effects on the immune system, it is recommended that patients taking immunosuppressive drugs avoid this herb systemically. Long-term systemic use should be avoided, especially in patients with autoimmune disorders, as should use in pregnant women and young children until more is known about the effects of the herb and its active principles.

One ingredient, taspine, did not show evidence of carcinogenic or tumor-promoting effect after 17 months of treatment in the mouse two-stage skin carcinogenesis model.[7]

■ REFERENCES

1. Williams JL. Review of antiviral and immunomodulating properties of plants of the Peruvian rainforest with a particular emphasis on una de gato and sangre de grado. *Altern Med Rev* 2001;6:567.

2. Holodniy M, Koch J, Mistal M, et al. A double-blind, randomized, placebo-controlled Phase II study to assess the safety and efficacy of orally administered SP-303 for the treatment of diarrhea in patients with AIDS. *Am J Gastroenterol* 1999;94:3267.

3. Orozco-Topete R, Sierra-Madero J, Cano-Dominguez C, et al. Safety and efficacy of Virend for topical treatment genital and herpes simplex lesions in patients with AIDS. *Antiviral Res* 1997;35:91.

4. Miller MJ, Vergnolle N, McKnight W, et al. Inhibition of neurogenic inflammation by the Amazonian herbal medicine sangre de grado. *J Invest Dermatol* 2001;117:725.

5. Miller MJ, MacNaughton WK, Zhang XJ, et al. Treatment of gastric ulcers and diarrhea with the Amazonian herbal medicine sangre de grado. *Am J Physiol Gastrointest Liver Physiol* 2000;279:G192.

6. Sandoval M, Okuhama NN, Clark M, et al. Sangre de grado Croton palanostigma induces apoptosis in human gastrointestinal cells. *J Ethnopharmacol* 2002;80:121.

7. Vaisberg AJ, Milla M, Planas MC, et al. Taspine is the cicatrizant principle in sangre de grado extracted from croton lechleri. *Planta Med* 1989;55:140.

SARSAPARILLA (THE SARSAPARILLAS)

■ SOURCE, DESCRIPTION, USES

Discussion of sarsaparilla can be very confusing because of the number of unrelated botanicals called "sarsaparilla" and the number of *Smilax* species, the true sarsaparillas, used in herbal medicine for diverse purposes. The name derives from the Spanish *zarzaparilla*, a combination of *zarza*, meaning bramble and *parra*, meaning vine—thus a thorny vine, an apt description of the true sarsaparillas. There are estimated to be over 225 species in this family (Smilacaeae),[1] but many are still classified as Liliaceae.[2] Some plants, such as bristly sarsaparilla and wild sarsaparilla, are actually members of the ginseng, or Araliaceae, family.[3] In all cases, it is the dried root (rhizome) that constitutes the herb.

■ PHARMACOLOGY

AMERICAN SARSAPARILLA

American sarsaparilla, or *Aralia nudicaulis*, also is known as wild sarsaparilla, shot bush, wild licorice, and by many other names. It is a plant resembling the Umbelliferae, with an umbel consisting of clusters of small, pale green flowers that produce small black berries.[4] Traditionally a treatment for cutaneous ulcers, shingles, and pulmonary infections,[4] it does not seem to be much used now.

JAMAICAN SARSAPARILLA

Smilax ornata or *S. medica* is a true sarsaparilla that grows in the Caribbean and Central America.[5] It was originally exported through Jamaica to Europe as a treatment for syphilis. Other traditional uses were as a tonic, and for skin conditions, rheumatism, and dropsy.

SMILAX GLABRA

This variant has been used extensively for centuries in Chinese medicine to treat bacterial dysentery, nephritis, and syphilis.[6] It contains a number of phenylpropanoid glycosides and has been shown to possess some hepatoprotective activity. It also has been shown to have some hypoglycemic effect in mice, possibly by increasing insulin sensitivity.[7] Other animal studies have shown *S. glabra* to have anti-inflammatory and immunomodulatory activity.[8]

Smilax extracts have been used in performance-enhancing nutritional supplements, but there are few studies testing their efficacy.[9] Numerous other properties have been attributed to various sarsaparillas, and animal studies have been conducted, but clinical evidence of efficacy is lacking as yet.

■ ADVERSE EFFECTS AND INTERACTIONS

The German Commission E monograph for sarsaparilla lists it as an unapproved herb and states that preparations lead to gastric irritation and temporary kidney impairment (diuresis) and may increase the absorption of some drugs, such as digitalis glycosides and bismuth. The monograph also states that it will accelerate the renal excretion of other drugs such as hypnotics.[10] However, no scientific data supporting these claims are presented. Reports that sarsaparilla may contain carcinogens also have appeared, without specific references.[11] There is one report of *S. campestris*, a Brazilian species, causing mutation in a *Salmonella*/microsome test.[12]

Part of the confusion regarding the efficacy and safety of sarsaparillas must surely relate to the multiplicity of plants given this name and from which herbal remedies are prepared. In India, for example, the name is applied to *Hemidesmus indicus*, from which a compound with adjuvant properties has been isolated.[13]

In summary, despite the widespread use of sarsaparilla plants in herbal medicine throughout the world, and the numerous pharmacological properties that have been demonstrated in animal studies, evidence for efficacy and safety in humans is notably lacking.

■ REFERENCES

1. Smilacaceae. BoDD—Botanical Dermatology database. Available at: http://bodd.cf.ac.uk/BotDermFolder/BotDermS/SMIL.html.
2. Peterson RT, McKenny M. *Northeastern Wildflowers: Roger Tory Peterson Field Guides.* Norwalk, Conn: Easton Press; 1984:370.
3. Peterson RT, McKenny M. *Northeastern Wildflowers: Roger Tory Peterson Field Guides.* Norwalk, Conn: Easton Press; 1984:50.
4. Sarsaparilla, American. In: Grieve M. *A Modern Herbal.* Botanical.com website. Available at: http://botanical.com/botanical/mgmh/s/sarame15.html.
5. Sarsaparilla, Jamaican. In: Grieve M. *A Modern Herbal.* Botanical.com website. Available at: http://www.botanical.com/botanical/mgmh/s/sar-jam17.html.
6. Chen T, Li J-X, Xu Q. Phenylpropanoid glycosides from Smilax glabra. *Phytochemistry* 2000;53:1051.
7. Fukunaga T, Miura T, Furuta K, Kato A. Hypoglycemic effect of the rhizomes of Smilax glabra in normal and diabetic mice. *Biol Pharm Bull* 1997;20:44.
8. Jiang J, Xu Q. Immunomodulatory activity of the aqueous extract from the rhizome of Smilax glabra in the late phase of adjuvant-induced arthritis in rats. *J Ethnopharmacol* 2003;85:53.
9. Bucci LR. Selected herbals and human exercise performance. *Am J Clin Nutr* 2000;72(suppl):624S.
10. German Commission E monographs. Available at: http://libux.utmb.edu/comme.
11. Fisher CR, Veronneau SJH. Herbal preparations: A primer for the aeromedical physician. *Aviat Space Environ Med* 2000;71:45.
12. de Sa Ferriera IC, Ferrao Vargas VM. Mutagenicity of medicinal plant extracts in Salmonella/microsome assay. *Phytother Res* 1999;13:397.
13. Alam MI, Gomes A. Adjuvant effects and antiserum action potentiation by a (herbal) compound 2-hydroxy-4-methoxy benzoic acid isolated from the root extract of the Indian medicinal plant "sarsaparilla" (Hemidesmus indicus R. Br.). *Toxicon* 1998;36:1423.

SASSAFRAS

■ SOURCE, DESCRIPTION, USES

Sassafras (*Sassafras albidum, S. officinale*) is a medium to large tree with reddish bark and three-lobed leaves. Twigs are green, often branched, and sometimes hairy.[1] Crushed leaves, twigs, and bark emit a spicy fragrance.

Sassafras grows widely throughout eastern and central North America. The root bark generally is used as the herbal remedy, and traditional uses include as a diaphoretic; for rheumatism, syphilis, and skin diseases; and to induce vomiting (oil of sassafras).[2] Abortion has been associated with sassafras use. It was previously used as a flavoring for soft drinks, candy, and cough remedies, often in conjunction with sarsaparilla.

■ PHARMACOLOGY

Sassafras contains several active principles, including tannins, mucilages, thymol, and the alkylbenzene safrole.[2,3] Isosafrole and dihydrosafrole are related to safrole. Sassafras has been reported to possess diuretic activity.[4]

■ ADVERSE EFFECTS AND INTERACTIONS

In 1978, because of concern that the incidence of cancer was high in areas where herbal remedies were used extensively, a study of aqueous extracts of several herbs was conducted to determine their carcinogenicty.[5] When sassafras extract was injected subcutaneously into rats, it elicited tumors in over 50% of the animals.[5] The U.S. Food and Drug Administration subsequently invoked the Delaney Amendment, which prohibits the use of any food additive that has been found to be carcinogenic. A shipment of sassafras was seized, and there was no further use of sassafras as a flavoring agent.[6] It is still available through Internet suppliers, however, and its relative ubiquity makes it easy to harvest by herbalists or individuals.

It is now recognized that the carcinogen in sassafras is the alkylbenzene safrole.[7,8] Safrole has been shown to form DNA adducts in a dose-dependent manner in mouse liver over a 10,000-fold dose range. The livers were examined up to 40 days after injection injection of female mice with safrole. A ten-fold dosage increase was associated with a ten-fold increase in DNA adducts.

Sassafras also may interact with diuretics.[4] In light of the carcinogenic potential of sassafras, use of this herb is ill advised.

■ REFERENCES

1. Petrides GA. *Trees and Shrubs: Roger Tory Peterson Field Guides.* Norwalk, Conn: Easton Press; 1984:208, 320.
2. Sassafras. In: Grieve M. *A Modern Herbal.* Botanical.com website. Available at: http://www.botanical.com/botanical/mgmh/s/sassaf20.html.
3. Carlson M, Thompson RD. Liquid chromatographic determination of safrole in sassafras-derived herbal products. *J AOAC Int* 1997;80:1023.

4. Fisher CR, Veronneau SJH. Herbal preparations: A primer for the aeromedical physician. *Aviat Space Environ Med* 2000;71:45.

5. Kapadia GL, Chung EB, Ghosh B, et al. Carcinogenicity of some folk medicinal herbs in rats. *J Natl Cancer Inst* 1978;60:683.

6. Miller L, Murray WJ, eds. *Herbal Medicinals: A Clinician's Guide.* New York, NY: Pharmaceuticals Products Press; 1998:147.

7. Vesselinovitch SD, Rao KVN, Mihailovich N. Transplacental and lactational carcinogenesis by safrole. *Cancer Res* 1979;39:4378.

8. Miller EC, Swanson AP, Phillips DH, Fletcher TL, Liem A, Miller JA. Structure-activity studies of the carcinogenicities in the mouse and rat of some naturally occurring and synthetic alkylbenzene derivatives related to safrole and estragole. *Cancer Res* 1983;43:1124.

9. Gupta KP, van Golen KL, Putnam KL, Randerath K. Formation and persistence of safrole-DNA adducts over a 10,000-fold dose range in mouse liver. *Carcinogenesis* 1993;14:1517.

SAW PALMETTO

■ SOURCE, DESCRIPTION, USES

The dried, powdered berries of the American dwarf palm (*Serenoa repens, Sabal serrulata, Serenoa serrulata*) have been used in folk medicine for generations to treat genitourinary tract problems as well as for sexual dysfunction and as a diuretic.[1]

■ PHARMACOLOGY

Current use is almost exclusively for the treatment of benign prostatic hypertrophy (BPH). Meta-analysis of a number of clinical trials suggests that saw palmetto is as effective as finasteride (Proscar),[1] and the incidence of adverse reactions is low. Active ingredients include essential and fixed oils, a liposterolic compound, and high-molecular-weight polysaccharides.[2] Common dosage is 160 mg twice daily of a standardized, fat-soluble extract containing 85% to 95% fatty acids and sterols.[2] The mechanism of action appears to be similar to that of finasteride; namely, inhibition of the enzyme 5-α reductase and, hence, the conversion of testosterone to its active form, dihydrotestosterone (DHT). Interference of binding of DHT to cytosolic receptors in prostate cells appears to play a role, as well.[3,4]

■ ADVERSE EFFECTS AND INTERACTIONS

Nausea and abdominal pain, hypertension, headache, urinary retention, and back pain have been reported but are rare.[2] The American Urological Association has expressed concern that self-medication with saw palmetto for symptoms associated with BPH could mask prostate cancer and delay treatment, with serious consequences. Inhibitors of 5-α reductase are known to lower prostate-specific antigen (PSA) levels, which could lead to false-negative results with the PSA test.[5] Because saw palmetto is a modulator of androgenic and estrogenic effects, it is contraindicated for patients with breast cancer and those receiving estrogen therapy for any reason. Women who take oral contraceptives should not use saw palmetto for urogenital problems, nor should pregnant or lactating women.[2] Effects of long-term use are unknown. Tannin-containing herbs such as saw palmetto may interfere with iron absorption.[6] This may not be a serious problem clinically but should be considered in anemic patients, and it is advisable to avoid taking iron and the herbal preparation together.

■ REFERENCES

1. Ernst E. The risk-benefit profile of commonly used herbal therapies: Ginkgo, St. John's wort, ginseng, echinacea, saw palmetto and kava. *Ann Intern Med* 2002;136:42.
2. Arizona Poison and Drug Information Center website. Saw palmetto. Available at: http://www.pharmacy.arizona.edu/centers/apdic/sawpalmetto.shtml.
3. Sultan C, Terraza A, Devillier C, et al. Inhibition of androgen metabolism and binding by a liposterolic extract of "Serenoa repens B" in human foreskin fibroblasts. *J Steroid Biochem* 1984;20:515.
4. Di Silverio F, Monti S, Sciarra A, et al. Effects of long-term treatment with Seranoa repens (Permixon) on the concentrations and regional distribution of androgens and epidermal growth factor in benign prostatic hyperplasia. *Prostate* 1998;37:77.
5. Trabucco AF. Saw palmetto warning: Problems with detecting prostate cancer? Available at: http://www.priory.com/med/saw.htm.
6. Miller LG. Herbal medicinals: Selected clinical considerations focusing on known or potential drug-herb interactions. *Arch Intern Med* 1998;158:2200.

SENNA

■ SOURCE, DESCRIPTION, USES

The stripped leaves of two species of *Cassia, C. senna* from the Nile valley and *C. angustifolia* from the Red Sea area, are used in teas and in extracts that may be used in over-the-counter cathartics.[1] Both are sometimes included in a single taxon, *Senna alexandrina*.[1] Senna contains anthraquinone glycosides as the active agents, and the toxicity, contraindications, and interactive potential are the same as those of aloe vera[2] (see ALOE VERA). In addition, senna has been associated with cases of toxic hepatitis.[3]

■ REFERENCES

1. Schulz V, Hansel R, Tyler VE. *Rational Phytotherapy: A Physician's Guide to Herbal Medicine.* New York, NY: Springer-Verlag; 1998:210.
2. Jafri S, Pasricha PJ. Agents used for diarrhea, constipation and inflammatory bowel disease; agents used for biliary and pancreatic disease. In: Hardman JG, Limbird L, Gilman AG, eds. *Goodman and Gilman's The Pharmacological Basis of Therapeutics.* 10th ed. New York, NY: McGraw-Hill; 2001:1046.
3. Haller CA, Dyer JE, Ko R, Olson KR. Making a diagnosis of herbal-related toxic hepatitis. *West J Med* 2002;176:39.

SITOSTEROL

See β-SITOSTEROL.

SILYBUM

See MILK THISTLE.

SILYMARIN

See MILK THISTLE.

SKULLCAP

■ SOURCES, DESCRIPTION, USES

Skullcap (*Scutalleria laterifolia*), or scullcap, is a member of the mint (Labiatae) family that is native to much of northeastern North America. It grows to a height of about 0.5 m, with violet or blue flowers and leaves that are arranged oppositely. The dried, aerial portions of the plant are used to prepare the herb.[1] Its common name, mad dog, derived from the belief that skullcap could cure rabies.[2] Other traditional uses were as a treatment for epilepsy, an antispasmodic, a diuretic, a sedative, and a tonic.[1] Current herbal use is as a tonic, a tranquilizer, and an antispasmodic.[3]

■ PHARMACOLOGY

Not much documentation exists regarding the pharmacology of skullcap. It contains assorted flavonoids and other compounds, such as butylated hydroxytoluene, that may account for the purported antispasmodic activity.[3] The central effects (tranquilizing, sedative) have not been confirmed.[3] The German Commission E monographs do not list skullcap.[4] It appears to be primarily a New World herbal remedy and was once used in Native American medicine.

■ ADVERSE EFFECTS AND INTERACTIONS

Concern about the hepatotoxicity of skullcap was noted as early as 1989. MacGregor and colleagues[5] discussed four cases, all women, in which toxic liver damage developed after taking herbal preparations containing skullcap. There have been more recent reports of hepatic failure, sometimes fatal, with skullcap, often used in combination with other herbal remedies.[6] One of these[7] involved a patient taking six tablets of skullcap daily for the preceding 6 months, along with pau d'arco at an unspecified dose. No other herbs apparently were involved, and other potential causes were ruled out. The patient developed progressive liver failure over the ensuing 5 weeks and died while awaiting liver transplantation. The causal agent in skullcap has not been identified but does not appear to be a pyrrolizidine.[8]

In view of the lack of demonstrable efficacy and safety of skullcap, one review[3] concluded that use of the herb should be avoided. I concur with that evaluation. See also Appendix III.

■ REFERENCES

1. Scullcaps. In: Grieve M. *A Modern Herbal.* Botanical.com website. Available at: http://www.botanical.com/botanical/mgmh/s/scullc34.html.
2. Peterson RT, McKenny M. *Northeastern Wildflowers: Roger Tory Peterson Field Guides.* Norwalk, Conn: Easton Press; 1984:346.
3. Cauffield JS, Forbes HJ. Dietary supplements used in the treatment of depression, anxiety, and sleep disorders. *Prim Care* 1999;3:290.
4. Keller K. Legal requirements for the use of phytopharmaceutical drugs in the Federal Republic of Germany. *J Ethnopharmacol* 1991;31:225.
5. MacGregor FB, Abernethy VE, Dahabra S, Cobden I, Hayes PC. Hepatotoxicity of herbal remedies. *BMJ* 1989;299:1156.
6. Haller CA, Dyer JE, Ko R, Olson KR. Making a diagnosis of herbal-related toxic hepatitis. *West J Med* 2002;176:39.
7. Hullar TE, Sapers BL, Ridker PM, Jenkins PL, Huth TS, Farraye FA. Herbal toxicity and fatal hepatic failure. *Am J Med* 1999;106:267.
8. Langmead L, Rampton DS. Review article: Herbal treatment in gastrointestinal disease-benefits and dangers. *Aliment Pharmacol Ther* 2001;15:1239.

SKULLCAP (CHINESE)

■ SOURCE, DESCRIPTION, USES

Chinese skullcap herb is prepared from *Scutellaria baikalensis,* a member of the mint (Labiatae) family. It is a native of Russia and China, the species name being derived from Baikal, the largest freshwater lake in Russia. The herb is used in traditional Chinese medicine to treat skin conditions, allergies, elevated plasma lipids, and hypertension.[1]

■ PHARMACOLOGY

The root contains a polyphenolic flavonoid, baicalin, which has been the subject of extensive research recently. Wartenberg and colleagues[2] examined several traditional Chinese herbs and their active principles for their ability to inhibit tumor-induced angiogenesis (and, hence, tumor proliferation) and found that baicalein significantly inhibited angiogenesis as did several other herbal ingredients. This effect was attributed to their antioxidant properties. Vitamin E also completely blocked tumor-induced angiogenesis.

A mixture of seven Chinese herbs, PC-SPES, has shown promise in clinical trials for the treatment of prostate cancer.[3] Two of the component herbs, *Glycyrrhiza uralensis* and *S. baicalensis*, inhibited cell growth and downregulated prostate-specific antigen in a human prostate cancer cell line, suggesting that at least some of the activity of the mixture could be a result of these herbs. Baicalein has been shown to be a 12-lipoxegenase inhibitor, to inhibit platelet-activating factor–induced platelet aggregation,[4] and to inhibit hepatic fibrosis.[5]

■ ADVERSE EFFECTS AND INTERACTIONS

No evidence was found regarding adverse effects and interactions. There is one report[6] that *S. baicalensis* can inhibit 11-β-hydroxysteroid dehydrogenase, leading to pseudohyperaldosteronism. Given the multiplicity of pharmacological actions attributed to baicalein, the possibility of drug interactions with anticancer and other prescription drugs such as antiplatelet agents cannot be discounted. Use in pregnant or nursing mothers and children should be discouraged.

■ REFERENCES

1. Chinese skullcap. Available at: http://www.hollandandbarrett.com/Herb/Skullcap_Chinese.htm
2. Wartenberg M, Budde P, De Marees M. Inhibition of tumor-induced angiogenesis and matrix-metalloproteinase expression in confrontation cultures of embryoid bodies and tumor spheroids by plant ingredients used in traditional Chinese medicine. *Lab Invest* 2003;83:87.
3. Hsieh T-C, Lu X, Chea J, Wu JM. Prevention and management of prostate cancer using PC-SPES: A scientific perspective. *J Nutrit* 2002;132:3513S.
4. Michibayashi T. Platelet aggregating response to platelet activating factor participates in activation of the 12-lipoxygenase pathway in platelets from rabbits. *Int Angiol* 2002;21:260.
5. Schuppan D, Porov Y. Hepatic fibrosis: From bench to bedside. *J Gastroenterol Hepatol* 2002;17(suppl):S300.
6. Miller LG, Murray WJ, eds. *Herbal Medicines: A Clinician's Guide.* New York, NY: Pharmaceutical Products Press; 1998:13, 23.

SUPEROXIDE DISMUTASE

■ SOURCE, DESCRIPTION, USES

Superoxide dismutase (SOD) is an enzyme, present in mammalian cells, that catalyses the dismutation of superoxide radical (O_2^-) to hydrogen peroxide (H_2O_2). The H_2O_2 is then degraded to H_2O and O_2 under the influence of another enzyme, catalase. The system is able to handle the small amounts of free radicals that are continuously generated by cell functions, but it may be overwhelmed in certain pathological situations.[1] This constitutes the rationale for SOD supplementation or therapy. Because animal studies have shown that the levels of SOD decline with age, SOD also has become fashionable as an anti-aging supplement.[2]

■ PHARMACOLOGY

SODs differ in their requirement for trace metals. Copper-zinc superoxide dismutase (CuZnSOD) is found in the cytosol and manganese superoxide dismutase (MnSOD) in mitochondria.[1] SOD also is present in serum in high concentrations and functions to protect the vascular endothelium against oxidative damage.[1] Exogenous SOD has been employed to prevent the development of chronic lung disease in premature infants. Although there was some evidence following discharge that treated infants had fewer respiratory problems and fewer chest abnormalities on X-ray, there were no differences in mortality before discharge between treated and untreated groups.[3] Erythrocyte SOD levels are reduced in low-birth-weight infants given iron supplementation, possibly because of altered copper metabolism resulting from the supplemental iron.[4] Oral administration of SOD is unreliable because of gastric digestion of the protein, and sublingual tablets are no more reliable.[2] There is no evidence to support recommending SOD as a nutritional supplement for anti-aging effects or any other purpose.

■ ADVERSE REACTIONS AND INTERACTIONS

The Cochrane review[3] found that SOD was well tolerated. No other information regarding side effects or interactions is available.

■ REFERENCES

1. Morikawa K, Morikawa S. Immunomodulatory effect of recombinant human superoxide dismutase (SOD) on human B lymphocyte function. *Cell Immunol* 1996;172:70.

2. Anti-aging products, Part 1: Can supplements rewind our body clocks? *Harvard Women's Health Watch* 2001;9:2.

3. Suresh GK, Davis JM, Soll RF. Superoxide dismutase for preventing chronic lung disease in mechanically ventilated infants (Cochrane Review). Cochrane Library issue 2; 2003. Available at: http://www.update-software.com/abstracts/ab001968.htm.

4. Barclay SM, Aggett PJ, Lloyd DJ, Duffty P. Reduced erythrocyte superoxide dismutase activity in low birth weight infants given iron supplements. *Pediatr Res* 1991;29:297.

TAMARIND

■ SOURCE, DESCRIPTION, USES

The Tamarind (*Tamarindus indica*) is a large tree native to India, although one variety is native to the West Indies.[1] It has fragrant, yellow-veined flowers and 6 to 12 seeds within a long pod. The pulp of the fruit is used as a laxative, and other traditional uses include as a febrifuge and an antiseptic.[1] It also has been used for stomachache and for gallbladder ailments.[2] The fruit is available as an extract, a syrup, or as molded cakes for oral consumption.[2]

■ PHARMACOLOGY

Tamarind contains tartaric acid, sugar, pectin, pyrazines, and thiazols.[2] Pectin and organic acids are believed to impart the laxative effect. Tamarind is one of a number of herbs and spices that have been shown to possess antibacterial action. It had potent inhibitory effect on several organisms.[3]

■ ADVERSE EFFECTS AND INTERACTIONS

There is one report of tamarind increasing the bioavailability of aspirin, leading to gastrointestinal bleeding.[2] No other information is available regarding interactions between tamarind and other nonsteroidal anti-inflammatory drugs (NSAIDs).

In one study of 20 healthy schoolboys who ate 10 g of tamarind daily with lunch for 18 days, urinary fluoride levels were significantly increased (4.8 versus 3.5 mg excreted per day).[4] The authors concluded that tamarind could be useful in delaying the progression of fluorosis. Conversely, it could interfere with water fluoridation programs by increasing urinary excretion and retarding deposition in dental enamel.

Tamarind frequently is used in the preparation of candy. There have been several cases of lead contamination of imported candies, leading to lead poisoning in children.[4,5]

In summary, the occasional use of tamarind as a laxative probably carries little risk. Habitual use probably should be avoided by persons who habitually use NSAIDs. Excessive consumption of candies by children should be discouraged if fluoridation for prevention of dental cares is in progress. Imported tamarind candy should be avoided. See also Appendix I.

■ REFERENCES

1. Tamarinds. In: Grieve M. *A Modern Herbal*. Botanical.com website. Available at: http://www.botanical.com/botanical/mgmh/t/tamari04. html.
2. Abebe W. Herbal medication: Potential for adverse interactions with analgesic drugs. *J Clin Pharm Ther* 2002;27:391.
3. Krishna De M, Banerjee AB. Antimicrobial screening of some Indian spices. *Phytother Res* 1999;13:616.
4. Childhood lead poisoning associated with tamarind candy and folk remedies—California 1999–2000. *Morbid Mortal Weekly Rep* 2002;51:684.
5. Lynch RA, Boatwright DT, Moss SK. Lead-contaminated candy and children's blood lead levels. *Pub Health Rep* 2000;115:537.

TRIPTERYGIUM WILDFORDII

■ SOURCE, DESCRIPTION, USES

Tripterygium wildfordii Hook F (TWHF) is a shrubby vine (family Celastraceae) native to much of Southeast Asia. It has glossy, light green leaves, small white flowers, and three-winged fruit. In Chinese herbal medicine it is known as lei gong teng, and it also is called yellow vine. It has been used for generations for treating arthritic as well as autoimmune and inflammatory diseases.[1] Currently, western medicine is investigating this herb for these and other applications.

■ PHARMACOLOGY

Several clinical trials have been conducted, generally with an ethanol-ethyl-acetate extract of TWHF root. In one study using 180 and 360 mg/day of herb extract and a placebo over 20 weeks, 4 of 10 subjects in a low-dose and 8 of 10 in a high-dose group showed appreciable clinical improvement, compared with none of 12 subjects in the placebo group. Clinically positive response was based on a 20% improvement in the criteria of the American Rheumatism Association.[1] Similar evidence of efficacy was observed in an open-label trial conducted at similar doses.[2] One group reviewed evidence for efficacy of several alternative remedies in the treatment of systemic lupus erythematosus (SLE) and found that only TWHF provided convincing evidence of significant improvement.[3]

One in vitro study examined the ability of TWHF and several other Chinese herbs to inhibit the release of prostaglandin E_2 and interleukin-2 from human monocytes. The researchers found that only TWHF did so at concentrations that could reasonably be achieved clinically, suggesting that this could be involved in its mechanism of action.[4]

Considerable research is ongoing on the potential immunosuppressive and anticancer activity of this herb.[5,6]

■ ADVERSE EFFECTS AND INTERACTIONS

One of the major drawbacks of this herbal preparation has been a relatively high incidence of adverse reactions, some serious. Common side effects include stomach upset, diarrhea, skin rash, and skin pigmentation.[3] These reactions tend to be dose related and transient. However, disturbances in both male and female reproductive function also have been reported, and overdose has been associated with myocardial and renal damage.[3] There is some interest in exploring the herb for use as a male contraceptive. In the study of rheumatoid arthritis,[1] mentioned earlier, there was little difference in the number of patients with one or more adverse effects among the three groups (including the placebo group). Several of these reactions occurred only in the high-dose group, however, including facial rash, tinnitus, abdominal pain, and vaginal spotting.

Drug interactions have not been reported, but given the broad range of pharmacological actions of this herb, there is a strong potential for these. Likely candidates would be cardiovascular drugs, nonsteroidal anti-inflammatory drugs, corticosteroids, and immunosuppressive drugs. In summary, TWHF may develop into a useful alternative for treating autoimmune diseases if toxicity can be controlled, and research may yield useful new agents from it in the future. See also Appendices VII and VIII.

■ REFERENCES

1. Tao X, Younger J, Fan FZ, Wang B, Lipsky PE. Benefit of an extract of Tripteygium wildfordii Hook F in patients with rheumatoid arthritis: A double-blind, placebo-controlled study. *Arthritis Rheum* 2002;46:1735.

2. Tao X, Cush JJ, Garret M, Lipsky PE. A phase I study of ethyl acetate extract of the Chinese antirheumatic herb Tripterygium wilfordii Hook F in rheumatoid arthritis. J Rheumatol 28: 2160, 2001.

3. Patavino T, Brady DM. Natural medicine and nutritive therapy as an alternative treatment in systemic lupus erythematosus. *Altern Med Rev* 2001;6:460.

4. Chou CT, Chang SC. The inhibitory effect of common traditional antirheumatic herb formulas on prostaglandin E and interleukin 2 in vitro: A comparative study with Tripterygium wilfordii. *J Ethnopharmacol* 1998;62:167.

5. Fidler JM, Ku GY, Piazza D, Xu R, Jin R, Chen Z. Immunosuppressive activity of the Chinese medicinal plant Tripterygium wilfordii. III. Suppression of graft-versus-host disease in murine allogenic bone marrow transplantation by the PG27 extract. *Transplantation* 2000;74:445.

6. Kiviharju TM, Lecane PS, Sellers RG, Peehl DM. Antiproliferative and proapoptotic activities of triptolide (PG-490), a natural product entering clinical trials, on primary cultures of human prostatic epithelial cells. *Clin Cancer Res* 2002;8:2666.

TRYPTOPHAN

See L-TRYPTOPHAN.

TURMERIC

■ SOURCE, DESCRIPTION, USES

Turmeric is the main ingredient in curry spice. It consists of the powdered root of *Curcuma longa*, which is widely cultivated throughout India, Asia, and Africa.[1] *C. longa* belongs to the family Zingiberaceae and is thus related to ginger. Although not used much as an herbal remedy now, the traditional use of turmeric included as a stimulant, and for treating jaundice.[1] More recently, it has been used to treat pain of arthritis, inflammation, and skin infections.[2] Several potentially useful biological activities have been identified in turmeric, and these are the subjects of ongoing research.

■ PHARMACOLOGY

Turmeric contains the volatile oils zingiberen and turmerone, which have antispasmodic and antibiotic actions.[2] Curcumin, another component, has anti-inflammatory and antiplatelet activity attributed to inhibition of prostaglandin and thromboxane synthesis.[2]

Curcumin also has been shown to induce apoptosis in a number of cell lines.[3] Of particular interest is the fact that curcumin was able to induce apoptosis in multiple drug–resistant (MDR) cancer cell lines. MDR cancer cells overexpress P-glycoprotein, which functions as a pump to exclude antineoplastic drugs from the cell, keeping intracellular levels below the therapeutic threshold. P-glycoprotein also appears to retard programmed cell death by inhibiting an enzyme, caspase-3. The fact that curcumin can induce apoptosis independent of caspase-3 could make it an important tool in the treatment of MDR cancers. In addition, curcumin has been shown to induce apoptosis in both androgen-dependent and androgen-independent prostate cancer cell lines.[4]

Curcumin, a component of tumeric, has been identified chemically as diferuloyl-methane and has been shown to enhance apoptosis in prostate cancer cells by a mechanism involving tumor necrosis factor.[5] Both turmeric and curcumin were shown to inhibit the growth of *Helicobacter pylori*, an organism responsible for peptic ulcer and a group 1 carcinogen.[6] Anti-inflammatory activity using a microsphere drug delivery system has been shown in a rat model of inflammation.[7]

Recently, experimental evidence was presented to suggest that curcumin can protect skin from radiation damage, apparently by reducing infiltration of inflammatory mononuclear leukocytes.[8]

Antioxidant and hepatoprotective properties also have been attributed to curcumin, but clinical usefulness may be limited by poor gastrointestinal absorption.[9]

■ ADVERSE REACTIONS AND INTERACTIONS

Fetal effects are unknown, and use during pregnancy, other than as a food spice, is probably best avoided. Prolonged use has been associated with gastrointestinal upset and may increase the risk of peptic ulcer.[9] Use in patients with biliary obstruction or gallstones is contraindicated by some authorities.[9] There is a potential for interaction with nonsteroidal anti-inflammatory drugs and platelet-inhibiting drugs because of the effect of tumeric on prostaglandin synthesis. See also Appendix I.

In summary, the clinical usefulness of curcumin remains to be established, but the experimental promise is significant and there is a reasonable expectation that new therapeutic agents will emerge in the future. Herbal usefulness is probably limited by poor gastrointestinal absorption.

■ REFERENCES

1. Turmeric. In: Grieve M. *A Modern Herbal.* Botanical.com website. Available at: http://www.botanical.com/botanical/mgmh/t/turmer30.html.
2. Abebe W. Herbal medication: Potential for adverse interactions with analgesics. *J Clin Pharm Ther* 2002;27:391.
3. Piwocka K, Bielak-Zmijewska A, Sikora E. Curcumin induces caspase-3-independent apoptosis in human multidrug-resistant cells. *Ann N Y Acad Sci* 2002;973:250.
4. Dorai T, Gehani N, Katz A. Therapeutic potential of curcumin in human prostate cancer-I. Curcumin induces apoptosis in both androgen-dependent and androgen-independent prostate cancer cells. *Prostate Cancer Prostatic Dis* 2000;3:84.
5. Deeb D, Xu YX, Jiang H, et al. Curcumin (diferuloyl-methane) enhances tumor necrosis factor-related apoptosis-inducing ligand-induced apoptosis in LNCaP prostate cancer cells. *Mol Cancer Ther* 2003;2:95.
6. Mahady GB, Pendland SL, Yun G, Lu ZZ. Turmeric (Curcuma longa) and curcumin inhibit the growth of Helicobacter pylori, a group 1 carcinogen. *Anticancer Res* 2002;22:4179.
7. Kumar V, Lewis SA, Mutalik S, Shenoy DB, Venkatesh UN. Biodegradable microspheres of curcumin for treatment of inflammation. *Indian J Physiol Pharmacol* 2002;46:209.
8. Kerr C. Curry ingredient protects skin against radiation. *Lancet Oncol* 2002;3:713. Available at: http://oncology.thelancet.com..
9. Miller LG, Murray WJ. *Herbal Medicinals: A Clinician's Guide.* New York, NY: Pharmaceutical Products Press; 1998:50, 99.

VALERIAN

■ SOURCE, DESCRIPTION, USES

This herb, produced from the dried, powdered root of the plant *Valeriana officinalis*, has been used as a sedative-hypnotic for decades. It originated in Europe and is an escapee from North American gardens. Growing up to 1 m in height, with tight clusters of pale pink flowers, it can be found along roadsides throughout much of north and central North America.[1] Also referred to as garden heliotrope and vandal, valerian is used as a sedative-hypnotic to treat insomnia and as a mild sedative, and it is present in many herbal sleep aids.[2]

■ PHARMACOLOGY

There are at least two chemical groups of pharmacological interest: valepo-triates and sesquiterpenes.[3] Both have sedative properties, but the former, often used to standardize preparations, is cytotoxic whereas the latter is not. Other chemical components may contribute to the pharmacological properties of valerian. Aqueous root extracts contain significant levels of γ-aminobutyric acid (GABA), which could directly induce sedation although its bioavailability is in question.[2] A -blind study on a preparation (Valerina Natt) containing mainly sesquiterpenes found that it significantly improved the quality of sleep for insomniacs.[3]

Valerian's effect is dose–dependent,[4] and its mechanism appears to involve effects on GABA neurotransmission, including possible effects on GABA receptors.[5,6] Inhibition of GABA breakdown also may play a role.[2]

■ ADVERSE EFFECTS AND INTERACTIONS

There is one case on record[7] of withdrawal symptoms following discontinuation of valerian. Following surgery, the patient developed delirium and cardiac symptoms, similar to those of benzodiazepine withdrawal, which were relieved by benzodiazepine administration. This observation lends further credence to a role for GABA neurotransmission as the site of action for valerian and raises the possibility that physical dependence to valerian could occur. Care should be taken when discontinuing valerian in any patient who has been consuming it regularly. Few data are available regarding valerian-drug interactions, but given its mechanism of action there is a potential for valerian to be additive or even synergistic with other central nervous system depressants, especially those that act on GABA receptors. Concomitant use with alcohol, barbiturates, benzodiazepines, anesthetics, and other sedative-hypnotics, including other herbal preparations, is not advisable.[8,9] Withdrawal, tapered if indicated, is advisable prior to surgery.[6] No information is available regarding valerian's effects on pregnancy, lactation, or reproduction. Valerian in combination with skullcap has been associated with a case of toxic hepatitis.[10] Tannin-containing herbs such as valerian may interfere with iron absorption.[11] This may not be a serious problem clinically but should be considered in anemic patients, and it is advisable to avoid taking iron and the herbal preparation together.

■ REFERENCES

1. Peterson RT, McKenny M. *Northeastern Wildflowers. Roger Tory Peterson Field Guides.* Norwalk, Conn: Easton Press; 1984:296.
2. Houghton PJ. The scientific basis for the reputed activity of valerian. *J Pharm Pharmacol* 1999;51:505.

3. Lindahl O, Lindwall L. Double blind study of a valerian preparation. *Pharmacol Biochem Behav* 1989;32:1065.

4. Hendriks H, Bos R, Allersma DP, Malingre TM, Koster AS. Pharmacological screening of valerenal and some other components of essential oil of *Valeriana officinalis*. *Planta Med* 1981;42:62.

5. Ortiz JG, Nieves-Natal J, Chavez P. Effects of *Valeriana officinalis* extracts on [^{3}H] flunitrazepam binding, synaptosomal [^{3}H] GABA uptake, and hippocampal [^{3}H] GABA release. *Neurochem Res* 1999;24:1373.

6. Santos MS, Ferriera F, Cunha AP, Carvalho AP, Ribeiro CF, Macedo T. Synaptosomal GABA release as influenced by valerian extract—involvement of the GABA carrier. *Arch Int Pharmacodyn Ther* 1994;327:220.

7. Garges HP, Varia I, Doraiswamy PM. Cardiac complications and delirium associated with valerian root withdrawal. *JAMA* 1998;280:1566.

8. Ang-Lee MK, Moss J, Yuan C-S. Herbal medicines and perioperative care. *JAMA* 2001;286:208.

9. Select "valerian" at: http://www.mcp.edu/herbal/

10. Haller CA, Dyer JE, Ko R, Olson KR. Making a diagnosis of herbal related toxic hepatitis. *West J Med* 2002;176:39.

11. Miller LG. Herbal medicinals: Selected clinical considerations focusing on known or potential herb-drug interactions. *Arch Intern Med* 1998;158:2200.

WILD CARROT

■ SOURCE, DESCRIPTION, USES

Wild carrot (*Daucus carota*, family Umbelliferae), also called Queen Anne's lace, is a native of Europe that has become well established in North America, growing extensively on waste ground and along fence-rows.[1] It can grow to 1 m in height and is topped by a flat cluster of lacy white flowers, which often are slightly depressed at the center, giving rise to another common name, bird's nest. Wild carrot is closely related to the vegetable carrot variety. It bears a resemblance to fool's parsley, poison hemlock, and hemlock parsley, all of which are highly toxic.[1] The central flower of the umbel (umbrella-like flower cluster) is often red or purple.[1,2]

Traditionally, the whole herb has been used as a diuretic and stimulant and the seeds as a carminative. It also was recommended for liver ailments such as jaundice.[2] In East Indian herbal medicine, extract of carrot has been used for many purposes, including kidney dysfunction, asthma, inflammation, and even as an aphrodisiac.[3]

■ PHARMACOLOGY

A volatile oil extracted from wild carrot is credited with the activity of this herb.[1] Little information is available regarding its constituents or pharmacokinetics. A water extract has been shown to possess hepatoprotective activity in mice challenged with carbon tetrachloride. Pretreatment with the extract significantly lowered serum enzyme levels compared with untreated controls.[3] Hypotensive and sedative properties have been attributed to wild carrot,[4] but there is little evidence of its efficacy in this regard.

■ ADVERSE EFFECTS AND INTERACTIONS

It has been suggested that wild carrot might potentiate the effect of diuretics used concomitantly[5]; however, no case reports of such an interaction are available. As with all members of the Umbelliferae family, there is a risk of contact phytophotodermatitis because of the presence of psoralens[6] and of contact allergic dermatitis. Cross-reactivity with other Umbelliferae is also possible. See AMMI for a more detailed description of photophytodermatitis. See also Appendix XIII.

In summary, at this time there is little scientific evidence to support the claims for wild carrot.

■ REFERENCES

1. Peterson RT, McKenny M. *Northeastern Wildflowers: Roger Tory Peterson Field Guides.* Norwalk, Conn: Easton Press; 1984:48.
2. Carrot, wild. In: Grieve M. *A Modern Herbal.* Botanical.com website. Available at: http://www.botanical.com/botanical/mgmh/c/carwil25.html.
3. Bishayee A, Sarkar A, Chatterjee M. Hepatoprotective activity of carrot (Daucus carota) against carbon tetrachloride intoxication in mouse liver. *J Ethnopharmacol* 1995;47:69.
4. Miller LG, Murray WJ. *Herbal Medicinals: A Clinician's Guide.* New York, NY: Pharmaceutical Products Press; 1998: 154, 230.
5. Fisher CR, Veronneau SJH. Herbal preparations: A primer for the aeromedical physician. *Aviat Space Environ Med* 2000;71:45.
6. Botanical Dermatology: Phytophotodermatitis. Available at: http://www.telemedicine.org/botanica5.htm. First select "Electronic Textbook of Dermatology" and then "Phytodermatitis"

WILD YAM

■ SOURCE, DESCRIPTION, USES

The root of *Dioscoria villosa*, wild yam, is used as a cream to retard aging of the skin because of its purported estrogenic activity.

■ PHARMACOLOGY

Wild yam root contains the active phytoestrogen diosgenin and possibly dehydroepiandrosterone (DHEA), purported precursors of progesterone.[1] Knowledge regarding transdermal absorption is lacking. In one report,[2] wild yam cream was studied for possible beneficial effects on menopausal symptoms, serum lipids, and plasma hormone levels. After 3 months of treatment, treated subjects showed no significant differences from control subjects in total serum levels of cholesterol, triglyceride, high-density lipoprotein cholesterol, follicle-stimulating hormone, glucose, estradiol, and progesterone. Both treated and placebo groups showed mild improvement in subjective symptoms, but there were no differences between them. No side effects were noted. The authors concluded that there was no demonstrated efficacy for short term-treatment of menopausal symptoms with wild yam cream. See also DHEA, and PHYTOESTROGENS AND PHYTOPROGESTINS.

■ ADVERSE EFFECTS AND INTERACTIONS

A pilot study[3] has shown that wild yam suppresses progesterone synthesis. Thus, there is a potential for interference with hormone replacement therapy and oral contraception in women if wild yam is taken orally.[1] As previously noted, topical application likely has no effect.

■ REFERENCES

1. Smolinske SC. Dietary supplement-drug interactions. *J Am Womens Med Assoc* 1999;54:191.
2. Komesaroff PA, Black CV, Cable V, Sudhir K. Effects of wild yam extract on menopausal symptoms, lipids and sex hormones in healthy menopausal women. *Climacteric* 2001;4:144.
3. Zava DT, Dollbaum CM, Blen M. Estrogen and progestin bioactivity of foods, herbs and spices. *Proc Soc Exp Biol Med* 1998;217:369.

WILLOW BARK

■ SOURCE, DESCRIPTION, USES

The bark of various species of willow tree (*Salix* species), of which there are upwards of 50 in North America alone,[1] has been used since the time of the 1st century Greek physician Diascorides for the treatment of fever and rheumatic conditions in various cultures around the world.[2] The weeping willow, *Salix babylonica* (family Salicaceae), with which most people are familiar, is an Old World native and an escapee in North America, where many native species, such as pussy willow, are low shrubs.[1] The herbal preparation is recommended for febrile diseases, rheumatic complaints, and headache.[2]

■ PHARMACOLOGY

Willow bark was probably the first botanical remedy to evolve into a pharmaceutical. The active ingredient, salicin, is a bitter alkaloid that was first isolated in pure form in 1829. After nearly 175 years, much research on salicin is still being conducted to determine is efficacy and safety as a nonsteroidal anti-inflammatory drug (NSAID). A recent in-depth study was conducted of salicin pharmacokinetics.[3] Several precursors in willow bark (tremulacin, salicortin, acetylsalicortin) are hydrolyzed chemically during the extraction process to salicin, which is metabolized to gentisic acid, salicylic acid, and salicyluric acid. These acids and their glucuronide conjugates are excreted via the kidneys. Serum total salicylate levels (salicylic, gentisic, and salicyluric acids) peak about 1 hour after a single oral dose of standard extract. The mechanism of action of salicin, like that of all NSAIDs, involves inhibition of cyclooxygenase (COX) and, hence, of prostaglandin and thromboxane synthesis.[4] Similar to all first-generation NSAIDs, salicin is not selective for COX-2. Although numerous pharmacological actions have been identified for salicylates, and debate over their precise mechanism of action continues, there is a clear correlation between their ability to inhibit COX and their anti-inflammatory activity.[4] In a study of six benzoic acid derivatives, a strong, positive correlation was noted between their ability to inhibit prostaglandin synthesis in rat and human platelets and their ability to inhibit platelet aggregation and carrageenin-induced rat paw edema.[5]

Several clinical trials of willow bark extract (WBE) have been conducted in recent years, generally with promising results. A randomized, double-blind study of recurrent low pack pain[6] found that 120 or 240 mg of WBE per day elicited a significant improvement that was evident after 1 week on the higher dose, and that became more pronounced as time progressed. Another study found that a commercial preparation containing 15% salicin (per 240 mg dose) was as effective as the COX-2 inhibitor rofecoxib (12.5 mg) at relieving low back pain when given once daily.[7] The incidence of side effects was similar in both groups. This same dose has been reported to lower the baseline Western Ontario and McMaster Universities (WOMAC) pain score by 14% in patients with osteoarthritis.[8] Conversely, the score increased by 2% in the placebo group. The cost of treatment was considerably lower with WBE than with prescription medicines.

■ ADVERSE EFFECTS AND INTERACTIONS

Potential adverse reactions and interactions are those that apply to all NSAIDs to varying degrees. These include gastrointestinal upset, activation of peptic ulcers, occult or frank blood loss from the gastrointestinal tract, and increased risk of bleeding in patients taking oral anticoagulants and, possibly, platelet-inhibiting drugs (see also Appendix I). A reduction in renal blood flow in patients with cardiac, hepatic, and renal disease also has been reported.[4] Allergic reactions, and possibly cross-sensitivity to other NSAIDs, also are possible. The important question is whether there is a substantial reduction in the incidence of untoward reactions with WBE or salicin compared with other similar drugs. In one placebo-controlled study, the incidence of reported adverse effects was actually higher in the placebo group (28 reported) than in the treated group (17 reported).[8] The incidence of gastrointestinal disorders was more than double in the placebo group (seven versus three). In the study comparing WBE to rofecoxib, the incidence of adverse reactions was about the same in both groups.[7] There were 13 gastrointestinal complaints in the WBE group versus 16 in the rofecoxib group and more allergic reactions in the former than in the latter. Of the 114 subjects in each group, 11 withdrew from the WBE group and 15 from the rofecoxib group as a result of untoward reactions.

There has been concern in the past that salicylate might interfere with the antithrombotic action of acetylsalicylic acid by competing at COX binding sites. Although such a competition has not been demonstrated in an animal model of thrombosis,[9] some evidence for it was seen in human platelets.[10] There would not seem to be much purpose in combining these agents, at least when acetylsalicylic acid is being used for its platelet-inhibiting property.

In summary, WBE (salicin) could be a much cheaper, and perhaps safer, alternative to prescription NSAIDs, at least for some indications. See also Appendices VII and VIII.

■ REFERENCES

1. Petrides GA. *Trees and Shrubs: Roger Tory Peterson Field Guides.* Norwalk, Conn: Easton Press; 1984:344..

2. Schulz V, Hansel R, Tyler VE. *Rational Phytotherapy: A Physician's Guide to Herbal Medicine.* New York, NY: Springer-Verlag; 1998:144.

3. Schmid B, Kotter I, Heide L. Pharmacokinetics of salicin after oral administration of a standardized willow bark extract. *Eur J Clin Pharmacol* 2001;57:387.

4. Roberts LJ, Morrow JD. Analgesic-antipyretic and antiinflammatory agents and drugs employed in the treatment of gout. In: Hardman JG, Limbird L, Gilman AG, eds. *Goodman and Gilman's The Pharmacological Basis of Therapeutics.* 10th ed. New York, NY: McGraw-Hill; 2001:687.

5. Cerkus I, Philp RB. Relationship of inhibition of prostaglandin synthesis in platelets to anti-aggregatory and anti-inflammatory activity of some benzoic acid derivatives. *Agents Actions* 1981;11:281.

6. Chrubasik S, Eisenberg E, Balan E, Weinberger T, Luzzati R, Conradt C. Treatment of low back pain exacerbations with willow bark extract: A randomized double-blind study. *Am J Med* 2000;109:9.

7. Chrunasik S, Kunzel O, Model A, Conradt C, Black A. Treatment of low back pain with a herbal or synthetic anti-rheumatic: A randomized controlled study. Willow bark extract for low back pain. *Rheumatology* 2001;40:1388.

8. Schmid B, Ludtke R, Selbmann HK, et al. Efficacy and tolerability of a standardized willow bark extract in patients with osteoarthritis: Randomized placebo-controlled, double blind clinical trial. *Phytother Res* 2001;15:344.

9. Philp RB, Paul ML. Non-interference by salicylate with aspirin inhibition of arterial thrombosis in rats. *Prostaglandins Med* 1981;7:91.

10. Philp RB, Paul ML. Salicylate antagonism of acetylsalicylic acid inhibition of platelet aggregation in male and female subjects: Influence of citrate concentration. *Haemostasis* 1986;16:369.

WINTERGREEN (OIL OF)

■ SOURCE, DESCRIPTION, USES

Oil of wintergreen is obtained from the berries of the wintergreen plant *Gaultheria procumbens*, which is native to northeastern North America and grows further south in mountainous regions.[1] The plant also is known as the checkerberry plant. Synonyms for oil of wintergreen include sweet birch oil, gaultheria oil, bethula oil, and teaberry oil.[2] Oil of wintergreen has been used for generations as a topical counterirritant to treat sprains, pulled muscles, and other local traumas.[3] It is present in many liniments and ointments sold for this purpose. It also is used in aromatherapy for its pleasant odor. One website describes it as "great tasting and useful internally and externally."

PHARMACOLOGY

Conventional wisdom has held that counterirritants such as oil of wintergreen work by increasing local blood flow to accelerate the removal of pain-inducing chemicals, such as bradykinin. It also has been suggested that stimulation of organ-associated areas of the skin (Head's areas) is involved, via spinal neurons.[3] More recent research reveals a more complex picture, possibly involving central inhibitory effects mediated by cold-sensitive nerve fibers, at least for some counterirritants.[3] The case of oil of wintergreen is further complicated by the presence of an analgesic, methyl salicylate, which is the active principle.

ADVERSE EFFECTS AND INTERACTIONS

The principle hazard associated with oil of wintergreen is salicylate poisoning resulting from accidental or deliberate ingestion, especially in children. As little as 4 mL of oil may be fatal to children.[2] Chan[4] reviewed 80 cases of attempted suicide resulting from the ingestion of either acetylsalicylic acid (ASA) tablets or topical medications. Although plasma salicylate levels were generally higher in the former group, the two highest levels were seen in subjects who had consumed a topical liquid preparation. Severe salicylism syndrome may include headache, dizziness, tinnitus, dimmed vision, hearing loss, mental confusion, drowsiness, lassitude, hyperventilation, sweating, thirst, nausea, and vomiting.[3] In extreme cases, coma and convulsions may occur. Disturbed acid-base balance is a hallmark of salicylate poisoning.

Salicylates may be absorbed transdermally, and medicated skin patches have been used this way. Whenever the integrity of the epidermis is compromised, absorption may be increased significantly. In one case, a 40-year-old male patient was using an herbal skin cream containing methyl salicylate to treat psoriasis. He presented at an emergency department with tinnitus, vomiting, tachypnea, and acid-base disturbance.[5] Toxicity was limited because the patient had washed off the treated area soon after he developed symptoms. The taste and flavor of oil of wintergreen may be associated with confections, because it is sometimes used as a flavoring agent, and children may be tempted to consume the oil. One case of fatal cardiopulmonary arrest following ingestion of oil of wintergreen was documented in an intellectually challenged 44-year-old man who consumed about 30 mL thinking it was castor oil.[6] The amount of salicylate was calculated to equate with that in 171 ASA tablets of 325 mg.

Allergic contact dermatitis and irritant dermatitis may occur following the application of oil of wintergreen.[2] One case of poisoning was recorded in a 21-month-old infant who took a swallow of oil of wintergreen oil that had been marketed as a flavoring agent for candy.[7] The infant was treated successfully. The mother had been unaware that oil of wintergreen was toxic and assumed that it was no different than oil of peppermint.

Drug interactions with oil of wintergreen are not common, but there is the possibility of additive effect if it is taken internally with other ASA-containing preparations. Because of transdermal absorption, oil of wintergreen has the potential to interact with warfarin and other oral anticoagulants and probably should be avoided by people with bleeding disorders.[8] See also Appendices VII and VIII.

Undiluted oil of wintergreen constitutes a major household hazard comparable to or greater than that of many cleaning agents, and its use should be discouraged, especially if there are small children in the house.

■ REFERENCES

1. Peterson RT, McKenny M. *Northeastern Wildflowers: Roger Tory Peterson Field Guides.* Norwalk, Conn: Easton Press; 1984:130.
2. Roberts LJ, Morrow JD. Analgesic-antipyretic and antiinflammatory agents and drugs employed in the treatment of gout. In: Hardman JG, Limbird L, Gilman AG, eds. *Goodman and Gilman's The Pharmacological Basis of Therapeutics.* 10th ed. New York, NY: McGraw-Hill; 2001:687.
3. Schulz V, Hansel R, Tyler VE. *Rational Phytotherapy: A Physician's Guide to Herbal Medicine.* New York, NY: Springer-Verlag; 1998:264.
4. Chan TY. The risk of severe salicylate poisoning following the ingestion of topical medicaments or aspirin. *Postgrad Med* 1996;72:109.
5. Bell AJ, Duggin G. Acute methyl salicylate toxicity complicating herbal skin treatment for psoriasis. *Emerg Med* 2002;14:188.
6. Cauthen WL, Hester WH. Accidental ingestion of oil of wintergreen. *J Fam Pract* 1989;29:679.
7. Howrie DL, Moriarty R, Breit R. Candy flavoring as a source of salicylate poisoning. *Pediatrics* 1985;75:869.
8. Chan TY. Potential dangers from topical preparations containing methyl salicylate. *Hum Exp Toxicol* 1996;15:747.

WITCH HAZEL

■ SOURCE, DESCRIPTION, USES

Witch hazel (*Hamamelis virginiana*) is a shrub or small tree with toothed, uneven-based leaves and hairy buds. It can grow to 8 m and is native to the south-central United States and eastern North America. Flowers appear in early fall and the fruits in late fall.[1] North American natives used the leaves and bark as a poultice for painful swellings, tumors, and injuries. Its astringent properties were also recognized.[2] In traditional folk medicine, a tea made from the leaves or bark was recommended for bleeding ulcers and "complaints of the bowels," and a rectal instillation was a treatment for hemorrhoids.[2] Pond's Extract of Witch Hazel was a common household topical remedy for burns, scalds, and inflammatory skin conditions.[2]

■ PHARMACOLOGY

Witch hazel contains numerous pharmacologically active principles, including quercetin, myricetin, kaemferol, gallic acid, tannins, and acetaldehyde.[3] Witch hazel is approved as an astringent by the U.S. Food and Drug Administration.[4] An extract of *H. virginiana* was shown to have significant anti-inflammatory activity in suppressing erythema induced by ultraviolet (UV) exposure in a study involving 40 volunteers, but it was not as effective as hydrocortisone preparations.[5] A major constituent of witch hazel, hamamelitannin, extracted from the roots and purified, has been shown to protect cultured endothelial cells against tumor necrosis factor-α–induced DNA fragmentation and cell death, a possible explanation for its UV-protective and antihemorrhagic activity.[6] A recent study found that witch hazel bark possessed significant antioxidant properties, being the most potent of several herbs in scavenging peroxynitrite ($ONOO^-$).[7]

■ ADVERSE EFFECTS AND INTERACTIONS

Witch hazel is a common ingredient in facial cosmetics, especially those claiming to be herbal preparations. Although such use is generally regarded as safe, contact dermatitis and a positive reaction to patch tests have been reported.[8,9] Witch hazel tea, taken internally, is still used in folk medicine, especially as a treatment for internal bleeding; however, gastrointestinal upset has been associated with such use. The concomitant use of oral medications is not advisable because there are some indications of interference with bioavailability.[10] Although there are no reported contraindications for internal use during pregnancy or breast-feeding, such use should be undertaken cautiously, if at all.

■ REFERENCES

1. Petrides GA. *Trees and Shrubs: Roger Tory Peterson Field Guides*. Norwalk, Conn: Easton Press; 1984:263.
2. Witch hazel. In: Grieve M. *A Modern Herbal*. Botanical.com website. Available at: http://www.botanical.com/botanical/mgmh/w/withaz27. html.

3. Witch hazel. Dr. Duke's phytochemical and ethnobotanical databases. Available at: http://ars-grin.gov/duke/plants.html.

4. Fisher CR, Veronneau SJH. Herbal preparations: A primer for the aeromedical physician. *Aviat Space Environ Med* 2000;71:45.

5. Hughes-Formella BJ, Filbry A, Gassmueller J, Rippke F. Anti-inflammatory efficacy of tonic preparations with 10% hamamelis distillate in a UV erythema test. *Skin Pharmacol Appl Skin Physiol* 2002;15:125.

6. Habtemariam S. Hamamelitannin from Hamamelis virginiana inhibits the tumour necrosis factor-α (TNF–α)-induced endothelial cell death in vitro. *Toxicon* 2002;40:83.

7. Choi HR, Choi JS, Han YN, Bae SJ, Chung HY. Peroxynitrite scavenging activity of herb extracts. *Phytother Res* 2002;16:364.

8. Granlund H. Contact allergy to witch hazel. *Contact Dermatitis* 1994;31:195.

9. Khanna N, Datta Gupta S. Rejuvenating facial massage—a bane or boon? *Int J Dermatol* 2002;41:407.

10. McGuffin MC, Hobbs C, Upton R, Goldberg A. *American Herbal Products Association Botanical Safety Handbook.* Boca Raton, Fla: CRC Press; 1997.

WORMWOOD

■ SOURCE, DESCRIPTION, USES

Wormwood is the source of absinthe, the liqueur of French impressionist fame. It comes from the plant *Artemisia absinthum* (family Compositae). There are about 150 members of the genus *Artemisia*, which includes the mugworts.[1] Many are under investigation for possible medicinal use. Wormwood is native to Europe and introduced to North America, where it now grows throughout the northeast.[1] It is an aromatic, weedy plant with clusters of tiny green flower heads similar to those of ragweed, to which it is related.[1] It can grow to about 0.6 m in height.

Traditional herbal use included as a nervine tonic, a stomachic, a febrifuge, and an anthelmintic.[2] The dried, whole plant served as the herb.

■ PHARMACOLOGY

It is generally agreed that the active principles of wormwood (absinthe) are α-and β-thujone. α-Thujone is the more potent of the two monoterpenoids, and it has been shown to be a modulator of γ-aminobutyric acid

(GABA) type A receptors by blocking chloride channels associated with the receptor.[3] It is biotransformed in mouse liver by cytochrome P450 enzymes to several metabolites.[3] Other than as a bitter carminative at low doses, there is no other legitimate use for wormwood essential oil. Actions attributed to absinthe, such as aphrodisiac, hallucinogenic, and mind-expanding effects, have not been confirmed by research.[4]

■ ADVERSE EFFECTS AND INTERACTIONS

During the latter half of the 19th century, absinthe achieved widespread popularity in France, especially Paris, as an alcoholic beverage. Workers rushed to their favorite bar to enjoy "l'heure verte," the emerald-green liqueur also known as the green fairy.[4] Many creative artists and writers adopted a bohemian lifestyle that centered on absinthe, which was supplied by the Swiss firm Pernod. Because absinthe potentiates the effects of alcohol, addiction became a major problem, leading to the banning of the wormwood oil–based drink before the Great War. α-Thujone is a convulsant, and excessive use of absinthe resulted in a syndrome called *absinthism,* characterized by visual and auditory hallucinations, gastrointestinal problems, epileptiform seizures, and psychiatric disturbances.[5] Because many of these effects, other than convulsions, also are characteristic of chronic alcoholism, it is difficult to determine which result exclusively from thujone. Certainly, thujone can induce seizures in experimental animals.[5,6]

Although there do not appear to be any reports specifically relating to drug interactions, there is obviously a great potential for interactions with any agent having central nervous system activity.

As a member of the Compositae family, wormwood carries a risk of contact dermatitis (see also Appendix IX). Other members of this group, especially of the genus *Artemisia,* are frequent causes of allergic rhinitis.

It should be noted that Pernod still makes an anise-flavored drink that does not contain oil of wormwood and, therefore, has no thujone. Oil of wormwood, however, is available from Internet sources or from plants harvested from the wild. There is concern that the original form of absinthe is making a comeback among young people in Europe and North America and that a reappearance of absinthism may be not far behind.

■ REFERENCES

1. Peterson RT, McKenny M. *Northeastern Wildflowers: Roger Tory Peterson Field Guides.* Norwalk, Conn: Easton Press; 1984:374.
2. Wormwoods. In: Grieve M. *A Modern Herbal.* Botanical.com website. Available at: http://www.botanical.com/botanical/mgmh/w/wormwo37.html.

3. Hold KM, Sirisoma NS, Ikeda T, Narahashi T, Casida JE. α-Thujone (the active component of absinthe): γ-Aminobutyric acid type A receptor modulation and metabolic detoxification. *PNAS* 2000;97:3826.
4. Gambelunghe C, Melai P. Absinthe: Enjoying a new popularity among young people? *Forensic Sci Intern* 2002;130:183.
5. Strang J, Arnold W. Absinthe: What's your poison? *BMJ* 1999;319:1590.
6. Olsen RW. Commentary: Absinthe and γ-aminobutyric acid receptors. *PNAS* 2000;97:4417.

YARROW

■ SOURCE, DESCRIPTION, USES

Yarrow (*Achillea millefolium*) is another member of the Compositae, or daisy, family (also known as Asteraceae).[1] It also is known as milfoil and soldier's woundwort.[2] White or pinkish multiple flowers top a single stem that can grow to nearly 1 m. The leaves are long, narrow, and fern-like, with serrated edges.[1] Traditionally, yarrow was used to stanch bleeding from wounds (hence, woundwort) and as an ointment for hemorrhoids and skin conditions. It also was used for gynecological disorders.[3] Internally, it was taken for colds and coughs. The aerial portion of the plant is dried to provide the herb.

The German Commission E currently approves yarrow for use in sitz baths for painful conditions of the pelvis in women and orally for dyspeptic complaints. The herb is reputed to be an antispasmodic.[3] Yarrow extract also has been used in a variety of other applications, including in cosmetics, and in the treatment of epilepsy, hemorrhage, and hypertension.[4]

■ PHARMACOLOGY

Rohloff and colleagues[4] analyzed yarrow essential oil obtained from the dried, crushed, aerial portion of the plant by steam distillation. A variety of monoterpenes and sesquiterpenes were identified, including camphor, α-thujone, and α-thugene. Most activities of yarrow are attributed to these terpenic volatiles. The relative concentration of some of these depended on the stage of growth at which the plants were harvested. Other researchers have identified polyacetylenes, simple coumarins, and flavonoids in yarrow.[5]

Clinical trials of yarrow for the various conditions for which it has been taken do not appear to have been conducted.

■ ADVERSE EFFECTS AND INTERACTIONS

A safety review of yarrow found evidence of weak genotoxicity of yarrow tea in a fruit fly test. Although no evidence of skin irritation was found in cosmetic preparations containing yarrow or in yarrow itself, the report concluded that data were insufficient to support the safety of yarrow in cosmetics and that further data were needed regarding topical and systemic toxicity.[5]

As a member of the Compositae family, yarrow has the potential to cause contact dermatitis and to be cross-reactive with other members of this family. See also Appendix IX.

■ REFERENCES

1. Peterson RT, McKenny M. *Northeastern Wildflowers: Roger Tory Peterson Field Guides.* Norwalk, Conn: Easton Press; 1984:47.
2. Yarrow. In: Grieve M. *A Modern Herbal.* Botanical.com website. Available at: http://www.botanical.com/botanical/mgmh/y/yarrow02.html.
3. Schulz V, Hansel R, Tyler VE. *Rational Phytotherapy: A Physician's Guide to Herbal Medicine.* New York, NY: Springer-Verlag; 1998:245.
4. Rohloff J, Skagen EB, Steen AH, Iversen TH. Production of yarrow (Achillea millefolium L.) in Norway: Essential oil content and quality. *J Agric Food Chem* 2000;48:6205.
5. Final report on the safety assessment of yarrow (Achillea millefolium) extract. *Int J Toxicol* 2001;20(suppl):79.

YOHIMBE

■ SOURCE, DESCRIPTION, USES

Yohimbe is an herbal preparation that comes from the bark of a tree or trees native to Africa (*Pausinystalia yohimbe, Corynanthe yohimbe*). It contains a number of alkaloids, one of which—yohimbine—also is found in the root of *Rauwolfia serpentina* and bears structural similarities to reserpine.[1] Yohimbe has been used for many years to treat erectile dysfunction and to increase libido, especially in older men.[2]

■ PHARMACOLOGY

Yohimbine, the principal active ingredient of yohimbe, is a presynaptic α-adrenergic blocking agent[1,3] and a serotonin (5-HT) antagonist.[1] It crosses the blood-brain barrier and acts centrally to increase blood pressure. Yohimbine is available as a prescription adrenergic blocking drug and has been prescribed for sexual dysfunction in men and also for postural hypotension and diabetic neuropathy.[1] It has been shown to enhance sexual activity in male rats.[1] The mechanism of yohimbine's effect in male sexual dysfunction is complex and appears to involve both central and peripheral vascular components.

■ ADVERSE EFFECTS AND INTERACTIONS

As would be expected, the main concern in using yohimbe herb is the potential for hypertension. High doses can cause a pressor response by themselves, and lower doses may potentiate the pressor effect of other drugs, particularly the tricyclic antidepressants.[4] This herb should be used cautiously, if at all, in patients with hypertension or cardiovascular disease because of the increased availability of norepinephrine. Hypertensive crisis has been reported in a man taking yohimbine for erectile dysfunction.[2]

Some authors record a perceived difference in the effects of *Coryanthe yohimbe*, which is believed to produce more hallucinations and have less anti-impotence activity, and *Pausinystalia yohimbe*, which causes more of the latter and fewer of the former effects.[5] However, both species are capable of causing hallucinations.

Yohimbine has been associated with a host of side effects unrelated to its hypertensive properties but possibly resulting in some cases from excess norepinephrine. These effects include piloerection, anxiety, cold sweaty hands, urge to void, rhinorrhea, bronchospasm, productive cough, shortness of breath, restlessness, manic symptoms, and other central nervous system disturbances.[6]

A variety of cutaneous reactions have been reported,[6,7] including pruritus, scaly skin, eruptions, and desquamation. Associated fever, chills, elevated erythrocyte sedimentation rate, and eosinophilia also have been reported.[6]

In summary, it is important to distinguish between yohimbine (the prescription drug) and yohimbe (the herbal remedy). Although many of the side effects discussed earlier were associated with the use of prescription yohimbine, their occurrence following consumption of yohimbe herb is not unheard of, and doubtless is related to the amount consumed and the concentration of active principle in the preparation. This herb should not be used by patients with hypertension, who are more sensitive to its pressor effects, or by patients taking tricyclic antidepressants, antihypertensive medications, or other centrally acting drugs. See also Appendices II, V, and VII.

■ REFERENCES

1. Hoffman BB. Catecholamines, sympathomimetic drugs and adrenergic receptor antagonists. In: Hardman JG, Limbird L, Gilman AG, eds. *Goodman and Gilman's The Pharmacological Basis of Therapeutics.* 10th ed. New York, NY: McGraw-Hill; 2001:249.
2. Ernst E. Herbal medications for common ailments in the elderly. *Drugs Aging* 1999;15:423.
3. Mansoor GA. Herbs and alternative therapies in the hypertension clinic. *Am J Hypertens* 2001;14:971.
4. Fugh-Berman A. Herb-drug interactions. *Lancet* 2000;355:134.
5. Fisher CR, Veronneau SJH. Herbal preparations: A primer for the aeromedical physician. *Aviat Space Environ Med* 2000;71:45.
6. Miller LG, Murray WJ. *Herbal Medicinals: A Clinician's Guide.* New York, NY: Pharmaceutical Products Press: 1998:140.
7. Ernst E. Adverse effects of herbal drugs in dermatology. *Br J Dermatol* 2000;143:923.

Section 3

Appendices

This section attempts to collect nutriceuticals and botanicals with common or similar purported uses, adverse effects or interactions. Review articles that cover several herbs are listed, when available, at the end of each appendix. The reader should also refer to the individual herb monographs. These lists should not be regarded as exhaustive.

Appendices

APPENDIX I:
DOCUMENTED AND POTENTIAL INTERACTIONS BETWEEN BOTANICALS/NUTRICEUTICALS AND ANTICOAGULANT/PLATELET-INHIBITING DRUGS

■ A. POSSIBLE POTENTIATION OF ANTICOAGULANT ACTION

An increased risk of bruising, bleeding, or interference with therapeutic response may result.

HERBS	PRESCRIPTION AND OTC DRUGS
Angelica root (coumarin-like)	abciximab (ReoPro)—platelet inhibitor
Anise (coumarin-like)	
Arnica flower (coumarin-like)	acetylsalicylic acid, ASA (numerous proprietary names)—platelet inhibitor
Asafoetida (coumarin-like)	
Bai zhi (*see* Angelica root)	anagrelide (Agrylin)—lowers platelet count
Bogbean (hemolytic)	
Borage seed oil (anticoagulant)	anisindione (Miradon)—anticoagulant
Bromelain (antiplatelet)	
Capsicum (anticoagulant)	clopidogrel (Plavix)— platelet inhibitor
Celery (coumarin-like)	
Chamomile (coumarin-like)	dicoumarol (Dicumarol)—anticoagulant
Clove (antiplatelet)	dipyridamole (Persantine)—platelet inhibitor
Danshen (antiplatelet, etc.)—documented	
	nicoumalone—anticoagulant
Devil's claw (anticoagulant?)—documented	sulfinpyrazone (Anturane)—platelet inhibitor
Dong quai (anticoagulant)—documented	ticlopidine (Ticlid)—platelet inhibitor

HERBS	PRESCRIPTION AND OTC DRUGS
Fenugreek (coumarin-like)	tirofiban (Aggrastat)—platelet inhibitor
Feverfew (antiplatelet)	warfarin (Coumadin) and related drugs—anticoagulant
Garlic (antiplatelet)—documented	
Ginger (antiplatelet)	
Ginkgo (antiplatelet)—documented	
Ginsana	
Horse chestnut (coumarin-like)	
Licorice root (coumarin-like)	
Lovage root (coumarin-like)	
Meadowsweet (salicylates)	
Motherwort (antiplatelet, lowers fibrinogen level in blood)	
Onion (antiplatelet)	
Papain	
Papaya extract	
Parsley (coumarin-like)	
Passionflower herb (coumarin-like)	
Pau d'arco (coumarin-like)	
Poplar (salicylates)	
Quassia (coumarin-like)	
Red clover (coumarin-like)	
Rue (coumarin-like)	
Sweet clover (coumarin-like)	
Tamarind (increases bioavailability of ASA)	
Turmeric (antiplatelet)	
Willow bark (salicylates)	

ASA, acetylsalicylic acid; OTC, over the counter.
Drug names are given as generic (lower case) followed by Trade name in parentheses.

■ B. POSSIBLE REDUCTION OF ANTICOAGULANT ACTION

- Coenzyme Q10, ginseng, green tea: There are documented reports of reduced anticoagulant activity (see Heck and colleagues).
- St. John's wort may *antagonize* warfarin and related drugs by accelerating biotransformation through cytochrome P450 enzyme induction.
- Goldenseal may *reduce* the action of anticoagulants and platelet inhibitors by an unknown mechanism.

■ REFERENCES

Fugh-Berman A, Ernst E. Herb-drug interactions: Review and assessment of report reliability. *Br J Clin Pharmacol* 2001;52:587.

Heck AM, Dewitt BA, Lukes AL. Potential interactions between alternative therapies and warfarin. *Am J Health Syst Pharm* 2000;57:1221.

APPENDIX II:
CONFIRMED AND THEORETICAL INTERACTIONS (POTENTIATIVE OR ADDITIVE) BETWEEN HERBS/NUTRICEUTICALS AND PSYCHOTROPIC/OTHER CENTRALLY ACTING DRUGS

HERBS	DRUGS
Balm	**Benzodiazepine Tranquilizers**
Betel nut	alprazolam (Xanax)
	clonazepam (Klonopin)
Calamus	chlordiazepoxide (Librium)
Cola beans	diazepam (Valium)
	flurazepam (Dalmane)
CoQ10	halazepam (Paxipam)
Danshen	lorazepam (Ativan)
	midazolam (Versed)
Evening primrose oil	oxazepam (Serax)
Fennel essential oil	prazepam (Centrax)
	sertraline (Zoloft)
Ginkgo	temazepam (Restoril)
Ginseng (Panax)	triazolam (Halcion)
Goldenseal	**Other Tranquilizers**
Henbane	meprobamate (Equanil, Miltown)
Jimsonweed	**Antidepressants**
Kava	fluoxetine (Prozac)
	paroxetine (Paxil)
L-tryptophan	
Lobelia	*MAO inhibitors*
	phenelzine (Nardil)
Mandrake (European)	tranylcypromine (Parnate)
Marijuana	*Tricyclic antidepressants*
	amitriptyline (Elavil)
Melatonin	imipramine (Tofranil)
Motherwort	nortriptyline (Pamelor)
	trimipramine (Surmontil)
St. John's wort	**Antipsychotics**
Sage essential oil	chlorpromazine HCl
	promazine HCl
Valerian	
Yohimbine	**Other Sedative-hypnotics**
	Barbiturates, chloral hydrate

HERBS	DRUGS

Herbs listed below are purported to be useful for depression; therefore, interactions are possible on theoretical grounds.

Basil

California poppy

Corydalis

Guarana

Jambolana

Lemon balm

Marjoram

Maté

Mugwort

Nux vomica

Passionflower

Scarlet pimpernel

Herbs listed below contain caffeine and other methylxanthines.

Gotu kola

Guarana

Kava

Kola nut

Maté

Miscellaneous
  Nasal decongestants (pseudoephedrine, other sympathomimetics)
  Sedative antihistamines, antinausea drugs

Drug names are given as generic (lower case) followed by Trade name in parentheses.

■ REFERENCES

Burkhard PR, Burkhardt K, Haenggeli CA, Landis T. Plant-induced seizures: Reappearance of an old problem. *J Neurol* 1999;246:667.

Fugh-Berman A, Ernst E. Herb-drug interactions: Review and assessment of report reliability. *Br J Clin Pharmacol* 2001;52:587.

Pies R. Adverse neuropsychiatric reactions to herbal and over-the-counter "antidepressants". *J Clin Psychiatry* 2000;61:815.

Appendix III:
Herbs/Botanicals That May Cause Hepatotoxicity

Many plants contain pyrrolizidine alkaloids (PAs) that cause hepatotoxic veno-occlusive (HVO) disease. Although not all of these alkaloids are hepatotoxic, as a group, PAs are responsible for most cases of plant-related hepatotoxicity and probably other forms of plant toxicity. Contamination of foodstuffs with plants that produce PAs has caused numerous outbreaks of HVO disease (see later discussion). The dominant feature of HVO disease is occlusion of the centrolobular veins of the liver lobules. Hepatotoxicity of a PA depends on its conversion by the liver to reactive electrophiles that can form adducts with macromolecules, leading to chronic toxicity after even a single exposure.

An *asterisk* (*) indicates that the presence of hepatotoxic PAs has been confirmed.

- Agrimony (Agrimonia eupatoria)
- Asian herbs for psoriasis (Dictamnus dasycarpus, Rehmannia glutimosa, Paeonia spp., Glycyrrhiza spp., Lophantherum spp.)
- Atractylis gummifera
- Black cohosh (Cimicifuga racemosa)
- Buchu (Agathosma betulina)
- Bush tea (Crotalaria asamica Benth, C. sessiflora)*
- Celandine (Chelidonium majus)
- Chaparral (Larrea trientata)
- Chinese herbal (*Paeonia* spp.)
- Coltsfoot (Tusilago farfara)*
- Comfrey (*Symphytum* spp.)
- Ephedra (Ma huang)
- Germander (Teucrium chamaedrys)
- Greater celandine (*Chelidonium majus*)
- Groundsels (*Senecio* spp.)*
- Herbal tea (Senecio and Crotolaria)
- Jin bu huan (shu ling) (Lycopodium serrata, Stephania spp., Corydalis spp.)
- Menispermum (Menispermum canadense, M. dauricum)
- Mistletoe (*Viscum album*)
- Packera candisissima
- Passionflower (Passiflora incantata)
- Pennyroyal oil (Mentha pulegium, Hedeoma pulegoides)
- Ragworts (*Senecio* spp.)*
- Sassafras (Sassafras albidum)
- Senecio (Senecio longilobus)*
- Senio chrysanthemoides*
- Senio scandens Buch-Hams*
- Senna (Cassia augustifolia)

- Skullcap and pau d'arco (*Tabebuia* spp.)
- Skullcap-valarian combination (Scutellaria lateriflora and Valeriana officinalis)
- Syo-saikoto-to (a mixture of seven herbs)

■ DIETARY SOURCES OF HEPATOTOXIC PAS

According to Prakash and colleagues, more than 200 PAs have been identified in over 300 plant species representing 13 families, and up to 3% of the world's flowering plants contain toxic PAs. The main sources are Boraginaceae (all genera, e.g. *Heliotropium*), Compositae (tribes *Sinecionae* and *Eupatoriae*), and Leguminosiae (*Crotalaria*).

PAs have been detected in honey from Oregon, where bees foraged on tansy ragwort (*S. jabonaea*), and Australia. Contamination of wheat with borages has caused outbreaks in the West Indies, parts of Russia, Uzbekistan, Afghanistan, and India.

■ REFERENCES

Haller CA, Dyer JE, Ko R, Olson KR. Making a diagnosis of herbal-related toxic hepatitis. *West J Med* 2002;176:39.

Ko RJ. Adverse reactions to watch for in patients using herbal remedies. *West J Med* 1999;171:181.

Langmead L, Rampton, DS. Review article: Herbal treatment in gastrointestinal and liver disease—benefits and dangers. *Aliment Pharmacol Ther* 2001;15:1239.

Luper S. A review of plants used in the treatment of liver disease: Part 1. *Altern Med Rev* 1998;3:410.

McDermott WV, Ridker PM. The Budd-Chiari syndrome and hepatic veno-occlusive disease. Recognition and treatment. *Arch Surg* 1990;125:252.

McRae CA, Agarwal K, Mutimer D, Bassendine MF. Hepatitis associated with Chinese herbs. *Eur J Gasteroenterol Hepatol* 2002;14:559.

Prakash AS, Pereira TN, Reilly PE, Seawright AA. Pyrrolizidine alkaloids in the human diet. *Mut Res* 1999;443:53.

Simon SR. Herbal toxicity and fatal hepatic failure. *Am J Med* 1999;106:267.

Stickler F, Egerer G, Seitz HK. Hepatotoxicity of botanicals. *Public Health Nutr* 2000;3:113.

Whiting PW, Clouston A, Kerlin P. Black cohosh and other herbal remedies associated with acute hepatitis. *Med J Austral* 2002;177:440.

Yeong ML, Swinburn B, Kennedy M, Nicholson G. Hepatic veno-occlusive disease associated with comfrey ingestion. *J Gastroenterol Hepatol* 1990;5:211.

APPENDIX IV:
HERBS AND FOODS THAT MAY CONTAIN PHYTOESTROGENS AND/OR PHYTOPROGESTINS

These levels may not by physiologically significant. See Zava and colleagues and Liu and colleagues, below, regarding estrogen and progesterone receptor binding.

FOODS	HERBS/SPICES
Alfalfa sprouts	
Barley	
Chick peas and other legumes	Black cohosh
Clover sprouts	Bloodroot
Kala chana seeds	Bluegrass
Lima bean seeds	Chaparral
Oats	Chasteberry
Oil seeds (eg flaxseed)	Dong quai
Pinto bean seeds	Fenugreek
Rice	Garlic
Rye	Hops
Soybean sprouts	Kudzu
Soy foods	Licorice
Split peas	Mandrake
Sunflower	Panax ginseng
Wheat	Red clover
	Spanish sage
The following are weakly estrogenic.	Thyme
Chenopodiacae (beets)	Toothed medic
Liliaceae (garlic)	Tumeric
Polygonaeae (rhubarb)	Verbena
Rosaceae (apple, cherry, plum)	Wild yam (may suppress progesterone synthesis)
Rubiaceae (coffee)	Yucca
Solanaceae (potato)	
Umbelliferae (parsley)	

■ REFERENCES

Golden RJ, Noller KL, Titus-Ernstoff L, et al. Environmental endocrine modulators and human health: an assessment of the biological evidence. *Crit Rev Toxicol* 1998;28:109.

Liu J, Burdette JE, Xu H, et al. Evaluation of estrogenic activity of plant extracts for the potential treatment of menopausal symptoms. *J Agric Food Chem* 2001;49:2472.

Philp RB. Environmental hormone disrupters. In: *Ecosystems and Human Health*. Boca Raton, Fla: CRC/Lewis Press; 2001:261.

Rudel R. Predicting health effects of exposure to compounds with estrogenic activity: methodological issues. *Environ Health Perspect* 1997;105(suppl):655.

Zava DT, Dollbaum CM, Blen M. Estrogen and progestin bioactivity of foods, herbs and spices. *Proc Soc Exp Biol Med* 1998;217:369.

Appendix V:
Herbal Preparations That May Cause Adverse Skin Reactions When Used Systemically, Topically for Skin Conditions, or in Cosmetics

It has been noted that the use of topical botanicals is rising dramatically and that many of these have been associated with allergic contact dermatitis. Many of these botanicals belong to the Compositae (Asteraceae) family and cross-sensitivity among members of this family can occur.

Compositae species are identified by an *asterisk* (*) in the listing below. See also Appendix IX.

- Aloe (*Aloe vera*)—contact dermatitis and contact urticaria, delayed and immediate hypersensitivity
- Anise (*Pimpinella anisum*)—contact dermatitis, possible cross-reactivity with other Umbelliferae (Apiaceae, e.g. fennel)
- Arnica (*Arnica montana*)*—bullous dermatitis, cross-sensitivity with sunflower
- Carrot family (*Apiaceae*)—may contain furocoumarins that cause phytophotodermatitis
- Centella (*Centella asiatica*)—vesicular dermatitis
- Chamomile (several species of *Matricaria* and other Compositae, Asteraceae)*—contact dermatitis
- Cucumber (*Cucumus* spp.)—contact dermatitis from handling
- Dandelion (Taraxacum officinale)*
- Fennel (*Foeniculum vulgare*, family Umbelliferae)
- Ginkgo (*Ginkgo biloba*)—may actually reduce contact dermatitis from other causes; fruit pulp, not present in cosmetics, may be allergenic
- Kava (*Piper methysticum*)—kava dermatopathy
- Lavender oil (*Lavandula* spp.)—contact dermatitis
- Peppermint oil (*Mentha piperita*)—contact dermatitis, stomatitis, orofacial granulomatosis
- Rosemary (*Rosmarinus officinalis*)—contact dermatitis
- Sage (*Salvia officinalis*)—contact dermatitis
- St. John's wort (*Hypericum perferatum*)—photosensitivity after ingestion, resulting from hypericin content
- Stinging nettle (*Urtica dioica*)—contact dermatitis
- Tea tree oil (*Melaleuca alternifolia*)—contact dermatitis, appears to be caused by sesquiterpenes
- Witch hazel (*Haemamelis virginiana*)—contact dermatitis
- Yohimbe (*Pausinystalia yohimbe, Corynanthe yohimbe*)—taken orally for erectile dysfunction

Numerous herbs are used in cosmetics and topical herbal remedies that have not yet been associated with dermatitis (see Kiken and Cohen, below). Other members of the daisy (Compositae) family that could be cross-allergenic include various daisies, feverfew, wild chamomile, and various asters.

■ REFERENCES

Ernst E. Adverse effects of herbal drugs in dermatology. *Br J Dermatol* 2000;143:923.

Kiken DA, Cohen DE. Contact dermatitis to botanical extracts. *Am J Contact Derm* 2002;13:148.

Pribitkin E deA, Boger G. Herbal therapy: What every plastic surgeon must know. *Arch Facial Plast Surg* 2001;3:127.

Peterson RT, McKenny M. *Northeastern Wildflowers: Roger Tory Peterson Field Guides.* Norwalk, Conn: Easton Press; 1984.

APPENDIX VI:
BOTANICALS THAT MAY ALTER DRUG BIOTRANSFORMATIONS

Many phytochemicals are capable of either inhibiting or inducing the microsomal cytochrome P450 (CYP450) mixed-function oxidase enzymes that are responsible for the biotransformation of many drugs. Inhibition of these enzymes generally results in higher blood levels of the drug and an increased risk of toxicity. Potentiation results in increased biotransformation of the drug, with therapeutic failure as a possible consequence. The phytochemicals responsible for this effect may be found in foods or herbal remedies.

BOTANICAL	MECHANISM	CONSEQUENCE
Bai zhi (*Angelica dahurica*); furocoumarins	Inhibition of CYP3A4 in rat and human cell cultures	Possible increased drug plasma levels and toxicity (see grapefruit juice)
Cat's claw (*Uncaria guianensis*)	Inhibition of CYP450 enzymes	Potentiation of several drugs
Chamomile (*Matricaria recutita*)	Chamomile tea significantly inhibited activity of CYPs 1A2 and 2E (rat liver)	Clinical significance not yet established
Cruciferous vegetables (e.g., broccoli, cauliflower) Due to indole-3-carbinol	Upregulation of several CYP enzymes, such as CYP1A2. May increase glutathione-S-transferase, downregulate flavin monooxygenase	Complex effects, may not be clinically important under most conditions
Dandelion (*Taraxacum officinale*)	Dandelion tea significantly inhibited activity of CYPs 1A2 and 2E (rat liver) but increased activity of UDP-glucuronosyl transferase	Clinical significance not established
Garlic (*Allium sativum*)	Suppression of CYP2E1 and increased expression of CYP2B, 3A, 1A in rat liver	Not confirmed for humans
Ginseng (*Panax ginseng*) Saponins	Inhibition of CYP2E1 and CYP3A in rat liver	Not confirmed in humans
Grapefruit juice Furocoumarins Bergamottin, naringinin	Inhibition of hepatic CYP3A4	Reduces first-pass metabolism of many drugs; increased plasma levels and toxicity (see below)

BOTANICAL	MECHANISM	CONSEQUENCE
Licorice (*Glycyrrhiza glabra*) Glycyrrhizin	Inhibits 11β hydroxysteroid dehydrogenase Inhibition of CYP3A4 (also 2B, 1A2, 2A1)	Potentiation of glucocorticoids Increased plasma levels and toxicity (see below)
Magnolol (*Magnolia officinalis*)	Inhibits 11β hydroxysteroid dehydrogenase	Potentiation of glucocorticoids
Milk thistle (*see* Silymarin)		
Peppermint (*Mentha piperita*)	Peppermint tea significantly inhibited activity of CYPs 1A2 and 2E (rat liver)	Clinical significance not yet established
Saibuku-to, Japanese herb, combination of licorice and magnolol	Inhibits 11β hydroxysteroid dehydrogenase	Potentiation of glucocorticoids
St. John's wort (*Hypericum perforatum*); hyperforin, hypericin, quercetin	Upregulates hepatic and duodenal CYP3A4 and P-glycoprotein transporter	Increased metabolism, therapeutic failure (fatal transplantation failure with cyclosporin); see also below
Silymarin (*Silybum marianum*); silybin, silybinin	Dose-dependent inhibition of CYP2D6, 2E1, 3A4, 2C9	Potential increase of plasma levels and toxicity of many drugs. See below regarding CYP3A4

Some Drugs Metabolized by CYP3A4 Enzyme
Cyclosporin, antiviral protease inhibitors (indinavir), antiretroviral drugs (nevirapine), ethinylestradiol, warfarin, carbamazapine, digoxin, benzodiazepines (alprazolam), amitriptyline, theophylline

■ REFERENCES

Beckmann-Knopp S, Rietbrock S, Weyhenmeyer R, et al. Inhibitory effect of silibinin on cytochrome P-450 enzymes in human liver microsomes. *Pharmacol Toxicol* 2000;86:250.

Buratti S, Lavine JE. Drugs and the liver: Advances in metabolism, toxicity, and therapeutics. *Curr Opin Pediatr* 2002;14:601.

Homma M, Oka K, Niitsuma T, Itoh H. Pharmacokinetic evaluation of traditional Chinese remedies. *Lancet* 1993;341:1595.

Ioannides C. Pharmacokinetic interactions between herbal remedies and medicinal drugs. *Xenobiotica* 2002;32:451.

Zuber R, Modriansky M, Ddvorak K, et al. Effect of Silybin and its congeners on human liver microsomal cytochrome P450 activities. *Phytother Res* 2002;16:632.

Appendix VII

■ A. BOTANICALS (HERBAL REMEDIES AND PLANT TOXINS) THAT CAN AFFECT CARDIOVASCULAR FUNCTION

For herbal remedies affecting hemostasis, see Appendix I.

BOTANICAL	MECHANISM	CONSEQUENCE
Aconite—monkshood, wolfsbane (*Aconitum* spp., e.g., *uncinatum*, *napellus*)	Aconitine and other aconitine alkaloids open fast sodium channels in myocardium Lappaconitine *blocks* Na^+ channels.	Tachycardia, ventricular fibrillation, potentially fatal Shown in isolated cell preparations
Belladonna alkaloids from deadly nightshade (*Atropa belladonna*); also present in jimsonweed (*Datura stramonium*), henbane (*Hyocyamus niger*), and mandrake (*Mandragora officinarum*)	Atropine, scopolamine Muscarinic blockade	Unopposed adrenergic activity leading to tachycardia, arrhythmias
Betel nut (*Areca catechu*)	Numerous alkaloids, including arecoline, with muscarinic and also sympathomimetic activity	Tachycardia, palpitations, hypertension, chest pain; ventricular fibrillation has occurred
Cardiac glycosides present in many plants; foxglove (*Digitalis lanata, D. purpurea*), oleander (*Nerium oleander*), broom (*Cystisus scoparius*), pheasant's eye (*Adonis vernalis*), star-of-Bethlehem (*Ornithogalum umbellatum*), lily-of-the-valley (*Convallaria majalis*), squill (*Urginea maritima*), strophanthus (*Strophanthus kombe*), and white squill (*Scilla maritima*)	Inhibition of Na^+ pump (Na^+-K^+-ATPase) $\rightarrow$ increased Na^+/Ca^{2+} exchange $\rightarrow$ increased Ca_i Other complex actions	In normal subjects ventricular tachyarrhythmia, bradycardia, heart block Therapeutically $\rightarrow$ improved cardiac efficiency

BOTANICAL	MECHANISM	CONSEQUENCE
Danshen (*Salvia miltiorrhiza*)	ACE inhibition + unknown pharmacological effects	Hypotension, positive inotropy, negative chronotropy.
Ephedra (*see* Ma huang)		
Devil's claw (*Harpagophytum procumbens*)	Mechanism unknown	Hypotension and bradycardia in animal studies
French maritime pine bark (*Pinus maritima*)	Inhibits lipid peroxidation, preserves capillary integrity	Useful in treating chronic venous insufficiency
Ginger (*Zingiber officinale*)	Pressor effects, may involve Ca^{2+} pump	Shown in animal studies only
Hawthorn (*Crataegus* spp.)	Cardioactive amines and terpenes	Positive inotropy, negative chronotropy; digoxin-like activity
Hellebore (*Veratrum* spp.)	Veratrum alkaloids increase Na^+ nerve conductivity	Stimulation of coronary baroreceptors $\rightarrow$ reflex vagal stimulation, hypotension, bradycardia
Horse chestnut (*Aesculus hippocastanum*)	Inhibits lipid peroxidation, preserves capillary integrity	Useful in treating chronic venous insufficiency
Indian snakeroot (*Rauwolfia serpentina*)	Source of reserpine, depletion of biogenic amines, reduced cardiac output and peripheral resistance	Hypotensive, orthostatic hypotension

Licorice (*Glycyrrhiza glabra*)	Inhibition of 11β-hydroxysteroid dehydrogenase	Hypercortisolism → Na^+ Retention, hypertension, congestive heart failure
Ma huang (ephedrine from *Ephedra sinica*, other species)	Adrenergic α and β agonist (sympathomimetic)	Severe hypertension → Cerebrovascular accidents, arrhythmias, myocardial infarction
Motherwort (*Leonurus cardiaca*)	Lavandulifolioside acts like quinidine; cardiac glycosides are also present	Changes in ECG, heart rate, blood pressure, etc.
Tripterygium wilfordii (TWHF; lei gong teng)	Unknown mechanism; has immunosuppressive, anti-inflammatory properties	Myocardial damage has been associated with overdose
Xin bao (Chinese herbal)	Stimulation of sinoatrial node (under investigation)	May be useful in treating so-called sick sinus syndrome
Yohimbine (from bark of *Pausinystalia yohimbe* and *Corynanthe yohimbe*)	Competitive $α_2$ antagonist (used for erectile dysfunction)	Hypertension, tachycardia, arrhythmias

ACE, angiotensin–converting enzyme; ECG, electrocardiogram.

■ B. HERBAL REMEDIES PURPORTED TO LOWER SERUM LIPIDS

HERBAL REMEDY*	PROPOSED MECHANISM
β-sitosterol (from *Hypoxis rooperi*)	Interferes with absorption of cholesterol
Cashew shoots (*Anacardium occidentale*)	Inhibits LDL oxidation, increases hepatic LDL receptors (cell cultures)
Cholestin (red yeast rice), contains natural statins	Inhibitor of HMG-CoA
French maritime pine bark (*Pinus maritima*)	Inhibits lipid peroxidation, Anticholesterolemic
Garlic (*Allium sativum*)	Lowers serum cholesterol and triglycerides 5%–15% (clinical, controversial)
Green tea	Inhibits LDL oxidation, increases hepatic LDL receptors (cell cultures)
Hawthorn (*Crataegus* spp.)	Lowers cholesterol, increases hepatic LDL receptors (animal studies, cell cultures)
Japanese mint (*Mentha arvensis*)	Inhibits LDL oxidation, increases hepatic LDL receptors (cell cultures)
Myrrh, gugulipid resin of tree (*Commiphora mukol*) native to India	Lowers serum lipids, mostly cholesterol; may increase liver metabolism of lipids (clinical trials show promise)
Papaya (*Carica papaya*)	Inhibits LDL oxidation (cell cultures)
Semambu leaf (*Calamus scipronum*)	Inhibits LDL oxidation, increases hepatic LDL receptors (cell cultures)
Soy protein	Alters cholesterol metabolism in liver, decreases serum lipids

HMG-CoA, β-hydroxy-β-methylglutaryl coenzyme A; LDL, low-density lipoprotein.
*Numerous plants have been identified as having hypotensive constituents (see Wang and Ng, below, for these).

■ REFERENCES

Deng JF, Ger J, Tsai WJ, Kao WF, Yang CC. Acute toxicities of betel nut: Rare but probably overlooked events. *Clin Toxicol* 2001;39:355.

Fisher CR, Veronneau SJH. Herbal preparations: A primer for the aeromedical physician. *Aviat Space Environ Med* 2000;71:45.

Guha S, Dawn B, Dutta G, Chakraborty T, Pain S. Bradycardia, reversible panconduction defect and syncope following self-medication with a homeopathic medicine. *Cardiology* 1999;91:268.

Mansoor GA. Herbs and alternative therapies in the hypertension clinic. *Am J Hypertens* 2001;14:971.

Mashour NH, Lin GI, Frishman WH. Herbal medicine for the treatment of cardiovascular disease. *Arch Intern Med* 1998;158:2225.

Morelli V, Zoorob R. Alternative therapies: Part II. Congestive heart failure and hypercholesterolemia. *Am Family Pract* 2000;62:1325.

Salleh MN, Runnie I, Roach PD, Mohamed S, Abeywardena MY. Inhibition of low-density lipoprotein oxidation and up-regulation of low-density lipoprotein receptor in HepG2 cells by tropical plant extracts. *J Agric Food Chem* 2002;50:3693.

Valli G, Giardina E-GV. Benefits, adverse effects and drug interactions of herbal therapies with cardiovascular effects. *J Am Coll Cardiol* 2002;39:1083.

Wang HX, Ng TB. Natural products with hypoglycemic, hypotensive, hypocholesterolemic and antithrombotic activities. *Life Sci* 1999;65:2663.

Appendix VIII:
Herbal Remedies and Nutriceuticals With Anti-inflammatory and Antirheumatic Properties

HERBAL REMEDY/NEUTRICEUTICAL*	ACTIVE PRINCIPLE AND MECHANISM (WHERE KNOWN)	USES
Arnica (*Arnica montana*)	Helenalin; antiedemic in rat paw test	Topical use for local swelling, inflammation
Ash bark (*Fraxinus* spp.)+	Salicylates; COX inhibition	Inflammatory and degenerative joint diseases
Avocado/soybean unsaponifiable residues (ASU) (Pliascledine)	Inhibit chemical mediators of pain and inflammation (cytokines)	Improvement of pain and motion in osteoarthritis
Barberry (*Berberis vulgaris*)+	Berberine; probably COX inhibition	Potent anti-inflammatory analgesic in rat studies, has been used as herbal remedy for lumbago and rheumatism
Birch bark (*Betula alba*)+	Salicylates; COX inhibition	Inflammatory and degenerative joint diseases
Bromelain	Cox inhibiton?	Anti-inflammatory action
Calendula (*Calendula officinalis*), common marigold	Triterpenoids; inhibition of inducible nitric oxide synthase	Topical use as a treatment for inflammation of the skin
Capsaicin (*Capsicum frutescens*)	Counterirritant, local vasodilator	Topical use for relief of local pain of arthritis
Comfrey (*Symphytum officinale*)	Pyrrolizidine alkaloids; mechanism unclear *Caution:* hepatotoxic	Topical use for sprains, bruises
Chondroitin sulfate	Supports synthesis of glycosaminoglycans	Rebuilding of cartilage in osteoarthritis
Devil's claw (*Harpagophytum procumbens*)	Harpagoside; mechanism unclear, but does not seem to involve COX inhibition	Degenerative and rheumatoid joint diseases

HERBAL REMEDY/NEUTRICEUTICAL*	ACTIVE PRINCIPLE AND MECHANISM (WHERE KNOWN)	USES
Feverfew (*Chrysanthemum parthenium*)+	Parthenolide; inhibition of prostaglandin synthesis but not by COX inhibition	Rheumatic diseases; modest efficacy
Ginger (*Zingiber officinale*)	May be related to inhibition of thromboxane synthase	Rheumatic problems; no controlled trials as yet
Glucosamine sulfate	Supports synthesis of glycosaminoglycans	Rebuilding of cartilage in osteoarthritis
Meadowsweet (*Filipendula imaria*)+	Contains salicylates; COX inhibition	May be enough salicylate for antipyresis but not for anti-inflammatory action
Motherwort (*Leonurus cardiaca*)	Active principle unknown, but anti-inflammatory activity claimed	May interact with NSAIDs
Nettle, stinging (*Urtica dioica*)	Several active components; anti-inflammatory activity shown experimentally	Rheumatic conditions; no controlled trials as yet
Omega-3 fatty acids	Inhibition of TX synthase	No trials yet
Poplar (aspen) bark (*Populus tremula*)+	Salicylates; COX inhibition	Inflammatory and degenerative joint diseases
Rosemary (*Rosemarinus officinalis*)	Unkown	"Rheumatism"
Salai guggal (gum extract of *Boswellia serrata*)	Boswellic acids	NSAID

Tripterygium wilfordii (TWHF), yellow vine, lei gong teng	Ethanol root extract; appears to be inhibition of release of PGE_2 from monocytes	Clinical studies have shown effectiveness in rheumatoid arthritis
Willow bark (*Salix* spp.)+	Salicin (salicylate); COX inhibition	Inflammatory and degenerative joint diseases
Wintergreen oil (*Gaultheria procumbens*)+	Methylsalicylate; topical counterirritant	Sprains, bruises; too toxic for oral use; transdermal absorption has been reported

COX, cyclooxygenase; NSAID, nonsteroidal anti-inflammatory drug; PGE_2, prostaglandin E_2; TX, thromboxane.
Conclusive evidence is not available for all of these substances. Refer also to individual listings in Section 2.
+Inhibitors of COX may also inhibit platelet function.

■ REFERENCES

Felson DT, Lawrence RC, Hochberg MC, et al. Osteoarthritis: New insights. Part 2: Treatment approaches. *Ann Intern Med* 2000;133:726.

Hauselmann HJ. Nutriceuticals for osteoarthritis. *Best Practice Res Clin Rheum* 2001;15:595.

See also individual monographs for additional references.

APPENDIX IX:
MEMBERS OF THE COMPOSITAE (DAISY OR ASTERACEAE) FAMILY, INCLUDING WILD AND GARDEN FLOWERS

Allergic contact dermatitis is fairly common with this family. Cross-sensitivity may occur but is not absolute, because not all members share the same allergens. Zeller and colleagues studied ether extracts of 20 Compositae for sensitizing properties in guinea pigs. Strong sensitizers were Cnicus benedictus (blessed thistle), Chrysanthemum leucanthemum (marguerite, ox-eye daisy), and Helianthus debelis (dwarf sunflower). Medium-strength sensitizers were Helenium amarum (bitterweed), Gaillardia ambylodon (blanket flower), Artimisia ludoviciana (prairie sage), Ambrosia trifida (giant ragweed), and Solidago virgaurea (goldenrod). Plants with little or no sensitizing capacity included cornflower, wormwood, coltsfoot, and dandelion. An immunological requisite was the presence of sesquiterpene lactones having an a-methylene group. Cross-reactivity was common among the species studied. See also Appendix V.

Many of these plants have been used traditionally as herbal remedies. Those that are used most commonly today are indicated by an *asterisk* (*).

COMMON NAME	LATIN NAME
Arnica*	Arnica montana
Asters (numerous species)	Aster spp.
Beggar-ticks, sticktight	Bidens frondosa
Black-eyed Susan	Rudbeckia hirta
Blazing star spp.	Liatris spp.
Boneset*	Eupatorium perfoliatum
Boneset (upland)	Eupatorium sessilifolium
Burdock*	Arctium minus
Butterbur	Petasites hydridus
Camphorweed	Heterotheca subaxillaris
Cat's-ear	Hypochoeris radicata
Chamomile*	Matricaria chamomilla and M.. maritima
Chicory*	Chicorium intybus
Chrysogonum	Chrysogonum virginianum

COMMON NAME	LATIN NAME
Clammy everlasting	*Gnaphalium macounii*
Climbing hempweed, climbing boneset	*Mikania scandens*
Clotburs, cockleburs	*Xanthium* spp.
Coltsfoot*	*Tussilago farfara*
Compass-plant	*Silphium laciniatum*
Coneflower (gray-headed)	*Ratibida pinnata*
Coneflower (green-headed)	*Rudbeckia laciniata*
Coneflower (orange)	*Rudbeckia fulgida*
Coneflower (showy)	*Rudbeckia speciosa*
Coneflower (sweet)	*Rudbeckia subtomentosa*
Coneflower (thin-leafed)	*Rudbeckia triloba*
Coneflower (purple)*	*Echinacea purpurea*
Coreopsis, tickseeds	*Coreopsis* spp.
Cup-plant	*Silphium perfoliatum*
Daisy fleabane	*Erigeron annuus*
Dandelion (common)*	*Taraxacum officinale*
Dandelion (fall)	*Leontodon autumnalis*
Dandelion (red-seeded)	*Taraxacum erythrospermum*
Dusty miller	*Artemisia stelleriana*
Elecampane	*Inula helenium*
European beggar-ticks	*Bidens tripartita*
False boneset	*Kuhnia eupatorioides*
Feverfew*	*Chrysanthemum parthenium*
Fine-leafed sneezeweed	*Helenium tenuifolium*
Galinsoga	*Galinsoga*
Gall-of-the-earth	*Prenanthes trifoliata*
Golden aster (Maryland)	*Chrysopsis mariana*
Golden aster (prairie)	*Chrysopsis camporum*
Golden aster (sickle-leafed)	*Chrysopsis falcata*
Goldenrod*	*Solidago* spp.
Grassed-leafed golden-aster	*Chrysopsis graminifolia*

COMMON NAME	LATIN NAME
Great Indian-plantain	*Cacalia muhlenbergii*
Groundsel (common)*	*Senecio vulgaris*
Groundsel (stinking)	*Senecio viscosus*
Groundsel-tree	*Baccharis halimifolia*
Gumweed	*Grindelia squarrosa*
Hawksbeard	*Crepis capillaris*
Hawkweed spp.	*Hieracium* spp.
Horseweed	*Erigeron canadensis*
Ironweed spp.	*Veronia* spp.
Jerusalem artichoke	*Helianthus tuberosus*
Joe-pye-weed spp.	*Eupatorium* spp.
King devil	*Hieracium pratense*
Knapweed spp.	*Centaurea* spp.
Lamb succory	*Arnoseris minima*
Large-flowered leafcup	*Polymnia uvedalia*
Leafy-bracted beggar-ticks	*Bidens comosa*
Lettuce (hairy)	*Lactuca hirsuta*
Lettuce (prickly)	*Lactuca scariola*
Lion's foot	*Prenanthes serpentaria*
Low cudweed	*Gnaphalium uliginosum*
Mayweed	*Anthemis cutola*
Mugworts	*Artemesia* spp.
Nipplewort	*Lapsana communis*
Ox-eye	*Heliopsis helianthoides*
Ox-eye daisy	*Chrysanthemum leucanthemum*
Pale Indian-plantain	*Cacalia atriplicifolia*
Pearly everlasting	*Anaphalis margaritacea*
Pilewort, fireweed	*Erechtites hieracifolia*
Pineapple-weed	*Matricaria matricarioides*
Prairie-dock	*Silphium terebinthinaceaum*
Pussytoes (field)	*Antennaria neglecta*

COMMON NAME	LATIN NAME
Pussytoes spp.	*Antennaria* spp.
Ragweed (common)	*Ambrosia artemisiifolia*
Ragwort (balsam)	*Senecio pauperculus*
Ragwort spp.*	*Senecio* spp.
Rattlesnake-weed	*Hieracium venosum*
Rosinweed spp.	*Silphium* spp.
Salt-marsh fleabane	*Pluchea purpurascens*
Scotch thistle	*Onopordum acanthium*
Silver-rod	*Solidago bicolor*
Small-flowered leafcup	*Polymnia canadensis*
Smooth white lettuce	*Prenanthes racemosa*
Sneezeweed	*Helenium autumnale*
Sneezeweed (purple-headed)	*Helenium nudiforum*
Sow-thistle spp.	*Sonchus* spp.
Spanish needles	*Bidens bipinnata*
Sunflower (common)	*Helianthus annuus*
Sunflower spp.	*Helianthus* spp.
Swamp beggar-ticks	*Bidens connata*
Sweet everlasting	*Gnaphalium obtusifolium*
Sweet-scented Indian-plantain	*Cacalia suaveolens*
Tall white lettuce	*Prenanthes altissima*
Tansy (Huron)	*Tanacetum huronense*
Tansy*	*Tanacetum vulgare*
Thistle (Barnaby's)	*Centaurea solstilialis*
Thistle (blessed)	*Cnicus benedictus*
Thistles	*Carduus* spp., *Cirsium* spp.
Thoroughwort spp.	*Eupatorium* spp.
Toothed white-topped aster	*Seriocarpus asteroides*
Tuberous Indian-plantain	*Cacalia tuberosa*
Two-flowered cynthia	*Krigia biflora*
White lettuce (rattlesnake root)	*Prenanthes alba*
White snakeroot	*Eupatorium rugosum*

COMMON NAME	LATIN NAME
White-topped aster (narrow-leafed)	*Seriocarpus linifolius*
Wild lettuce	*Lactuca canadensis*
Wild quinine	*Parthenium integrifolium*
Wormwoods	*Artemesia* spp.
Yarrow (sneezeweed)	*Achillea ptarmica*
Yarrow*	*Achillea millefolium*
Yellow goat's beard	*Tragopogon pratensis*

◼ REFERENCES

Peterson RT, McKenny M. *Northeastern Wildflowers: Roger Tory Peterson Field Guides.* Norwalk, Conn: Easton Press; 1984.

Zeller W, de Gols M, Hausen BM. The sensitizing capacity of Compositae plants. VI. Guinea pig sensitization experiments with ornamental plants and weeds using different methods. *Arch Dermatol* 1985;277:28.

APPENDIX X:
HERBAL AND OTHER ALTERNATIVE REMEDIES PURPORTED TO HAVE HYPOGLYCEMIC OR ANTIDIABETIC PROPERTIES

In most cases, only the results of animal studies are available. Use in folk and herbal medicine may have occurred, but experimental and clinical evidence may be lacking.

REMEDY*	LATIN NAME (IF APPLICABLE)	ANIMAL STUDIES	CLINICAL STUDIES
Agrimony Oral infusion/decoction	*Agrimonia eupatoria*	Streptozotocin-induced diabetes in mice (+)	None found
Alfalfa Oral infusion/decoction	*Medicago sativa*	Streptozotocin-induced diabetes in mice (+)	One case study (+)
α-Lipoic acid (thioctic acid)	NA Antioxidant	Prevented nerve dysfunction, increased nerve regeneration	May reduce symptoms of diabetic neuropathy
Black plumb, black berry, jamun	*Eugenia jambolama* Aqueous extract	Moderate alloxan diabetes in rats (+); severe (+,−)	None found
Blackberry Oral infusion/decoction	*Rubus fructicosus*	Streptozotocin-induced diabetes in mice (−)	None found
Celandine Oral infusion/decoction	*Chelidonium majus*	Streptozotocin-induced diabetes in mice (−)	None found
Chromium	NA	May increase insulin secretion	Some efficacy; needs more study
Coriander seeds Oral infusion/decoction	*Coriandrum sativum*	Streptozotocin-induced diabetes in mice (+)	None found

REMEDY*	LATIN NAME (IF APPLICABLE)	ANIMAL STUDIES	CLINICAL STUDIES
Cowitch	*Mucuna pruriens*	Alloxan diabetic rabbits (++)	Used in Ayurvedic medicine in India; no controlled trials performed (+,−)
Damiana	*Turnera diffusa*	Diabetic rabbits and mice	Herbal use in Latin America; no clinical trials performed
Eucalyptus Oral infusion/decoction	*Eucalyptus globulus*	Streptozotocin-induced diabetes in mice (+)	None found
Fenugreek	*Trigonella foenum-graecum*	High in soluble fiber; 4-hydroxyisoleucine increases glucose-stimulated insulin release; trigonelline is hypoglycemic	Clinical studies confirm effect (++)
Garlic bulbs Oral infusion/decoction	*Allium sativum*	Streptozotocin-induced diabetes in mice (+,−)—reduced hyperphagia, polydipsia, not hyperglycemia)	None found
Ginseng (Asian)	*Panax ginseng*	Ginsenosides (triterpenoid saponin claimed, along with many other actions but clinical studies are few (+,−)	Hypoglycemic activity (glycosides) thought to be active principle
Gymnema	*Gymnema sylvestre*	Ethanol extract has insulin-sparing properties; increased release of insulin from β cells	Clinical studies confirm hypoglycemic effect (++)—small studies
Juniper berries Oral infusion/decoction	*Juniperus communis*	Streptozotocin-induced diabetes in mice (+)	None found

		Alloxan and streptozotocin diabetes in rodents (++)	
Karela Oral infusion/decoction	*Momordica charantia*		Some clinical studies performed; also used in Ayurvedic medicine in India (++)
Lady's mantle Oral infusion/decoction	*Alchemilla vulgaris*	Streptozotocin-induced diabetes in mice (−)	None found
Licorice	*Glycyrrhiza glabra*	Streptozotocin-induced diabetes in mice (+,−)—reduced hyperphagia, polydipsia, not hyperglycemia	None found
Lily-of-the-valley Oral infusion/decoction	*Convallaria majalis*	Streptozotocin-induced diabetes in mice (−)	None found
Marigold Methanol extract	*Calendula officinalis*	Hyperglycemia in glucose-loaded rats (++)	None found
Nopal (nopales, nopalitos), prickly pear cactus	*Opuntia fulingosa,* *O. streptacantha*	High soluble fiber content plus unknown mechanism	Clinical studies in Mexico indicate hypoglycemic action (++)
Spices: cinnamon, bay leaf (flowering plant)	Family Lauraceae	Compared with insulin with respect to CO_2 production by rat adipocytes	(++)
Spices: clove, allspice (flowering plant)	Family Myrtaceae	Compared with insulin with respect to CO_2 production by rat adipocytes	(++)

REMEDY*	LATIN NAME (IF APPLICABLE)	ANIMAL STUDIES	CLINICAL STUDIES
Spices: oregano, sage (flowering plant)	Family Labiatae	Compared with insulin with respect to CO_2 production by rat adipocytes	(++)
Teas (green and black)	Family Theaceae	Compared with insulin with respect to CO_2 production by rat adipocytes	(++)
Tinospora, glunchanb, giloe, ambervel Aqueous extract	Tinospora cordifolia	Moderate alloxan diabetes in rats (+); severe (−)	None found
Tronodora (yellow elder)	Tecoma stans	Animal studies inconclusive (−)	Used in Mexico for treatment of diabetes, but human studies are lacking -
Witch hazel (flowering plant)	Hamamelis virginiana	Compared with insulin with respect to CO_2 production by rat adipocytes	(++)

(+), (++) indicates positive findings and the (subjective) relative efficacy; (−) indicates negative findings.
*Many vegetables, such as cabbage, broccoli, green leafy vegetables, beans, and tubers, have been shown to be hypoglycemic in animal and human studies. Diet may have a preventative role. Further study is required.

Broadhurst and colleagues surveyed 49 aqueous extracts of herbs, spices, and medicinal plants for insulin-like activity using a rat epididymal adipocyte assay in which glucose oxidation is measured by released $^{14}CO_2$ and compared the results with those obtained using insulin. Only a few of the more potent substances are listed in this Appendix. Grover and colleagues discussed some 15 plants from India, some of which demonstrated efficacy as hypoglycemic agents. Not all are listed in the preceding table. Shapiro and Gong reviewed clinical and experimental evidence of several herbal preparations used for diabetes.

■ REFERENCES

Alarcon-Aguilara FJ, Roman-Ramos R, Perez-Gutierrez S, Aguilar-Contreras A, Contreras-Weber CC, Flores-Saenz JL. Study of the anti-hyperglycemic effect of plants used as antidiabetics. *J Ethnopharmacol* 1998;61:101.

Broadhurst CL, Polansky MM, Anderson RA. Insulin-like activity of culinary and medicinal plant aqueous extracts in vitro. *J Agric Food Chem* 2000;48:849.

Chattopadhyay RR. A comparative evaluation of some blood sugar lowering agents of plant origin. *J Ethnopharmacol* 1999;67:367.

Grover JK, Vats V, Rathi SS. Anti-hyperglycemic effect of Eugenia jambolana and Tinospora cordifolia in experimental diabetes and their effects on key metabolic enzymes involved in carbohydrate metabolism. *J Ethnopharmacol* 2000;73:461.

Grover JK, Yadav S, Vats V. Medicinal plants of India with anti-diabetic potential. *J Ethnopharmacol* 2002;81:81.

Miller LG. Herbal medicinals: Selected clinical considerations focusing on known or potential drug-herb interactions. *Arch Intern Med* 1998;158:2200.

Morelli V, Zoorob RJ. Alternative therapies: Part I. Depression, diabetes, obesity. *Am Fam Physician* 2000;62:1051.

Platel K, Srinivasan K. Plant foods in the management of diabetes mellitus: Vegetables as potential hypoglycemic agents. *Nahrung* 1997;41:68.

Shapiro K, Gong WC. Natural products used for diabetes. *J Am Pharmaceut Assoc* 2002;42:217.

Swanston-Flatt SK, Day C, Bailey CJ, Flatt PR. Traditional plant treatments for diabetes. Studies in normal and streptozotocin diabetic mice. *Diabetologica* 1990;33:462.

Yoshikawa M, Murakami T, Kishi A, Kageura T, Matsuda H. Medicinal flowers. III. Marigold. (1): Hypoglycemic, gastric emptying inhibitory, and gastroprotective principles and new oleanane-type triterpene oligoglycosides, calendasaponins A, B, C, and D, from Egyptian Calendula officinalis. *Chem Pharm Bull* 2001;49:863.

Appendix XI:
Herbs and the Kidney: Diuretic and Nephrotoxic Herbs

COMMON NAME(S)*	LATIN NAME	EFFECT
Agrimony	*Agrimonia eupatoria, A. pilosa, A. procera*	Diuretic, could potentiate other diuretics
Aristolochia	*Aristolochia* spp.	Interstitial nephritis
Bearberry	*Arctostaphylos uva-ursi*	Diuretic, could potentiate other diuretics
Broom, Scotch broom	*Cysticus scoparius, Sarothemanus scoparius*	Diuretic, could potentiate other diuretics
Buchu, bucco	*Barosma betulina*	Diuretic, could potentiate other diuretics
Celandine	*Chelidonium majus*	Diuretic, could potentiate other diuretics
Centaury	*Centaurium erythraea*	Diuretic, could potentiate other diuretics
Chinese slimming herbal	*Stephania tetrandra and Magnolia officinalis*	Fibrosing interstitial nephritis
Couchgrass	*Agropyrum repens*	Diuretic, could potentiate other diuretics
Dandelion	*Taraxacum officinale*	Diuretic, could potentiate other diuretics
Goosegrass	*Galium aparine*	Diuretic, could potentiate other diuretics
Ground holly	*Chimaphilia umbellata*	Diuretic, could potentiate other diuretics
Hydrangea	*Hydrangea paniculata, H. arborescens*	Diuretic, could potentiate other diuretics
Juniper	*Juniperus communis*	May be nephrotoxic with prolonged use
Lady's mantle	*Alchemilla* spp.	Diuretic, could potentiate other diuretics
Larch	*Larix americana*	Diuretic, could potentiate other diuretics

COMMON NAME(S)*	LATIN NAME	EFFECT
Lavender	*Lavandula officinalis*	Diuretic in rat studies
Licorice	*Glycyrrhiza glabra*	May cause sodium and water retention
Pansy	*Viola tricolor*	Diuretic, could potentiate other diuretics
Pareira brava root	*Chondodendron tormentosum*	Diuretic, could potentiate other diuretics
Parsley	*Petroselenium crispum*	Diuretic, could potentiate other diuretics
Pellitory	*Anacyclus pyrethrum*	Diuretic, could potentiate other diuretics
Pheasant's eye	*Adonis vernalis*	Diuretic, could potentiate other diuretics
Ragwort	*Senecio* spp.	Diuretic, could potentiate other diuretics
Rosemary	*Rosmarinus officinalis*	Diuretic, could potentiate other diuretics
Rupture wort	*Herniariea glabra*	Diuretic, could potentiate other diuretics
Sassafras	*Sassafras albidum*	Diuretic, could potentiate other diuretics
Shepherd's purse	*Capsella bursa-pastoris*	Diuretic, could potentiate other diuretics
Stone root	*Collinsonia canadensis*	Diuretic, could potentiate other diuretics
Water plantain	*Alisma plantago*	Diuretic, could potentiate other diuretics
Wild carrot	*Daucus carota*	Diuretic, could potentiate other diuretics
Wood sorrel	*Oxalis acetosella*	Diuretic, could potentiate other diuretics

*A USDA database website (discontinued) listed over 200 botanicals that have been used for various purposes related to the kidney; see Miller and Murray, below, for these.

■ REFERENCES

Dahl NV. Herbs and supplements in dialysis patients: Panacea or poison? *Semin Dialysis* 2001;14:186.

Fisher CR, Veronneau SJH. Herbal preparations: A primer for aeromedical physicians. *Aviat Space Environ Med* 2000;71:45.

Haloui M, Louedec L, Michel JB, Lyoussi B. Experimental diuretic effects of Rosmarinus officinalis and Centaurium erythraea. *J Ethnopharmacol* 2000;71:465.

Miller LG, Murray WJ, eds. *Herbal Medicines: A Clinician's Guide.* New York, NY: Pharmaceutical Products Press; 1998:27.

Vanherweghem J-L, Depierreux M, Tielemans C, et al. Rapidly progressive interstitial renal fibrosis in young women: Association with slimming Chinese herbs. *Lancet* 1993;341:387.

APPENDIX XII:
HERBS/BOTANICALS AND CANCER: CARCINOGENIC AND ANTINEOPLASTIC HERBS

◼ A. HERBS SHOWN TO BE CARCINOGENIC IN LABORATORY STUDIES

COMMON NAME	LATIN NAME
Borage	*Borago officinalis*
Calamus	*Acorus calamus*
Coltsfoot	*Tussilago farfar*
Comfrey	*Symphytum officinale*
Life root	*Senecio aureus*
Rosemary	*Rosmarinus officinalis*
Sassafras	*Sassafras albidum*

◼ REFERENCES

Johnson BM, Bolton, JL, van Breeman RB. Screening botanical extracts for quinoid metabolites. *Chem Res Toxicol* 2001;14:1546.

Klepser TB, Klepser ME. Unsafe and potentially safe herbal therapies. *Am J Health Syst Pharm* 1999;56:125.

◼ B. HERBS/BOTANICALS SHOWN TO BE ANTINEOPLASTIC IN LABORATORY STUDIES

ACTIVE PRINCIPLE	SOURCE	MECHANISM
Baicalein (a trihydroxyflavone)	Scutellaria baicalensis, *an herb found in sho-saikoto (a Japanese hormonal mixture)*	Inhibits 12-lipoxygenase; HETEs play role in cancer progression
Crude extract	Coptis groenlandica	Inhibits growth in 5 hepatoma cell lines
Diallyl sulfide	Garlic (*Allium sativum*)	Inhibits cytochrome P450 2E1; involved in metabolic activation of some carcinogens

ACTIVE PRINCIPLE	SOURCE	MECHANISM
D-Limonene (a monoterpene)	Citrus fruits (peels), also present in many trees and shrubs	Cytostatic (mechanism unclear)
Lapachol (a naphthoquinone)	Present in pau d'arco, derived from *Tabebuia*	Active against cultured cancer cells; no confirmation in human studies.
Lycopene (a carotinoid)	Tomatoes	Retards tumor growth; blocks expression of HMG-CoA reductase, required for cell to enter S-phase
Polyphenols, especially epigallocatechin gallate	Green tea, red grapes, tumeric	Anti-initiating, anti-promotional
Quercetin, rutin (flavonoids)	Present in hundreds of preparations (e.g., buckwheat tea)	Epidemiological studies suggest anticancer properties
Salai guggal *Boswellia serrata*	Resinous extract of	Inhibits 5-lipoxygenase; HETEs play role in cancer progression
Silymarin	Milk thistle (*Silybum marianus*)	Inhibits tumor progression
Tocotrienols	Whole grains, palm oil	Retard tumor growth; blocks expression of HMG-CoA reductase, required for cell to enter S-phase

HMG-CoA, β-hydroxy-β-methylglutaryl coenzyme A; HETE, hydroxyecosatetraeinoic acid.

■ REFERENCES

American Cancer Society. Questionable methods of cancer management: 'Nutritional' therapies. *CA Cancer J Clin* 1993;43:309.

Bhatia N, Agarwal C, Agarwal R. Differential responses of skin cancer-chemopreventive agents silibinin, quercetin, and epigallocatechin 3-gallate on mitogenic signaling and cell cycle regulators in human epidermoid carcinoma A431 cells. *Nutrit Cancer* 2001;39:292.

Johnson BM, Bolton JL, van Breeman RB. Screening botanical extracts for quinoid metabolites. *Chem Res Toxicol* 2001;14:1546.

Knekt P, Jarvinen R, Seppanen R, et al. Dietary flavonoids and the risk of lung cancer and other malignant neoplasms. *Am J Epidemiol* 1997;146:223.

Lin LT, Liu LT, Chiang LC, Lin CC. In vitro anti-hepatoma activity of fifteen natural medicines from Canada. *Phytother Res* 2002;16:440.

McCarty MF. Current prospects for controlling cancer growth with non-cytotoxic agents—nutrients, phytochemicals, herbal extracts, and available drugs. *Med Hypotheses* 2001;56:137.

Wargovich MJ, Woods C, Hollis DM, Zander ME. Herbals, cancer prevention and health. *J Nutrit* 2001;131:3034S.

APPENDIX XIII:
PSORALEN-CONTAINING BOTANICALS CAPABLE OF CAUSING PHYTOPHOTODERMATITIS

Four main families of plants are implicated in most cases of phytophoto-dermatitis. They are the Umbelliferae (Apiaceae), Leguminoseae (Fabaceae), Moraceae, and Rutaceae. Herbal remedies, common foodstuffs, and common garden plants and wildflowers are all represented in these groups. Phytophotodermatitis following the oral ingestion of natural plants in their unconcentrated form appears to be rare. Most cases occur after contact with the skin.

An *asterisk* (*) indicates a botanical used as an herb and appearing in the alphabetical list of monographs in Section 2.

■ FAMILY UMBELLIFERAE (ALSO KNOWN AS APIACEAE, CARROT, OR PARSLEY FAMILY)

- Ammi majus (ammi)*
- Angelica archangelica (angelica)
- *Angelica atropurpurea* (Alexander's angelica)
- Angelica dahurica (bai zhi)*
- Angelica sinensis (dong quai)*
- Angelica sylvestris (wild angelica)
- Anthriscus sylvestris (cow parsley)
- Apium graveolens (edible celery)
- *Conium maculatum* (poison hemlock)
- *Daucus carota* (wild carrot, Queen Anne's lace)
- Foeniculum vulgare (fennel)*
- Heracleum maximum (cow-parsnip)
- *Pastinaca sativa* (edible parsnip)
- Petroselinum crispum (edible parsley)
- Pimpinella anisum (anise)

■ FAMILY RUTACEAE

- *Citrus aurantifolia* (lime)
- *Citrus aurantium* (bitter orange)
- *Citrus bergamia* (bergamot orange)
- *Citrus limetta* (sweet lemon)
- *Citrus limon* (lemon)

- *Citrus paradisii* (grapefruit)
- *Citrus sinensis* (sweet orange)
- *Ruta graveolens* (rue)*

▮ FAMILY MORACEAE (MULBERRY)

Many trees belong to this family.

- *Ficus carica* (fig); other *Ficus* species
- *Morus alba* (white mulberry)
- *Morus rubrus* (red mulberry)
- *Sassafras albidum* (sassafras)

▮ LEGUMINOSEAE (FABACEAE, PEA FAMILY)

More than 7000 members of this family of pod-bearing plants exist world-wide, including all peas, beans, and lentils.

▮ REFERENCES

Botanical Dermatology: Phytophotodermatitis. Available at: http://www.telemedicine.org. Select "Electronic Textbook" then "Phytophotodermatitis."

Peterson RT, McKenny M. *Northeastern Wildflowers: Roger Tory Peterson Field Guides.* Norwalk, Conn: Easton Press; 1984.

APPENDIX XIV:
SOME USEFUL WEBSITES

- Botanical Dermatology: Phytophotodermatitis. Available at: http://www.telemedicine.org. Select "Electronic Textbook" then "Phytophotodermatitis."
- Chemical Safety Information for Intergovernmental Organizations. World Health Organization, United Nations Environment Programme, International Labour Organization. Available at: http://www.inchem.org.
- Dr. Duke's phytochemical and ethnobotanical databases. Available at: http://www.ars-grin.gov/duke/plants.html.
- Serrano E, Anderson J. Herbs for Health? Colorado State University. Available at: http://www.ext.colostate.edu/pubs/foodnut/09370.html.
- Stehlin IB. An FDA guide to choosing medical treatments. *FDA Consumer* June 1995. U.S. Food and Drug Administration website. Available at: http://www.fda.gov/oashi/aids/fdaguide.html.
- U.S. Food and Drug Administration, Center for Food Safety and Applied Nutrition. Listing of Botanical Ingredients of Concern. Available at: http://vm.cfsan.fda.gov/~dms/csds-bo2.html.

Appendix XV:
Glossary of Botanical Latin Names and Common Equivalents Used for Alphabetical Listing of Herbal Monographs in Text and Appendices

Wild and garden plants not used as herbs are not included. See Appendix IX for some of these. An *asterisk* (*) indicates that a monograph for that herb can be found in Section 2.

LATIN NAME	COMMON EQUIVALENT
Achillea millefolium*	Yarrow
Aconitum napellus*	Aconite
Acorus calamus	Calamus
Adonis vernalis	Pheasant's eye
Aesculus hippocastanum*	Horse chestnut
Agrimonia eupatoria*	Agrimony
Alchemilla vulgaris	Lady's mantle
Allium sativum*	Garlic
Aloe barbadensis*	Aloe vera
Aloe vulgari*	Aloe vera
Althaea officinalis*	Marsh mallow
Ammi majus*	Ammi
Ananas comosus*	Bromelain (pineapple)
Angelica dahurica*	Bai zhi
Angelica sinensis*	Dong quai
Arctium minus	Burdock
Areca catechu*	Betel nut
Aristolochia spp.*	Aristolochia
Arnica montana*	Arnica
Artemisia absinthum*	Wormwood
Atropa mandragora*	Mandrake (European)
Avena sativa*	Avena sativa
Barosma betulina*	Buchu

LATIN NAME	COMMON EQUIVALENT
*Berberis vulgaris**	Barberry
*Betula alba**	Birch (common)
*Borago officinalis**	Borage
*Boswellia serrata**	Salai guggal
*Calendula officinalis**	Calendula (marigold)
*Capsicum frutescens**	Capsaicin
*Cassia angustifolia**	Senna
*Cassia senna**	Senna
*Catraria icelandica**	Moss (Iceland)
*Centella asiatica**	Kola (gotu)
*Chelidonium majus**	Celandine (greater)
*Chrysanthemum parthenium**	Feverfew
*Cimicifuga racemosa**	Black cohosh
*Cola acuminata**	Kola nut (African)
*Cola nitada**	Kola nut (African)
*Colchicum autumnale**	Colchicum
*Commiphora myrrha**	Myrrh
Convalaria majalis	Lily-of-the-valley
Coptis groenlandica	Crude extract
Coriandrum sativum	Coriander
*Corynanthe yohimbe**	Yohimbe
*Craetagus spp**	Hawthorn
*Croton lechleri**	Sangre de grado
*Cuminum nigrum**	Cumin
*Curcuma longa**	Turmeric
*Cyamposis tetragonolobus**	Guar gum
*Daucus carota**	Wild carrot
*Datura stramonium**	Jimsonweed
Digitalis lanata	Digitalis (white foxglove)
Digitalis purpura	Digitalis (purple foxglove)
*Dioscoria villosa**	Wild yam

LATIN NAME	COMMON EQUIVALENT
*Echinacea purpurea**	Echinacea
Eleutherococcus senticosis	Ginseng
*Ephedra equisetina**	Ephedra
*Ephedra intermedia**	Ephedra
*Ephedra sinica**	Ephedra
*Eucalyptus globus**	Eucalyptus
Eugenia jambolana	Jamun
*Eupatorium perfoliatum**	Boneset, feverwort
*Filipendula ulmaria**	Meadowsweet
*Foeniculum vulgare**	Fennel
*Fraxinus spp.**	Ash bark
*Fucus vesiculosis**	Kelp
*Garcinia kola**	Kola (garcinia)
*Garcinia mangostana**	Kola (garcinia)
*Garcinia pedunculata**	Kola (garcinia)
*Gaultheria procumbens**	Wintergreen oil
*Ginkgo biloba**	Ginkgo biloba
*Glycyrrhiza glabra**	Licorice
*Gossypium herbaceum**	Cotton root
*Gymnema sylvestre**	Gymnema
*Gossypium hirsutum**	Gossypol
*Hamamelis virginiana**	Witch hazel
*Harpagophytum procumbens**	Devil's claw
*Hedeoma pulegoides**	Pennyroyal
*Hedera helix**	Ivy leaf
*Humulus lupulus**	Hops
*Hydrastis canadensis**	Goldenseal
*Hyocyamus niger**	Henbane
*Hypericum perforatum**	St. John's wort
*Hypoxis rooperi**	β-Sitosterol
*Ilex araguariensis**	Maté

LATIN NAME	COMMON EQUIVALENT
*Ilex paraguayensis**	Maté
*Illicium anisatum**	Anise (star)
*Illicium verum**	Anise (star)
Juniperus communis	Juniper
*Laminaria spp.**	Kelp
*Larrea tridentata**	Chaparral
*Lavandula spp.** (L. angustifolia, L. stoechas, L. latifolia)*	Lavender
*Lobelia inflata**	Lobelia
*Mandragora officinarum**	Mandrake (European)
*Matricaria recutita**	Chamomile
*Medicago sativa**	Alfalfa
*Melissa officinalis**	Balm
*Menispermum spp.**	Menispermum
*Mentha piperita**	Peppermint
*Mentha pulegium**	Pennyroyal
*Momordica charantia**	Karela
*Monascus purpureus**	Cholistin
*Morinda citrifolia**	Noni
*Mucuna pruriens**	Cowitch
*Nepeta cataria**	Catnip
*Oenothera biennis**	Evening primrose
*Panax ginseng**	Ginseng
*Panax japonicus**	Ginseng
*Panax quinquefolius**	Ginseng
*Passiflora incarnata**	Passionflower
*Paullinia cupana**	Guarana
*Pausinystalia yohimbe**	Yohimbe
*Picramnia antidesma**	Cascara amarga
*Pimpinella anisum**	Anise
*Pinus maritima**	French maritime pine bark
*Pinus pinaster**	French maritime pine bark
*Piper betle**	Betel nut

LATIN NAME	COMMON EQUIVALENT
Plantago major*	Plantain
Podophyllum peltatum*	Mandrake (American)
Pogostemon patchouli*	Patchouli
Piper methysticum*	Kava
Populus tremuloides*	Poplar (trembling)
Pueraria lobata*	Kudzu
Pulegium regium*	Pennyroyal
Pyrethrum parthenium*	Feverfew
Ranunculus ficaria*	Celandine (lesser)
Rauwolfia serpentina	Indian snakeroot
Rhamnus purshianus*	Cascara
Rosmarinus officinalis*	Rosemary
Rubus fructicosus	Blackberry
Ruta graveolens*	Rue
Sabal serrulata*	Saw palmetto
Saccharomyces boulardii* (S. cervisiae)	Saccharomyces
Salix babylonica*	Willow bark
Salix spp.*	Willow bark
Salvia lavanduaefolia*	Sage
Salvia miltiorrhiza*	Danshen
Salvia officinalis*	Sage
Sassafras albidum*	Sassafras
Scilla maritima	White squill
Scutellaria baicalensis	Baicalein
Scutallaria laterifolia*	Skullcap
Senecio spp.*	Groundsels, ragworts
Senna alexandria*	Senna
Serenoa repens*	Saw palmetto
Serenoa serrulata	Saw palmetto
Silybum marianus*	Milk thistle
Smilax species*	Sarsaparillas
Solanum dulcamara*	Bittersweet
Solidago altissima, other Solidago spp.	Goldenrod

LATIN NAME	COMMON EQUIVALENT
*Spiraea alba**	Meadowsweet
*Spiraea latifolia**	Meadowsweet
*Spiraea ulmaria**	Meadowsweet
*Stellaria media**	Chickweed
*Stephania spp.**	Jin bu huan
Strophanthus kombe	Strophanthus
*Symphytum officinale**	Comfrey
*Tabebuia avellanedae**	Pau d'arco
*Tamarindus indica**	Tamarind
*Tanacetum parthenium**	Feverfew
Tanacetum vulgare	Tansy
*Taraxacum officinale**	Common dandelion
*Teucrium chamaedrys**	Germander
*Teucrium polium**	Germander
Tinospora cordifolia	Tinospora
*Trifolium pratense**	Red clover
*Trigonella foenum-graecum**	Fenugreek
*Tripterygium wilfordii**	Tripterygium wilfordii
*Turnera diffusa**	Damiana
*Tussilago farfara**	Coltsfoot
*Uncaria guianensis**	Cat's claw
Urginea maritima	Squill
*Urtica dioica**	Nettle (stinging)
*Vaccinium macrocarpon**	Cranberry
*Vaccinium myrtillus**	Bilberry
*Valeriana officinalis**	Valerian
*Viscum album**	Mistletoe (European)
*Vitex agnus-castus**	Chasteberry
*Zingiber officinale**	Ginger
*Zingiberis rhizoma**	Ginger

Index